Bile Acids and Lipids

FALK SYMPOSIUM 29

Bile Acids and Lipids

EDITED BY

G. Paumgartner
Department of Internal Medicine II
University of Munich
West Germany

A. Stiehl
Department of Internal Medicine
University of Heidelberg
West Germany

W. Gerok
Department of Internal Medicine
University of Freiburg/Br.
West Germany

Proceedings of the 6th Bile Acid Meeting (Falk Symposium 29) held at Freiburg im Breisgau, West Germany, October 9–11, 1980

MTP PRESS LIMITED
International Medical Publishers

Published by
MTP Press Limited
Falcon House
Lancaster, England

ISBN: 0–85200–389–7

Typeset, printed and bound in Great Britain by
REDWOOD BURN LIMITED
Trowbridge & Esher

Contents

SECTION 3 Biliary Secretion

SECTION 4 Bile Acids, Lipids and Lipoproteins

List of Contributors

H. ABBERGER
Chemisches Laboratorium
Universität Freiburg
D-7800 Freiburg i. Br., West Germany

J. AHLBERG
Department of Surgery
Danderyd's Hospital
S-182 03 Danderyd, Sweden

M. ALAVI
Department of Internal Medicine
Division of Metabolism, Nutrition and Gastroenterology
University of Ulm
D-7900 Ulm, West Germany

R. ALDINI
Clinica Medica 3
University of Bologna
Bologna, Italy

E. ANDERSEN
Department of Medicine
St Erik's Hospital
S-112 82 Stockholm, Sweden

B. ANGELIN
Department of Medicine
Huddinge University Hospital
S-141 86 Huddinge, Sweden

N. K. N. AYENGAR
Lipid Research Laboratory
Department of Surgery
Beth Israel Medical Center
New York, NY 10003, USA

L. BARBARA
Clinica Medica 3
University of Bologna
Bologna, Italy

C. A. BARTH
Forschergrüppe Ernährung
Medicinische Poliklinik der Universität München
D 8000 München 2, West Germany

M. C. BATESON
Department of Medicine
Ninewells Hospital and Medical School
Dundee DD1 9SY, United Kingdom

H. BAUMGÄRTEL
Center of Internal Medicine
Department of Gastroenterology
University Hospital
D-6000 Frankfurt 70, West Germany

F. BAZZOLI
Clinica Medica 3
University of Bologna
Bologna, Italy

Z. H. BEG
Molecular Disease Branch
National Heart, Lung and Blood Institute
National Institutes of Health
Bethesda, Maryland, USA

F. BEGEMANN
I. Medizinische Klinik
Universitäts-Krankenhaus Eppendorf
D-2000 Hamburg 20, West Germany

G. D. BELL
Department of Therapeutics
City Hospital
Nottingham NG5 1PB, United Kingdom

L. J. BENNION
Department of Internal Medicine
Sunnyvale Medical Clinic
Sunnyvale, California, USA

K. von BERGMANN
Medical University Clinic
D-5300 Bonn, West Germany

U. BICKEL
Chemisches Laboratorium
Univerität Freiburg
D-7800 Freiburg i. Br., West Germany

G. G. BONORRIS
Department of Gastroenterology
Cedars-Sinai Medical Center
Los Angeles, CA 90048, USA

T. BOSCH
Medical University Clinic
D-5300 Bonn, West Germany

H. BOSTRÖM
Department of Pharmaceutical Biochemistry
University of Uppsala, Box 578
S-751 23 Uppsala, Sweden

J. L. BOYER
Liver Study Unit
Yale University School of Medicine
New Haven, CT 06510, USA

A. BREMMELGAARD
Department of Clinical Chemistry
Rigshospitalet
Copenhagen, Denmark

H. B. BREWER Jr.
Molecular Disease Branch
National Heart, Lung and Blood Institute
National Institutes of Health
Bethesda, Maryland, USA

S. BURSTEIN
Division of Hepatic Diseases
New York Hospital
Cornell Medical Center
New York, NY 10021, USA

H-P. BUSCHER
Department of Internal Medicine
University of Freiburg
D-7800 Freiburg i. Br., West Germany

M. C. CAREY
G. I. Medicine, RB 013
Brigham and Women's Hospital
Harvard Medical School
Boston, Massachusetts, USA

N. CARULLI
Istituto di Clinica Medica II
Università di Modena
Modena, Italy

D. CHAPMAN
Department of Biochemistry
Royal Free Hospital School of Medicine
London WC1B 1BP, United Kingdom

P. CZYGAN
Medizinische Klinik
Universität Heidelberg
D-6900 Heidelberg, West Germany

H. DANIELSSON
Department of Pharmaceutical Biochemistry
University of Uppsala, Box 578
S-751 23 Uppsala, Sweden

B. DEMARK
Division of Biological and Medical Research
Argonne National Laboratory
Argonne, Illinois, USA

J. M. DIETSCHY
Department of Internal Medicine
The University of Texas Health Science Center
Dallas, Texas, USA

H. DITSCHUNEIT
Department of Internal Medicine
Division of Metabolism, Nutrition and Gastroenterology
University of Ulm
D-7900 Ulm, West Germany

R. H. DOWLING
Gastroenterology Unit
Guy's Hospital and Medical School
London SE1 9RT, United Kingdom

M. DUBIN
Instituto de Quinica Biologica
Universidad de Buenos Aires
Buenos Aires 1121, Argentina

M. DUMONT
Unité de Recherches de Physiopathologie Hépatique
INSERM U-24
Hôpital Beaujon
92118 Clichy Cedex, France

K. EINARSSON
Department of Medicine
Huddinge University Hospital
S-141 86 Huddinge, Sweden

S. ERLINGER
Unité de Recherches de
Physiopathologie Hépatique
INSERM U-24
Hôpital Beaujon
92118 Clichy Cedex, France

G. EVERSON
Division of Gastroenterology
University of Colorado School of Medicine
Denver, Colorado, USA

S. EWERTH
Department of Surgery
Huddinge University Hospital
S-141 86 Huddinge, Sweden

D. FESTI
Clinica Medica 3
University of Bologna
Bologna, Italy

M. M. FISHER
University of Toronto
Clinical Science Division
Medical Sciences Building
Toronto M5S 1A8, Canada

H. FROMM
Department of Medicine
School of Medicine
Montefiore Hospital
Pittsburgh, Pennsylvania 15213, USA

K. FUCHTE
Chemisches Laboratorium
Universität Freiburg
D-7800 Freiburg i. Br., West Germany

W. GEROK
Medizinische Universitätsklinik
D-7800 Freiburg i. Br., West Germany

I. T. GILMORE
Gastroenterology Unit
Royal Liverpool Hospital
Liverpool L7 8XP, United Kingdom

R. GÖTZ
Medizinische Klinik
Universität Heidelberg
D-690 Heidelberg, West Germany

D. GURANTZ
Department of Medicine (H-811D)
U.C.S.D. Medical Center
San Diego, CA 92103, USA

M. GUT
Worcester Foundation for Experimental Biology
Shrewsbury, MA 01545, USA

R. HANSSON
Department of Pharmaceutical Biochemistry
University of Uppsala, Box 578
S-751 23 Uppsala, Sweden

K. W. HEATON
University Department of Medicine
Bristol Royal Infirmary
Bristol, United Kingdom

K. HELLSTRÖM
Department of Medicine
St Erik's Hospital
S-11282 Stockholm, Sweden

I. HILLMAR
Forschergrüppe Ernährung
Medizinische Poliklinik der Universität München
D-800 München 2, West Germany

A. F. HOFMANN
Department of Medicine (H-811D)
U.C.S.D. Medical Center
San Diego, CA 92103, USA

S. HOTTINGER
Medizinische Klinik II
Klinikum Grosshadern
D-800 München 70, West Germany

B. V. HOWARD
Phoenix Clinical Research Section
National Institute of Arthritis, Metabolism and Digestive Diseases
Phoenix, Arizona, USA

K. E. HOWELL
European Molecular Biology Laboratory
Meyerhofstrasse 1 Postfach 10.2209
D-6900 Heidelberg, West Germany

H. IGIMI
1st Department of Surgery
Fukuoka University School of Medicine
Fukuoka, Japan

J. ISER
Department of Veterans' Affairs
Repatriation General Hospital
Heidelberg West 3081, Australia

N. B. JAVITT
Division of Hepatic Diseases
New York Hospital
Cornell Medical Center
New York, NY 10021, USA

I. KALLES
Department of Pharmaceutical Biochemistry
University of Uppsala, Box 578
S-751 23 Uppsala, Sweden

F. KERN Jr.
Division of Gastroenterology
University of Colorado School of Medicine
Denver, Colorado, USA

P. KLEIN
Division of Biological and Medical Research
Argonne National Laboratory
Argonne, Illinois, USA

E. KOK
Division of Hepatic Diseases
New York Hospital
Cornell Medical Center
New York, NY 10021, USA

B. KOMMERELL
Medizinische Klinik
Universität Heidelberg
D-6900 Heidelberg, West Germany

W. KRAMER
Chemisches Laboratorium
Universität Freiburg
D-7800 Freiburg i. Br., West Germany

G. KURZ
Chemisches Laboratorium
Universität Freiburg
D-7800 Freiburg i. Br., West Germany

J. M. LACHIN
Biostatistics Center
George Washington University
Bethesda, Maryland, USA

N. F. LARUSSO
Department of Gastroenterology
Mayo Medical School
Rochester, Minnesota, USA

B. LEIJD
Department of Medicine
St Erik's Hospital
S-112 82 Stockholm, Sweden

O. LEISS
Medical University Clinic
D-5300 Bonn, West Germany

U. LEUSCHNER
Center of Internal Medicine,
Department of Gastroenterology
University Hospital
D-6000 Frankfurt 70, West Germany

B. LIDSTRÖM
Department of Pharmaceutical Biochemistry
University of Uppsala, Box 578
S-751 23 Uppsala, Sweden

I. A. MACDONALD
Clinical Research Center
Faculty of Medicine
Dalhouse University
Halifax NS., Canada

CH. MÄNNER
Medizinische Klinik
Universität Heidelberg
D-6900 Heidelberg, West Germany

J. W. MARKS
Department of Gastroenterlogy
Cedars-Sinai Medical Center
Los Angeles, CA 90048, USA

S. MATERN
Medizinische Universitätsklinik
D-7800 Freiburg i. Br., West Germany

P. N. MATON
Gastroenterology Unit
Hammersmith Hospital
London W12 0HS, United Kingdom

D. P. MAUDGAL
Department of Medicine II
St. George's Hospital
Medical School
London SW17 0RE, United Kingdom

P. S. MAY
Lipid Research Laboratory
Department of Surgery
Beth Israel Medical Center
New York, NY 10003, USA

N. MAZER
Department of Medicine
Harvard Medical School
Division of Gastroenterology
Brigham and Women's Hospital
Boston, MA 02115, USA

LIST OF CONTRIBUTORS

G. MAZZELLA
Clinica Medica 3
University of Bologna
Bologna, Italy

C. K. McSHERRY
Lipid Research Laboratory
Department of Surgery
Beth Israel Medical Center
New York, N.Y. 10003, USA

E. MESSALE
Clinica Medica 3
University of Bologna
Bologna, Italy

T. A. MIETTINEN
2nd Department of Medicine
University of Helsinki
SF-00290 Helsinki 29, Finland

P. F. MISKOVITZ
Division of Hepatic Diseases
New York Hospital
Cornell Medical Center
New York, NY 10021, USA

G. MÖCKEL
Med.- und Röntgenabteilung
Krankenhaus Tabea
2000 Hamburg 55, West Germany

A. M. MORSELLI
Clinica Medica 3
University of Bologna
Bologna, Italy

E. H. MOSBACH
Lipid Research Laboratory
Department of Surgery
Beth Israel Medical Center
New York, NY 10003, USA

D. M. MOTT
Phoenix Clinical Research Section
National Institute of Arthritis,
Metabolism and Digestive Diseases
Phoenix, Arizona, USA

G. M. MURPHY
Gastroenterology Unit
Guy's Hospital and Medical School
London SE1 9RT, United Kingdom

S. NIELSEN
I. Medizinische Klinik
Universitäts-Krankenhaus Eppendorf
D-2000 Hamburg 20, West Germany

T. C. NORTHFIELD
St. George's Hospital
Medical School
University of London
London S.W.17 0RE, United Kingdom

J. D. OSTROW
Northwestern University Medical
School
Veterans Administration
Lakeside Hospital,
Chicago, Illinois 60611, USA

M. PAPENHAGEN
I. Medizinische Klinik
Universitäts-Krankenhaus Eppendorf
D-2000 Hamburg 20, West Germany

G. PAUMGARTNER
Department of Internal Medicine II
Klinikum Großhadern
University of Munich
8000 Munich 70, West Germany

B. J. PEARLMAN
Department of Gastroenterology
Cedars-Sinai Medical Center
Los Angeles, CA 90048, USA

J. R. POLEY
Department of Pediatrics
Division of Metabolism, Nutrition and
Gastroenterology
University of Ulm
D-7900 Ulm, West Germany

M. PONZ DE LEON
Istituto di Clinica Medica II
Università de Modena
Modena, Italy

R. PREISIG
Department of Clinical Pharmacology
University of Berne
CH-3010 Berne, Switzerland

R. RAEDSCH
Medizinische Klinik
Universität Heidelberg
D-6900 Heidelberg, West Germany

C. J. RESTALL
Department of Biochemistry
Royal Free Hospital School of Medicine
London WC1N 1BP, United Kingdom

A. REUBEN
Liver Study Unit
Yale University Medical School
New Haven, CT 06510, USA

A. RODA
Istituto di Scienze Chimiche
Facoltà di Farmacia
University of Bologna
Bologna, Italy

E. RODA
Clinica Medica 3
University of Bologna
Bologna, Italy

W. RÖSCH
Medizinische Universitätsklinik
D-8520 Erlangen, West Germany

G. SALEN
Department of Digestive Diseases
CMDNJ-New Jersey Medical School
Newark, NJ 07013, USA

C. SAMA
Department of Gastroenterology
University of Bologna
Bologna, Italy

T. SCHERSTEN
University of Göteborg
Department of Surgery III
41345 Göteborg, Sweden

A. SCHNEIDER
Department of Internal Medicine
Division of Metabolism, Nutrition and Gastroenterology
University of Ulm,
D-7900 Ulm, West Germany

L. J. SCHOENFIELD
Department of Gastroenterology
Cedars-Sinai Medical Center
Los Angeles, CA 90048, USA

C. C. SCHWARTZ
Department of Medicine
Medical College of Viginia
Virginia Commonwealth University
Richmond, Virginia, USA

S. SHEFER
Department of Digestive Diseases
CMDN-New Jersey Medical School
Newark, NJ 07013, USA

A. K. SINGHAL
Lipid Research Laboratory
Department of Surgery
Beth Israel Medical Center
New York, NY 10003, USA

J. SJÖVALL
Department of Physiological Chemistry
Karolinska Institutet
Stockholm, Sweden

D. M. SMALL
Biophysics Institute
Departments of Medicine and Biochemistry
Boston University School of Medicine
Boston, MA 02118, USA

R. A. SMALLWOOD
Gastroenterology Unit
Department of Medicine
University of Melbourne Austin Hospital
Heidelberg, Victoria 3084, Australia

E. F. STANGE
Department of Internal Medicine
Division of Metabolism, Nutrition and Gastroenterology
University of Ulm
D-7900 Ulm, West Germany

A. STIEHL
Medizinishce Klinik
Universität Heidelberg
D-6900 Heidelberg, West Germany

K. STOKES
Department of Medicine (H-811D)
U.C.S.D. Medical Center
San Diego, CA 92103, USA

S. O. SUE
Straub Clinic
888 South King Street
Honolulu, Hawaii 96813, USA

L. SWELL
Lipid Research Laboratory
VA Hospital
Richmond, Virginia, USA

P. A. SZCZEPANIK
Division of Bioligical and Medical Research
Argonne National Laboratory
Argonne, Illinois, USA

J. L. THISTLE
Division of Gastroenterology
Mayo Clinic and Mayo Foundation
Rochester, MN 55901, USA

J. R. THORNTON
University Department of Medicine
Bristol Royal Infirmary
Bristol, United Kingdom

G. S. TINT
GI Research Laboratory
VA Medical Center
East Orange, NJ 07019, USA

S. D. TURLEY
Department of Internal Medicine
University of Texas Health Science Center
Dallas, Texas, USA

P. VARADY
Cedars-Sinai Medical Center and UCLA
Los Angeles CA 90048, USA

D. VERGA
GI Research Laboratory
VA Medical Center
East Orange, NJ 07019, USA

Z. VLAHCEVIC
Department of Medicine
VA Hospital and Medical College of Virginia
Virginia Commonwealth University
Richmond, Virginia, USA

S. WALKER
Medizinische Klinik
Universität Heidelberg
D-6900 Heidelberg, West Germany

E. E. WEIS
Medizinische Poliklinik
Universität München
D-8000 München 2, West Germany

H. J. WEIS
II. Medizinische Klinik
des Allgemeinen Krankenhauses
8600 Bamberg, West Germany

H. WIETHOLTZ
Department of Clinical Pharmacology
University of Berne
CH-3010 Berne, Switzerland

K. WIKVALL
Department of Pharmaceutical Biochemistry
University of Uppsala, Box 578
S-751 23 Uppsala, Sweden

C. N. WILLIAMS
Clinical Research Center
Faculty of Medicine
Dalhousie University
Halifax N.S., Canada

C. WOLPERS
Department of Internal Medicine
Medicinische Hochschule
Lübeck, West Germany

Preface

It was ten years ago that a small group of scientists who had a strong interest in bile acids first met in Freiburg. The meeting, called Bile Salt Monday, was organized by Peter Back and Wolfgang Gerok and lasted only one day. The chairmen were Jan Sjövall, Henry Danielsson and Alan Hofmann. It was an exciting meeting with many new ideas and much heated discussion. Its success derived from excellent science with obvious clinical relevance. The meeting was so successful that Herbert Falk decided to sponsor a bile acid meeting every two years.

The 'genius loci' of Freiburg has been most favourable for bile acid and cholesterol research in the past. Among those who have laid the foundations of knowledge about the chemistry and physiological chemistry of bile acids and cholesterol, the chemists Wieland and Windaus and the physiological chemist Schönheimer have lived in Freiburg and have made many of their discoveries in Freiburg. The 'genius loci' also had a good influence on the communication of science in the bile acid field. In the ten years since their existence the Bile Acid Meetings exhibited a rapid growth.

The second Bile Acid Meeting in 1972 had the title 'Bile Acids in Human Diseases'. It was at this meeting that the first instance of gallstone dissolution by chenodeoxycholic acid was reported by the groups from the Mayo Clinic in Rochester and from the Hammersmith Hospital in London. From then on it was clear that bile acid research had great clinical relevance, and interest especially in chenodeoxycholic acid and later also in ursodeoxycholic acid increased.

The last Bile Acid Meetings in 1976 and 1978 dealt with both metabolic and pharmacodynamic aspects of bile acids. Within the framework of these topics the important interrelations between bile acids and lipids became apparent. It appeared important to examine the current understanding of these relationships because bile acid formation is the major catabolic pathway for cholesterol removal from the body and cholesterol is implicated in several diseases such as atherosclerosis and cholesterol cholelithiasis. Therefore, it was considered appropriate by many participants of the last meeting and by the organizers to devote the 6th Bile Acid Meeting to the study of the interrelationships between bile acids and lipids. Interest in this topic obviously has been great. More than 500 scientists from 33 countries have participated. This book comprises the contributions to this Meeting as well as a Workshop on Dissolution of Gallstones which was held jointly with the 6th Bile Acid Meeting.

Sincere appreciation is expressed to the contributors who made the 6th Bile Acid Meeting another success. The editors are deeply indebted to Dr Herbert Falk, whose generous support made the meeting possible. We also wish to thank Mr D. G. T. Bloomer, Managing Director of MTP Press Limited, for superb cooperation in publishing these proceedings.

The Editors

1
Presentation of the Adolf Windaus Prize

W. GEROK

It is a special honour for me today to present the Adolf Windaus Prize for the first time. The prize is to be awarded for exceptional work in the field of bile acid research carried out in the last few years. It has been donated by the Falk Foundation and the donator, Dr Falk, deserves our very special thanks.

First of all let me say a few words about Adolf Windaus (Figure 1) after whom the prize has been named. Adolf Windaus started his scientific career with studies on the structure of cholesterol here in Freiburg. The structural formula for cholesterol proposed by Windaus in 1912 (Figure 2) shows how far he still was from his goal, the definitive solution of the structure of

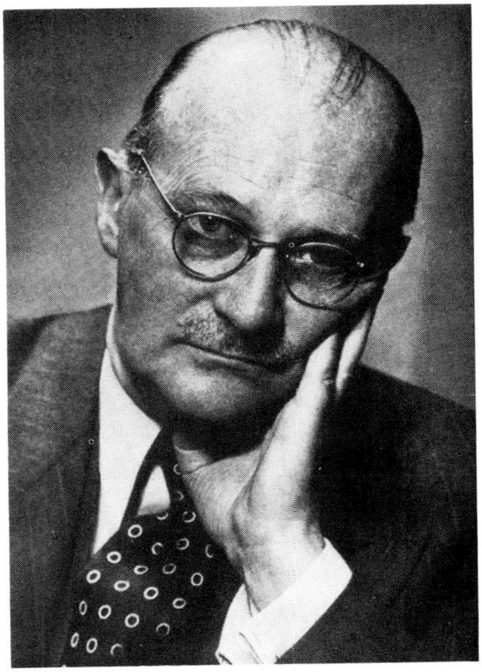

Figure 1 Adolf Windaus

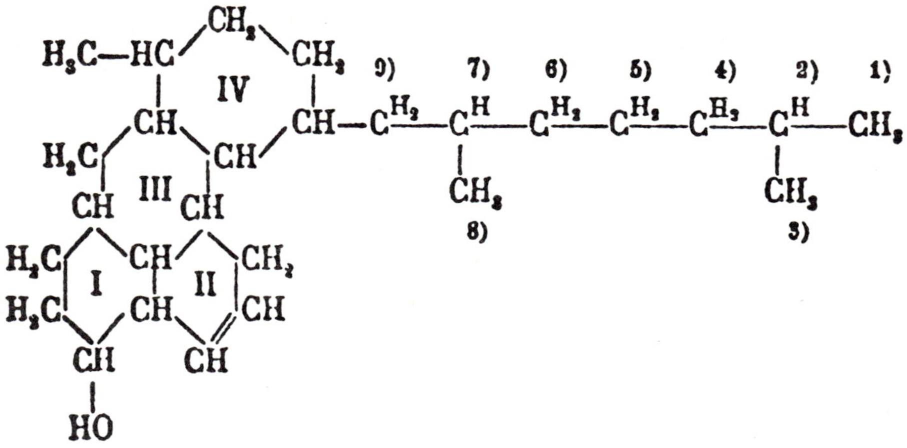

Figure 2 Formula for cholesterol proposed by Windaus in 1912

cholesterol. Windaus later carried on these studies in Göttingen, and it was there that he made a very important discovery in 1919. He showed that Coprostan could be oxidized to cholanic acid and therefore proved the close structural relationship between cholesterol and bile acids.

The second father of bile acid research, Heinrich Wieland, also worked here in Freiburg in the early 1920s, before moving to the University of Munich in 1924. With tenacious work and close cooperation the two groups, Windaus in Göttingen and Wieland in Munich, were able in 1927 to provide the definitive structure of cholesterol and bile acids. A further pinnacle of the work of Adolf Windaus was the discovery of the structure of the D vitamins and the solving of the mechanism of photoactivation of the provitamins.

In 1928 Windaus was awarded the Nobel Prize for chemistry.

Adolf Windaus was able to draw together a group of talented colleagues and to stimulate them. I only need to mention Adolf Butenandt, who received the Nobel Prize in 1939 for his work on the structure and synthesis of sexual hormones.

Colleagues of Adolf Windaus describe him as a scientist with great energy, concentration, clarity and determination. He was able through experiments to convert the right questions into clear answers. Major scientific achievements were combined with humility and human kindness. His life's work warrants great significance in biology and medicine. However, Adolf Windaus always emphasized that the aim of research was not the application, but the elucidation, of knowledge.

The committee was aware that the connection of the prize with the name of

Adolf Windaus meant a special responsiblity. The selection was extremely difficult. Mainly work of the last three years was considered by the committee, but earlier scientific achievements were also considered. Following a long and intensive exchange of opinions, the committee decided to confer the Adolf Windaus Prize for 1980 on Dr Kjell Hellström and Dr Kurt Einarsson.

Dr Kjell Hellström was born in 1930 in Stockholm. He received his medical training at the Karolinska Institute there. Following work in the Department of Medicine of the Serafiner Lasarett Stockholm from 1958 until 1964, he served as a post-doctoral fellow in the team of Professor Marvin Siperstein at the Dallas Medical School until 1966. In 1975 he was appointed Assistant Professor of Medicine in the Department of Medicine of the St Erik's Hospital in Stockholm.

Dr Kurt Einarsson was born in 1940 in Kristianstad (Sweden). He worked from 1962 until 1969 in the Karolinska Institute, Department of Chemistry, with Dr Henry Danielsson as immediate supervisor, leading to an assistant professorship in biochemistry. In 1969 he moved to the Department of Medicine of the Karolinska Institute, where he worked in close cooperation with Dr Hellström. In 1977 and 1978 he was NIH International Research Fellow in the team of Scott M. Grundy. In 1980 Dr Einarsson was appointed assistant professor in the Department of Medicine, Huddinge University Hospital, Stockholm.

The scientific work of both prizewinners is so closely linked that I would like to present their findings together.

Both have worked in the bile acid field for many years. In the work for which the Windaus Prize was awarded they present evidence for a tight regulation of the metabolism of lipoproteins and bile acids in hyperlipoproteinaemia types II and IV.

The first indication of a relationship between the metabolism of very-low-density-lipoproteins and bile acids emerged from a study demonstrating that the formation of bile acids was enhanced in more than 50% of patients with hyperlipoproteinaemia type IV; also the cholesterol biosynthesis and the activity of hepatic HMG-CoA reductase were abnormally high.

Subsequent work was devoted to studies of bile acid and triglyceride kinetics under various experimental conditions. The formation of bile acids was found to be closely correlated to that of triglycerides in very-low-density-lipoproteins. When bile acid biosynthesis was stimulated by administration of cholestyramine, the formation of triglycerides increased. The opposite effect was obtained with chenodeoxycholic acid which is known to inhibit bile acid formation. It was also possible to stimulate bile acid biosynthesis by giving a diet rich in carbohydrates that primarily may stimulate production of triglycerides.

Hyperlipoproteinaemia type II and IV also differed with regard to biliary lipid composition. Cholesterol saturation being abnormally high in type IV. The latter findings may offer an explanation of the increased prevalence of cholesterol gallstone disease in distinct hyperlipoproteinemia.

So the studies of Dr Hellström and Dr Einarsson have given important insights into the metabolism of bile acids, cholesterol, and triglycerides and have great significance for medicine.

ADOLF WINDAUS PRIZE LECTURE

2
Bile acid metabolism in hyperlipoproteinaemia

K. HELLSTRÖM

Professor Gerok, Dr Falk, ladies and gentlemen: Kurt Einarsson and myself are very proud of being selected for the Adolf Windaus Prize. The scientific contribution of Adolf Windaus was indeed outstanding and I think we all agree that the pioneer work performed by him and his colleagues is the basis for current research concerning steroids and steroid metabolism. For a clinician such as myself it is hard to believe that they were able to solve complicated biochemical problems with the analytical methods available at that time.

To be honest we were most of all surprised when we were informed about the decision of the prize committee. We did not, and do still not, understand how it was possible to select a winner among the many highly qualified researchers working in the bile acid field. Anyhow, we are very happy and we want to express our sincere gratitude to Dr Falk, the Falk Foundation and the prize committee for the honour they have shown us. We also want to thank Jon Ahlberg, Eva Andersén, Bo Angelin, Mora Kallner and Barbro Leijd who are the young colleagues we have had the privilege of working with during the past years. Their enthusiastic contribution has been of major importance in all the advances made. On an occasion like this we are very pleased to see Professor Jan Sjövall and Professor Henry Danielsson among the audience. Once upon a time they introduced us to this field, and they were our teachers in biochemical research.

The principal topic of our studies over the last few years has been to characterize bile acid and cholesterol metabolism under conditions known to influence the plasma lipoproteins. The subjects investigated were healthy controls and patients with primary HLP (hyperlipoproteinaemia). The results of one of the first studies[1] are summarized in Figure 1. Mainly due to an enhanced formation of cholic acid (CA) the total bile acid production was found to be increased in about two-thirds of the patients with HLP type IV (elevated plasma levels of VLDL, very low density lipoproteins). A different pattern was observed in HLP type IIa (increased plasma levels of LDL, low density lipoproteins) and HLP type IIb (increased plasma levels of both VLDL and LDL). In these disorders the biosynthesis of bile acids remained within normal limits but the formation of CA was slightly subnormal, a defect

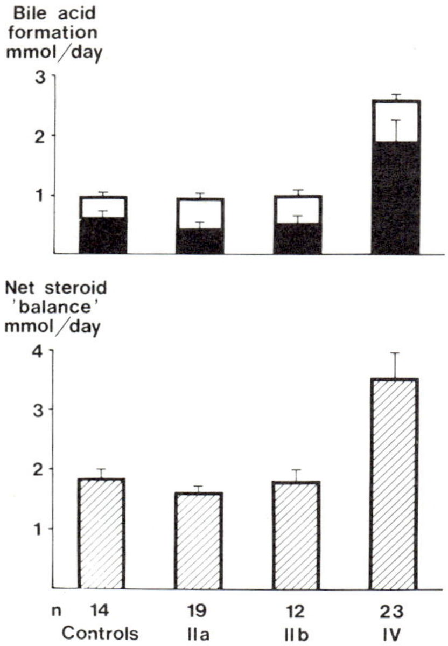

Figure 1 Upper panel demonstrates the formation of cholic acid (solid bars) and chenodeoxycholic acid (open bars) in control subjects and in patients with HLP type IIa, IIb and IV[1]. Lower panel shows net steroid balance (bile acid production plus faecal excretion of cholesterol and neutral cholesterol metabolites minus cholesterol intake) in the same subjects[2]. Data are presented as mean ± SEM

often compensated for by a slight rise in the production of CDCA (chenodeoxycholic acid). Net steroid balance (defined as bile acid formation plus faecal excretion of neutral steroids of cholesterol origin minus cholesterol intake) is also shown in Figure 1. This variable, which was supposed to equal total cholesterol synthesis, turned out to be normal in HLP type II but supranormal in about half of the patients with the type IV pattern[2].

In evaluating the data presented above it must be emphasized that any type of HLP may represent a collection of disorders rather than a single disease entity. A consistent finding in our study was the wide variations in bile acid formation among the patients with HLP type IV. Large fluctuations have also been observed with regard to VLDL production, and the type IV pattern may be explained by both overproduction and/or decreased clearance of the VLDL particles[3]. Considering the possibility of a linkage between the biosynthesis of bile acids and VLDL triglycerides these variables were characterized simultaneously in patients with different types of HLP[4]. Triglyceride kinetics were determined by the [^{3}H]glycerol method[5]. In accordance with our previous observations the formation of bile acids was higher in HLP type IV than in HLP type IIa. The synthesis ranged within wide limits, particularly in patients with the type IV pattern. However, in both types of HLP, as well as in the total series of patients, the production of bile acids and serum triglycerides correlated significantly (Figure 2).

Further indications of parallel changes in the metabolism of bile acids and triglycerides were obtained in subjects studied under various experimental conditions. Administration of cholestyramine that enhances bile acid production in HLP type II[6] also results in an increased production of serum triglyceride[7] (Figure 3). Feeding with CDCA, known to depress the synthesis of CA and probably also the total bile acid production,[8] was found to inhibit the rate of serum triglyceride formation[7] (Figure 3). The reduced biosynthesis of serum triglycerides reported by others upon treatment of HLP type IV with clofibrate[5] or nicotinic acid[9] was in our hands reflected by an inhibited conversion of cholesterol to bile acid[10,11] (Figure 4). A reduction of both bile acid production and plasma triglyceride concentration was observed after moderate weight reduction in patients with hypertriglyceridaemia[1] (Figure 5). Finally, the increased formation of serum triglycerides observed upon the shift from a fat-rich to a carbohydrate-rich diet was associated with a rise in

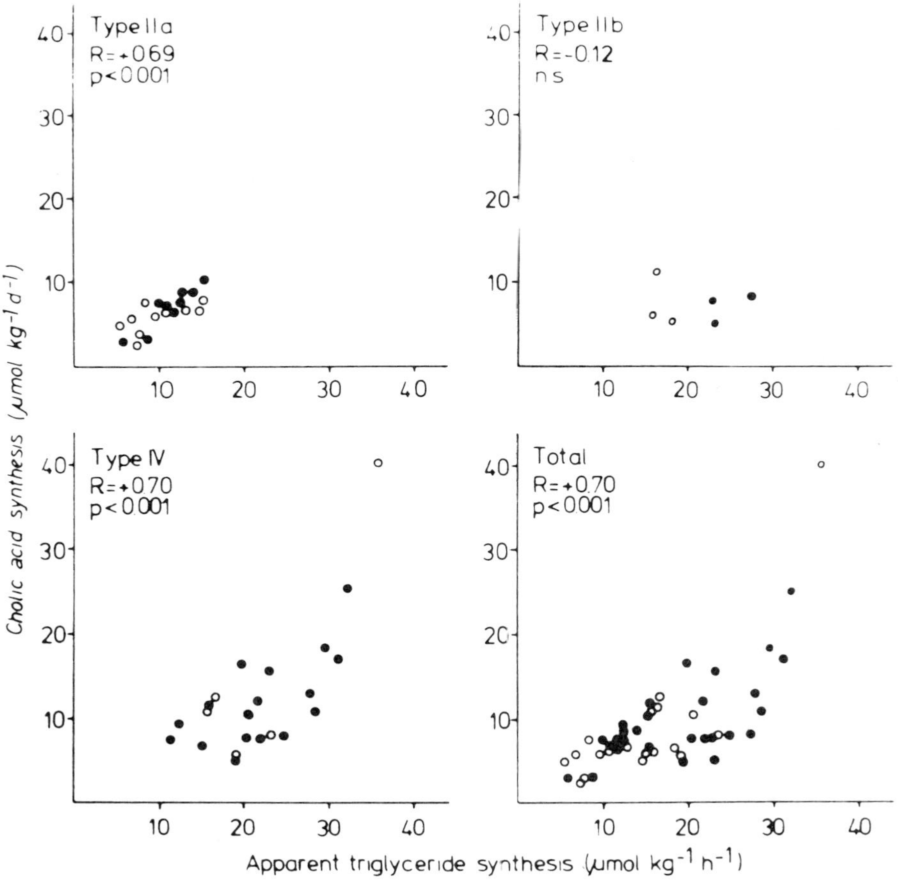

Figure 2 Cholic acid production and apparent triglyceride synthesis in patients with HLP type IIa, IIb and IV[4]

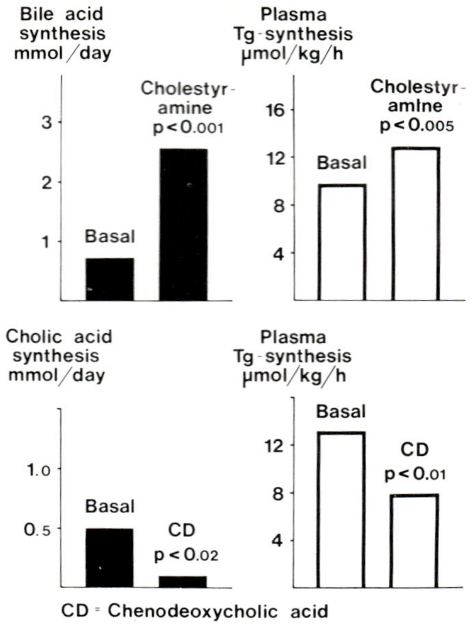

Figure 3 Upper panel demonstrates total bile acid formation[6] and apparent triglyceride synthesis[7] before and during treatment of cholestyramine in HLP type IIa. Lower panel shows cholic acid production[8] and apparent plasma triglyceride biosynthesis[7] in HLP type II before and during treatment with chenodeoxycholic acid

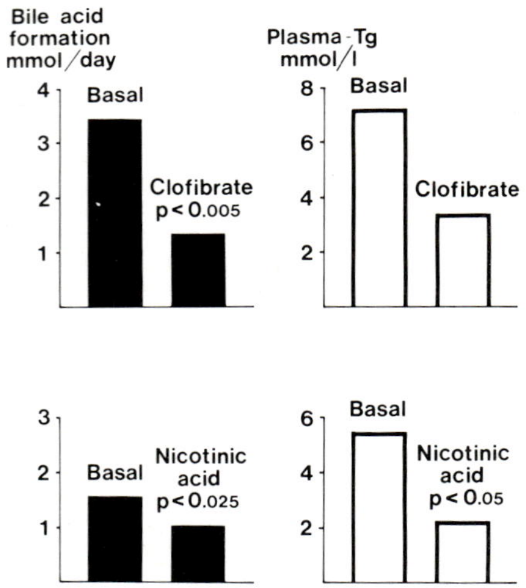

Figure 4 Bile acid formation and plasma triglyceride level before and during treatment with clofibrate[10] and nicotinic acid[11] in HLP type IV

bile acid production[12] (Figure 5). Due to a decline in the excretion of neutral steroids the net steroid balance seemed to be the same. A similar result, i.e.

an unchanged steroid balance, was also recorded in the type IV patients treated with nicotinic acid as the decreased formation of bile acids tended to be compensated for by a rise in the elimination of cholesterol as neutral products[11].

The parallel changes in the production of bile acids and plasma triglycerides observed under various circumstances suggest that the regulation of these variables is interrelated. VLDL and the bile acids are both synthesized in the liver. One regimen (cholesteryramine), that stimulates primarily bile acid biosynthesis and secondarily hepatic cholesterogenesis[13], appeared to be associated with an enhanced production of triglycerides. The primary action of all other regimens mentioned above remains uncertain. However, there are reasons for believing that factors primarily influencing VLDL formation may cause analogous changes of the bile synthesis.

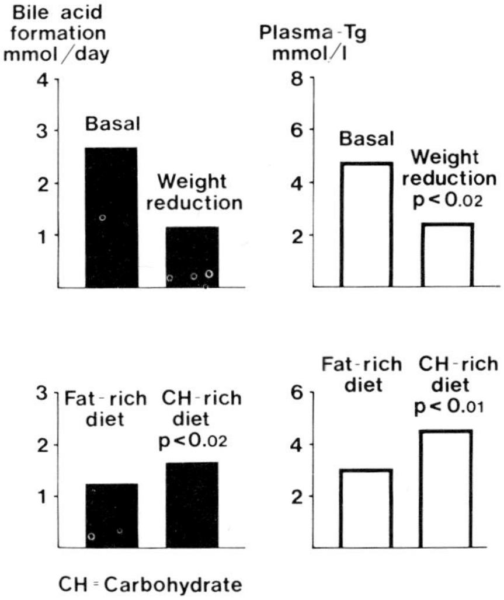

Figure 5 Bile acid formation and plasma triglyceride level before and after weight reduction in hypertriglyceridaemic patients[1] (upper panel) and before and after the shift from a fat-rich to a carbohydrate-rich diet given to hyperlipidaemic patients[12] (lower panel)

CA is the major bile acid in most healthy subjects. As mentioned above the CA/CDCA ratio of the bile acid synthesized was in general subnormal in HLP type II and supranormal in HLP type IV. A low CA/CDCA ratio was also found in patients with portal liver cirrhosis – a disorder often characterized by an impaired formation of CA[14]. In contrast to the patients with liver cirrhosis[15] those with HLP type II responded to cholestyramine with a marked rise of the CA/CDCA ratio of the bile acid produced[6]. A slight increase of the CA/CDCA ratio was also observed in healthy controls treated in a similar way[16]. The dramatic effects observed in HLP type II (Figure 6) indicate that the subnormal formation of CA under basal conditions is caused by homeostatic factors rather than inability to produce CA. This finding initiated another investigation in which we studied

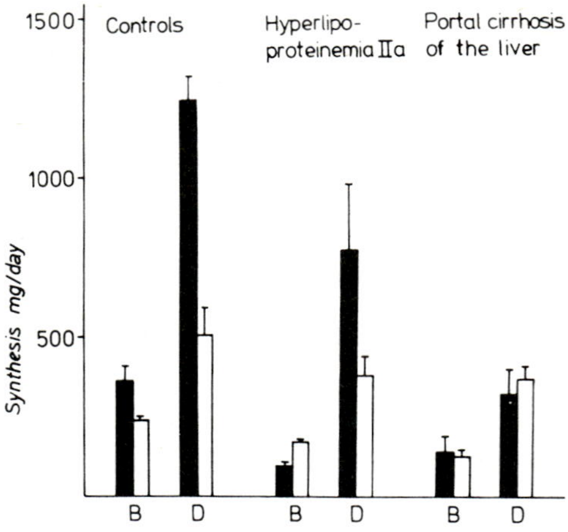

Figure 6 The synthesis of cholic acid (solid bars) and chenodeoxycholic acid (open bars) before and during administration of cholestyramine to healthy controls[16] and to patients with HLP type II[6] and portal cirrhosis[15], respectively

the effect of cholesterol feeding on bile acid kinetics[17]. With the cholesterol-rich diet the plasma cholesterol in the LDL fraction increased in the normolipidaemic subjects studied. Total bile acid formation remained constant but the CA/CDCA ratio of the bile acids produced showed a slight but significant decrease (Figure 7). Considering this response it is speculated that the high concentration of LDL cholesterol in HLP type II under basal conditions continuously stimulates the feedback inhibition of hepatic cholesterogenesis. If so, a supranormal part of the body cholesterol in this disorder might originate from extrahepatic sources, as the total cholesterol biosynthesis remains within normal limits[2]. However, further experiments are required to establish the existence of such a relationship.

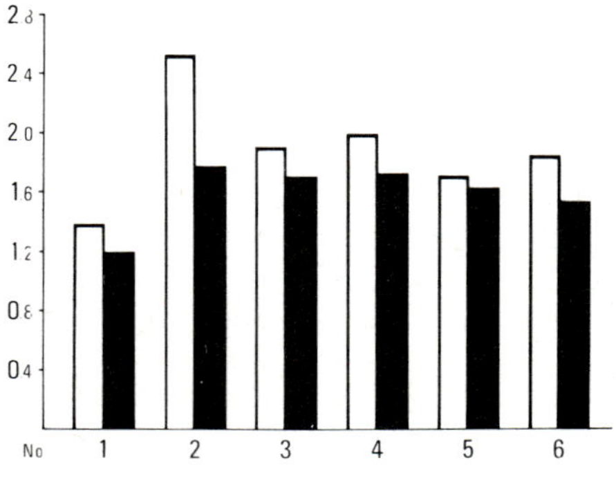

Figure 7 The effect of cholesterol feeding on the CA/CDCA ratio of bile acids synthesized in normolipidaemic controls[17]. Open bars, before cholesterol feeding; solid bars, during cholesterol feeding

References

1. Einarsson, K., Hellström, K. and Kallner, M. (1974). Bile acid kinetics in relation to sex, serum lipids, body weights and gallbladder disease in patients with various types of hyperlipoproteinaemia. *J. Clin. Invest.*, **54,** 1301
2. Angelin, B., Einarsson, K., Hellström, K. and Kallner, M. (1976). Elimination of cholesterol in hyperlipoproteinaemia. *Clin. Sci. Mol. Med.*, **51,** 393
3. Hellström, K. and Einarsson, K. (1977). Bile acid metabolism in hyperlipoproteinaemia. *Clin. Gastroenterol.*, **6,** 103
4. Angelin, B., Einarsson, K., Hellström, K. and Leijd, B. (1978). Bile acid kinetics in relation to endogenous triglyceride metabolism in various types of hyperlipoproteinaemia. *J. Lipid Res.*, **19,** 1004
5. Nikkilä, E. A. and Kecki, M. (1972). Plasma endogenous triglyceride transport in hypertriglyceridaemia and effect of a hypolipidaemic drug (SU-13437). *Eur. J. Clin. Invest.*, **2,** 231
6. Einarsson, K., Hellström, K. and Kallner, M. (1974). The effect of cholestyramine on the elimination of cholesterol as bile acids in patients with hyperlipoproteinaemia type II and IV. *Eur. J. Clin. Invest.*, **4,** 405
7. Angelin, B., Einarsson, K., Hellström, K. and Leijd, B. (1978). Effects of cholestyramine and chenodeoxycholic acid on the metabolism of endogenous triglyceride in hyperlipoproteinaemia. *J. Lipid Res.*, **19,** 1017
8. Kallner, M. (1975). The effect of chenodeoxycholic acid feeding on bile acid kinetics and faecal neutral steroid excretion in patients with hyperlipoproteinaemia types II and IV. *J. Lab. Clin. Med.*, **86,** 595
9. Kissebah, A. H., Alforsi, S., Adams, P. W. and Wynn, V. (1974). The mechanism of action of clofibrate and tetranicotinoylfructose (Bradilan) on the kinetics of plasma free fatty acid and triglyceride transport in type IV and type V hypertriglyceridaemia. *Eur. J. Clin. Invest.*, **4,** 163
10. Einarsson, K., Hellström, K. and Kallner, M. (1973). The effect of clofibrate on the elimination of cholesterol as bile acids in patients with hyperlipoproteinaemia type II and IV. *Eur. J. Clin. Invest.*, **3,** 1973
11. Einarsson, K., Hellström, K. and Leijd, B. (1977). Bile acid kinetics and steroid balance during nicotinic acid therapy in patients with hyperlipoproteinaemia types II and IV. *J. Lab. Clin. Med.*, **90,** 613
12. Andersén, E. and Hellström, K. (1980). Influence of fat-rich versus carbohydrate-rich diets on bile acid kinetics, biliary lipids and net steroid balance in hyperlipidaemic subjects. *Metabolism*, **29,** 400
13. Grundy, S. M., Ahrens, E. H. Jr. and Salen, G. (1971). Interruption of the enterohepatic circulation of bile acids in man: comparative effects of cholestyramine and ileal exclusion on cholesterol metabolism. *J. Lab. Clin. Med.*, **78,** 94
14. Einarsson, K., Hellström, K. and Schersten, T. (1975). The formation of bile acids in patients with portal liver cirrhosis. *Scand. J. Gastroenterol.*, **10,** 1975
15. Angelin, B., Einarsson, K. and Hellström, K. (1978). Effect of cholestyramine on bile acid kinetics in patients with portal cirrhosis of the liver. Evidence of a selective defect in the formation of cholic acid. *Am. J. Dig. Dis.*, **23,** 1115
16. Andersén, E. (1979). The effect of cholestyramine on bile acid kinetics in healthy controls. *Scand. J. Gastroenterol.*, **14,** 657
17. Andersén, E. and Hellström, K. (1979). The effect of cholesterol feeding on bile acid kinetics and biliary lipids in normolipidaemic and hypertriglyceridaemic subjects. *J. Lipid Res.*, **20,** 1020

ADOLF WINDAUS PRIZE LECTURE

3
Hepatic and biliary lipid metabolism in hyperlipidaemia

K. EINARSSON

INTRODUCTION

Hepatic cholesterol can be derived from plasma lipoproteins and from the liver itself by endogenous synthesis. A simplified schedule of cholesterol metabolism in the liver is presented in Figure 1. The rate-determining enzyme is HMG-CoA reductase which converts HMG-CoA to mevalonic acid. The mechanisms of the regulation for this enzyme in human liver are still incompletely known. Cholesterol can be removed from the liver via secretion

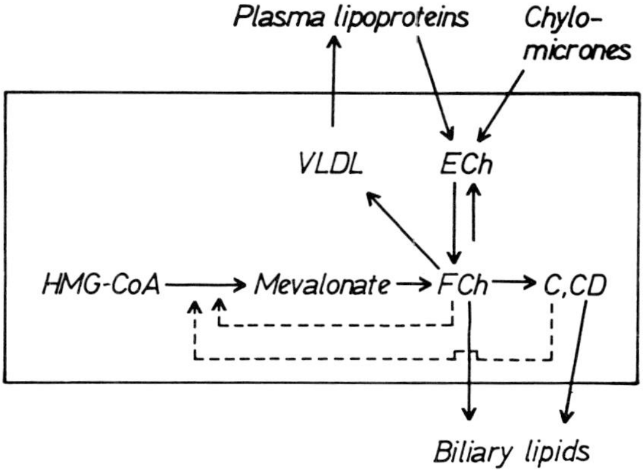

Figure 1 Metabolism of hepatic cholesterol. C, cholic acid; CD, chenodeoxycholic acid; ECh, esterified cholesterol; FCh, free cholesterol; VLDL, very low density lipoproteins

into the bile as free cholesterol or after conversion to the two primary bile acids cholic acid (CA) and chenodeoxycholic acid (CDCA) and by secretion into plasma as lipoproteins. This presentation will mainly focus on the hepatic HMG-CoA reductase and hydroxylases involved in bile acid synthesis in hyperlipoproteinaemia (HLP), the biliary lipid composition in HLP, and the influence of perturbations of bile acid metabolism on the triglyceride synthesis in the liver.

CHOLESTEROL AND BILE ACID SYNTHESIS

The HMG-CoA reductase activity was assayed in the microsomal fraction of liver biopsies obtained peroperatively from normolipidaemic and hyperlipidaemic gallstone patients undergoing cholecystectomy[1]. The assay system used was essentially the same as that described by Dr Mosbach's group[2]. There was a wide range of enzyme activities in the normolipidaemic group (Figure 2). This pattern is, however, similar to that seen for *in vivo* determina-

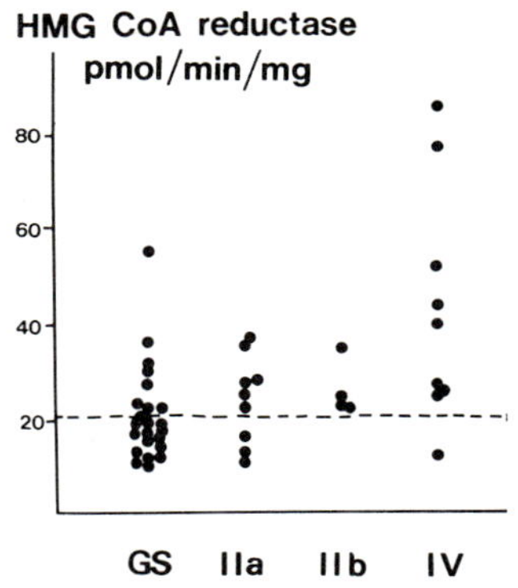

Figure 2 HMG-CoA reductase activities in normolipidaemic (GS) and hyperlipidaemic gallstone patients. Dotted line indicates mean value of HMG-CoA reductase activities in GS

tions of the net steroid balance in healthy subjects[3]. In the present study patients with HLP type IIa and IIb all had normal HMG-CoA reductase activity. This is in accordance with our previous finding that these patients have a normal endogenous cholesterol formation[3]. In HLP type IV, on the other hand, the mean value of HMG-CoA reductase activity was about twice that seen in normolipidaemic subjects. Four of the patients had activities within the normal range. These data agree fairly well those obtained for the net steroid balance in HLP type IV[3]. Thus about 50% of these patients had a steroid balance above the normal range.

Patients with HLP type II often display a low synthesis of CA relative to CDCA[4]. This might be explained by a reduction or deficiency of an enzyme, selective of CA formation. To test this hypothesis we assayed two hydroxylases involved in CA synthesis, namely the 12α-hydroxylase which is specific for CA formation and the 25-hydroxylase, whose role has not been finally established[1]. However, the 12α-hydroxylase and 25-hydroxylase activities were similar in all groups of patients (Figure 3). Subsequently these results gave no support for a selective deficiency of enzyme activities in HLP type II.

HYPERLIPOPROTEINAEMIA AND GALLSTONE DISEASE

In a series of investigations we have given evidence for an association between hypertriglyceridaemia and gallstone disease. Firstly, the frequency of gallstone

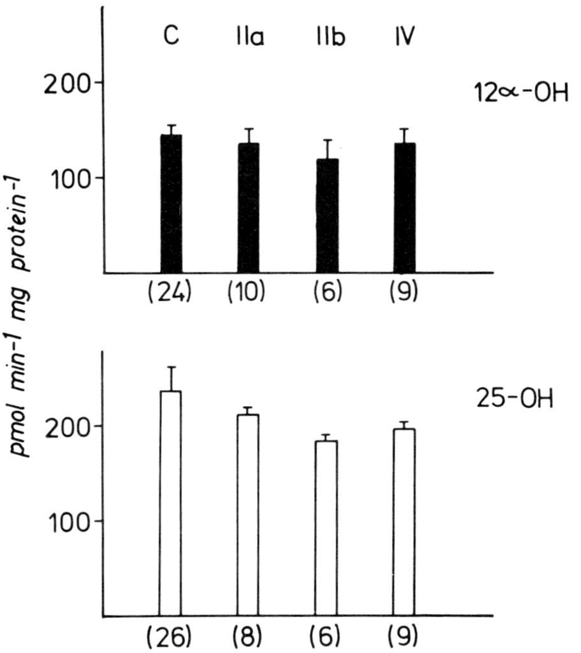

Figure 3 12α- and 25-hydroxylase activities in normolipidaemic (C) and hyperlipidaemic gallstone patients. Number of subjects within parentheses

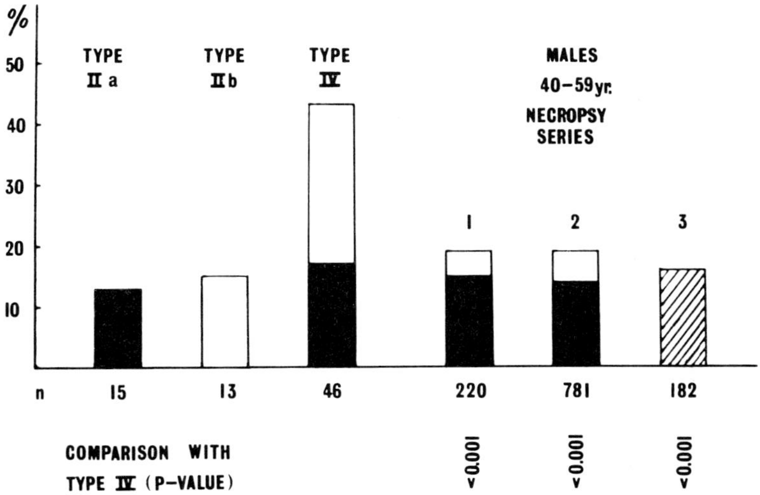

Figure 4 Prevalence of gallstone disease in 40–59-year old males with hyperlipoproteinaemia compared to that recorded for males of the same age in three reported necropsy series[6–8]. □ cholecystectomy; ■ cholelithiasis, cholecystitis; ▨ cholelithiasis, cholecystitis, cholecystectomy

disease was determined in 210 consecutive patients with HLP and compared to the prevalence in the general Swedish population as judged from three necropsy series[5]. Among 40–59-year-old patients the prevalence of gallstone disease was increased in males with HLP type IV (Figure 4) as well as females with HLP type IV (Figure 5). Although not significant on a statistical basis the occurrence of gallstone disease tended to be supranormal also in females with HLP type IIb. Overweight and impaired glucose tolerance, which are recognized as factors related to the development of gallstone disease, are often encountered in patients with type IV HLP. However, the exclusion of such patients did not change the obtained results. Secondly, serum lipid levels and prevalence of HLP in a consecutive series of gallstone patients were compared to a control series[9]. Serum cholesterol values were the same in the two series, while serum triglyceride levels were increased in the gallstone series. Among patients over 50 years there was a significant overrepresentation of HLP type IV among the gallstone patients.

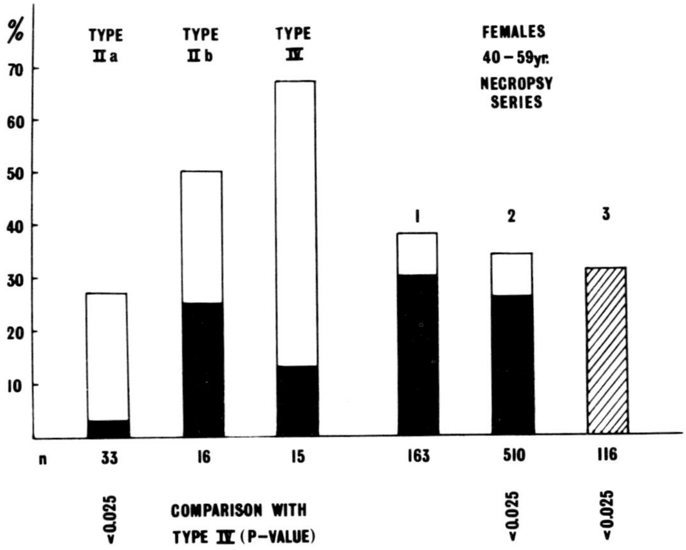

Figure 5 Prevalence of gallstone disease in 40–59-year-old females with hyperlipoproteinaemia compared to females of the same age in three reported necropsy series[6–8]. □ cholecystectomy; ■ cholelithiasis; cholecystitis; ▨ cholelithiasis, cholecystitis, cholecystectomy

Thirdly, the biliary lipid composition of fasting gallbladder bile has been investigated in a series of non-obese, healthy controls and in patients with HLP without gallstones[10]. A normal biliary cholesterol saturation was found in patients with HLP type IIa (Figure 6). All patients with type IIb and 10 of 12 with type IV had saturated bile. These results may explain the previous finding of an increased prevalence of gallstone disease in patients with HLP type IV. The mechanisms responsible for the development of supersaturated gallbladder bile in HLP type IV cannot be decided at present. Cholesterol

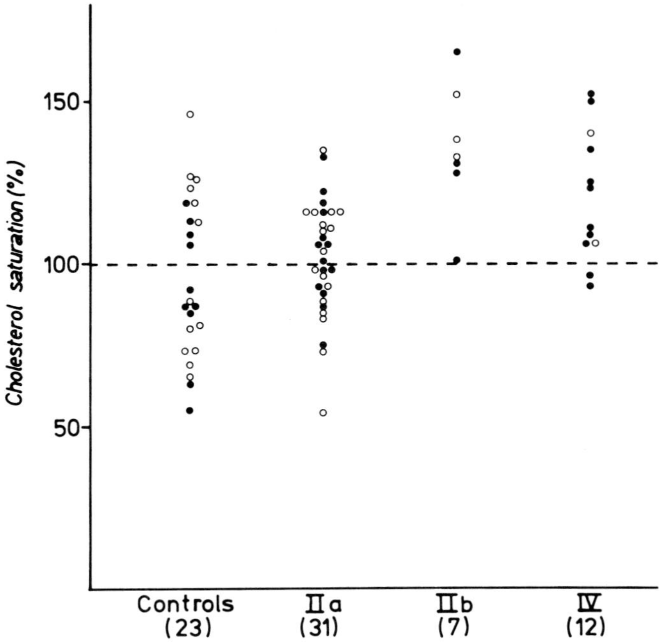

Figure 6 Cholesterol saturation of gallbladder bile in controls and patients with various types of hyperlipoproteinaemia without gallstone disease. Number of subjects within parentheses. Horizontal line indicates 100% saturation of bile; filled circles indicate males; open circles indicate females. (From Ahlberg *et al.*[10] reproduced with permission)

saturation may be changed by factors disproportionally influencing the hepatic secretion of bile acids, phospholipids and cholesterol. Since HLP type IV patients often have an enlarged pool size and an enhanced synthesis of bile acids[4], it seems more likely to suppose that the hepatic secretion of cholesterol is increased rather than that the bile acid secretion is deficient. Studies on the secretion rates of biliary lipids in HLP type IV are in progress in our laboratory.

HYPOLIPIDAEMIC DRUGS MAY INFLUENCE CHOLESTEROL SATURATION

Treatment with hypolipidaemic drugs may also influence the biliary secretion of cholesterol. We have investigated the effect of treatment with nicotinic acid, clofibrate and cholestyramine on the biliary lipid composition in HLP patients[11]. Nicotinic acid treatment was associated with a slight (about 20%) increase in biliary cholesterol concentration relative to biliary total lipids (Figure 7). Clofibrate raised the molar percentage of cholesterol about 40%, which is in accordance with the clinical finding that this drug increases the risk for gallstone formation. The addition of cholestyramine to clofibrate normalized the biliary composition. It has been suggested that the increased

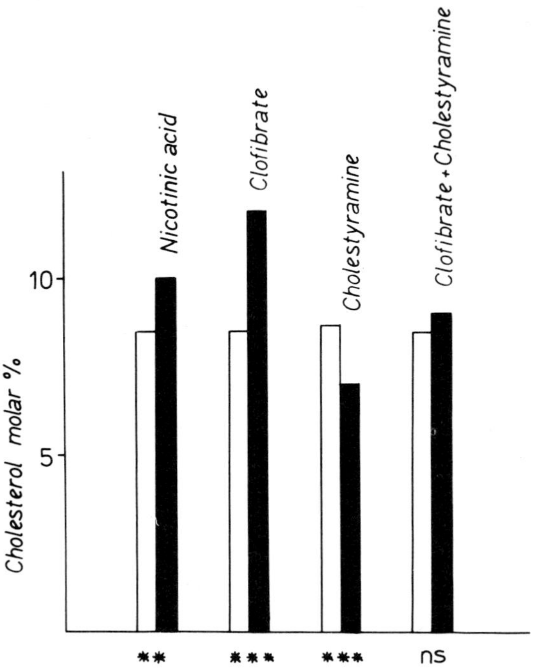

Figure 7 Relative cholesterol concentration in bile before □ and during ■ treatment with nicotinic acid, clofibrate, cholestyramine and combination of clofibrate and cholestyramine. **Significantly different from pretreatment values, $p < 0.01$; *** significantly different from pretreatment values, $p < 0.001$

biliary secretion of cholesterol during clofibrate treatment is a transient effect[12]. However, recent data from our laboratory show that most HLP patients still had an increased cholesterol saturation of bile after 2 years of treatment with clofibrate[13]. Although some patients may normalize their bile composition during long-term treatment the average value of the cholesterol saturation was the same after long-term as after short-term treatment.

BILE ACIDS AND TRIGLYCERIDE SYNTHESIS

In prelimiary studies we have assayed the activity of the hepatic soluble phosphatidic acid phosphatase, which is a rate-determining enzyme in triglyceride synthesis in rat[14]. Several experimental groups of animals have been studied. Bile fistula rats and rats pretreated with cholestyramine displayed an increased enzyme activity. Bile acid feeding, especially with chenodeoxycholic acid, on the other hand, was associated with a decreased enzyme activity. These results lend further support to our finding in man, that bile acid metabolism and triglyceride production seem to be integrated with each other[15–17]. We now also have an assay system for the soluble phosphatidic acid phosphatase in human liver, and attempts to assay this enzyme under various conditions in man are in progress.

Acknowledgment

This work was supported by grants from the Swedish Medical Research Council (Project no 19x-04793).

References

1. Ahlberg, J., Angelin, B., Björkhem, I., Einarsson, K. and Leijd, B. (1979). Hepatic cholesterol metabolism in normo- and hyperlipidemic patients with cholesterol gallstones. *J. Lipid Res.*, **20**, 107
2. Nicolau, G., Shefer, S., Salen, G. and Mosbach, E. H. (1974). Determination of hepatic 3-hydroxy-3-methylglutaryl CoA reductase activity in man. *J. Lipid Res.*, **15**, 94
3. Angelin, B., Einarsson, K., Hellström, K. and Kallner, M. (1976). Elimination of cholesterol in hyperlipoproteinaemia. *Clin. Sci. Mol. Med.*, **51**, 393
4. Einarsson, K., Hellström, K. and Kallner, M. (1974). Bile acid kinetics in relation to sex, serum lipids, body weight and gallbladder disease in patients with various types of hyperlipoproteinemia. *J. Clin. Invest.*, **54**, 1301
5. Ahlberg, J., Angelin, B., Einarsson, K., Hellström, K. and Leijd, B. (1979). Prevalence of gallbladder disease in hyperlipoproteinemia. *Am. J. Dig. Dis.*, **24**, 459
6. Sternby, N. H. (1968). Atherosclerosis in a defined population. An autopsy survey in Malmö, Sweden. *Acta Pathol. Microbiol. Scand.*, **194** (Suppl.)
7. Zahor, Z., Sternby, N. H., Kagan, A., Uemura, K., Vanecek, R. and Vichert, A. M. (1974). Frequency of cholelithiasis in Prague and Malmö. *Scand. J. Gastroenterol.*, **9**, 3
8. Lindström, C. H. (1977). Frequency of gallstone disease in a well-defined Swedish population. A prospective necropsy study in Malmö. *Scand. J. Gastroenterol.*, **12**, 341
9. Ahlberg, J. (1979). Serum lipid levels and hyperlipoproteinaemia in gallstone patients. *Acta Chir. Scand.*, **145**, 373
10. Ahlberg, J., Angelin, B., Einarsson, K., Hellström, K. and Leijd, B. (1980). Biliary lipid composition in normo- and hyperlipoproteinemia. *Gastroenterology*, **79**, 90
11. Angelin, B., Einarsson, K. and Leijd, B. (1979). Biliary lipid composition during treatment with different hypolipidaemic drugs. *Eur. J. Clin. Invest.*, **9**, 185
12. Grundy, S. M. (1979). Biliary lipids, gallstones and treatment of hyperlipidaemia. (Editorial). *Eur. J. Clin. Invest.*, **9**, 179
13. Angelin, B., Einarsson, K. and Leijd, B. (1981). Clofibrate treatment and bile cholesterol saturation: short-term and long-term effects and influence of combination with chenodeoxycholic acid. *Eur. J. Clin. Invest.* (In press)
14. Angelin, B., Björkhem, I. and Einarsson, K. (1981). Influence of bile acids on the rate-limiting step in biosynthesis of triglycerides in rat liver. (In preparation)
15. Angelin, B., Einarsson, K., Hellström, K. and Leijd, B. (1978). Bile acid kinetics in relation to endogenous triglyceride metabolism in various types of hyperlipoproteinemia. *J, Lipid Res.*, **19**, 1004
16. Angelin, B., Einarsson, K., Hellström. and Leijd, B. (1978). Effects of cholestyramine and chenodeoxycholic acid on the metabolism of endogenous triglyceride in hyperlipoproteinemia. *J. Lipid Res.*, **19**, 1017
17. Angelin, B. and Leijd, B. (1980). Effects of cholic acid on the metabolism of endogenous plasma triglyceride and on biliary lipid composition in hyperlipoproteinemia. *J. Lipid Res.*, **21**, 1

SECTION 1
Biosynthesis and Metabolism

4
Short-term regulation of cholesterol biosynthesis

H. B. BREWER AND Z. H. BEG

INTRODUCTION

During the last few years a great deal of interest has focused on the regulation of cholesterol biosynthesis. Hepatic cholesterol biosynthesis is regulated by the enzymic activity of 3-hydroxy-3-methylglutaryl coenzyme A reductase (HMG-CoA reductase, EC 1.1.1.34)[1-3]. Modulation of the enzymic activity of HMG-CoA reductase is achieved by two general mechanisms, long-term and short-term regulation. Long-term regulation involves changes in enzyme synthesis and/or degradation[1-3]. Short-term regulation is achieved by isosteric and allosteric effectors and covalent modification[4-8]. Of particular interest has been the elucidation of the role of covalent modification in the regulation of the enzymic activity of HMG-CoA reductase. This report reviews the results obtained in our laboratory which established that HMG-CoA reductase undergoes covalent modification by reversible phosphorylation *in vitro* and *in vivo*[4,6-8]. The enzyme which catalyses the phosphorylation of HMG-CoA reductase, reductase kinase, also undergoes reversible phosphorylation. The phosphorylated form of reductase kinase is active, whereas the dephosphorylated form of HMG-CoA reductase is the active species. These studies have established that the enzymic activity of HMG-CoA reductase is modulated by a bicyclic cascade system. This mechanism may represent a major method for the short-term regulation of cholesterol biosynthesis.

Materials and methods

The purification of HMG-CoA reductase, reductase kinase, and phosphoprotein phosphatase have been reported previously[6-8]. HMG-CoA, agarose-hexane-HMG-CoA, ATP were obtained from PL Biochemicals, [γ^{32}P] ATP, [^{32}P]phosphoric acid and [^{14}C]HMG-CoA from New England Nuclear; NADPH, glucose-6-phosphate, glucose-6-phosphate dehydrogenase, and NADP were purchased from Sigma. Glucagon was a gift of Eli Lilly and Company. Assay of HMG-CoA reductase and reductase kinase were performed as previously described[6-8]. Sodium dodecylsulphate electrophoresis

(5.6% acrylamide, pH 7.4) and production of antibodies to HMG-CoA reductase were performed as previously reported[6–8].

RESULTS

Purification of HMG-CoA reductase

HMG-CoA reductase has been solubilized from rat liver microsomes, and purified to homogeneity by the procedure detailed in Table 1[8]. HMG-CoA reductase was purified approximately 6000-fold with an overall yield of 35% in less than 24 h. The isolated enzyme demonstrated a single electrophoretic band on SDS gel electrophoresis with an apparent monomer molecular weight of 51 000 ± 1800. On aqueous polyacrylamide gel electrophoresis > 98% of HMG-CoA reductase activity was associated with the single electrophoretic band[6,8]. Antibodies prepared in a goat against purified rat liver HMG-CoA reductase formed a single immunoprecipitin line of identity with purified, solubilized, and microsomal HMG-CoA reductase[8].

Table 1 Purification of HMG-CoA reductase from rat liver microsomes

*Fraction**	*Protein* (mg)	*Activity* (units)	*Specific activity*† (units/mg)	*Purification* (*fold*)	*Yield* (%)
Microsomes	3028	2516	0.83	1	100
Solubilized fraction	198	2164	10.9	13	86
NH_4 sulphate precipitation (35–50%)	64	1761	27.5	33	70
Heat treatment (65 °C, 30 min) + NH_4 sulphate precipitation (0–50%)	4.97	1432	288	347	57
HMG-CoA affinity chromatography	0.171	890	5205	6271	35

* Isolated from 100 g of liver.
† One unit is definedas the amount of enzyme that catalyses 1/nmol of HMG-CoA to mevalonate in 1 min.

Reversible phosphorylation–dephosphorylation of HMG-CoA reductase *in vitro*

Incubation of electrophoretically homogeneous HMG-CoA reductase, reductase kinase, [γ-^{32}P]-ATP plus $MgCl_2$ was associated with a progressive decrease in enzyme activity and increase in ^{32}P-bound radioactivity[6,8]. A 78% decrease in HMG-CoA reductase activity was observed with a 30-min incubation containing 1 mM [γ^{32}P]-ATP. Radiolabelled [^{32}P]HMG-CoA reductase was analysed by SDS gel electrophoresis (Figure 1). Greater than 98% of the radioactivity was associated with the electrophoretic position of purified HMG-CoA reductase. Based on an assumed tetramer molecular weight of 200 000, an average of 3.68 ± 0.56 (n = 8) mol of phosphate were incorporated per tetramer[8]. Incubation of ^{32}P-labelled HMG-CoA reductase with phosphoprotein phosphatase resulted in >90% loss of protein-bound

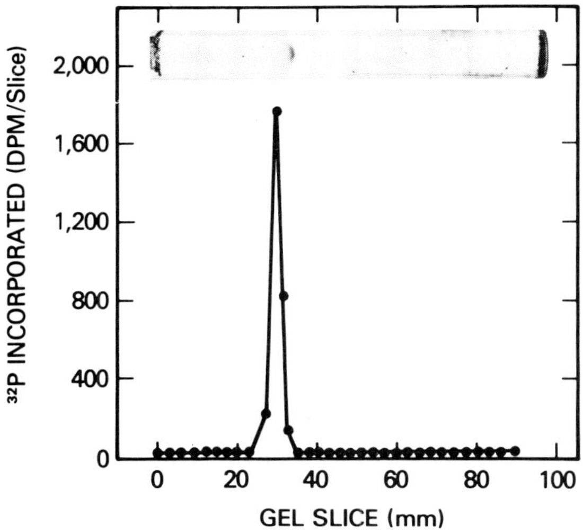

Figure 1 SDS gel electrophoresis of purified HMG-CoA reductase phosphorylated *in vitro*. HMG-CoA reductase, isolated by the method outlined in Table 1, was incubated for 1 h with 4 mM $MgCl_2$ + 0.2 mM [γ-^{32}P]ATP in a medium containing 2 mM DTT, 50 mM β-glycerophosphate (pH 7.0) and purified reductase kinase (0.08 mg/ml). Following incubation 1% SDS, 40 mM DTT, 1 mM EDTA, 10 μg pyronin Y, and 10 mM Tris-HCl (pH 8.0) were added, and the reaction mixture heated at 70 °C for 30 min. The electrophoretic band in the reference gel denotes the position of the 51 000 molecular weight subunit of HMG-CoA reductase

^{32}P radioactivity[6,8]. These results have established that purified HMG-CoA reductase undergoes a reversible phosphorylation–dephosphorylation reaction sequence *in vitro*.

Reversible phosphorylation–dephosphorylation of reductase kinase *in vitro*

The enzyme, reductase kinase, responsible for the phosphorylation of HMG-CoA reductase has been isolated to electrophoretic homogeneity[7]. Incubation of solubilized or purified reductase kinase, [γ^{32}P]ATP plus $MgCl_2$, and a partially purified kinase, designated reductase kinase kinase, resulted in a time-dependent increase in both protein-bound radioactivity and ability to catalyse the phosphorylation of HMG-CoA reductase[7]. Analysis of the incubation mixture by polyacrylamide gel electrophoresis revealed that >95% of the ^{32}P radioactivity was present in the electrophoretic position of purified reductase kinase (Figure 2). Dephosphorylation of ^{32}P-labelled reductase kinase with phosphoprotein phosphatase was associated with >70% loss of radioactivity of the protein band. cAMP and calmodulin have no effect on the enzymic activity of microsomal reductase kinase, and this kinase has been designated as the cAMP-independent reductase kinase. A cAMP-dependent reductase kinase, however, has been recognized and is currently being characterized in our laboratory[7].

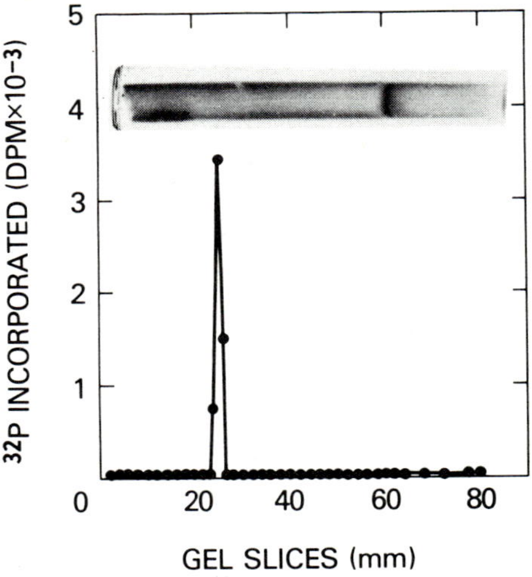

Figure 2 SDS gel electrophoresis of reductase kinase phosphorylated *in vitro*. Reductase kinase was incubated for 1 h with 4 mM $MgCl_2$ + 0.2 mM [γ-^{32}P]ATP with partially purified reductase kinase kinase. Following incubation samples were treated as outlined in Figure 1. The electrophoretic band in the reference gel indicates the electrophoretic position of purified reductase kinase

These combined results provided evidence for the *in vitro* modulation of the enzymic activity of HMG-CoA reductase and reductase kinase by reversible phosphorylation–dephosphorylation.

In vivo phosphorylation of HMG-CoA reductase

The *in vivo* phosphorylation of HMG-CoA reductase was studied in rats by injection of ^{32}P, followed by isolation of liver microsomes, and purification of HMG-CoA reductase by immunoprecipitation or to homogeneity by affinity chromatography as outlined in Table 1. Examination of the ^{32}P-labelled immunoprecipitates and purified enzyme by SDS gel electrophoresis revealed a single peak of radioactivity coincident with the migration of purified HMG-CoA reductase[8] (Figure 3). These results have established that HMG-CoA reductase undergoes phosphorylation *in vivo*.

Modulation of hepatic HMG-CoA reductase by glucagon

In order to evaluate the modulation of the enzymic activity of HMG-CoA reductase by change in degree of phosphorylation, rats were injected with glucagon, ^{32}P, and HMG-CoA reductase isolated by immunoprecipitation or affinity chromatography. The administration of glucagon was associated with a 35–40% decrease in enzymic activity of HMG-CoA reductase, a 10–12-fold increase in hepatic cyclic AMP content, a 2-fold increase in the incorporation of ^{32}P into HMG-CoA reductase, and no change in hepatic ATP specific activity (Table 2)[8].

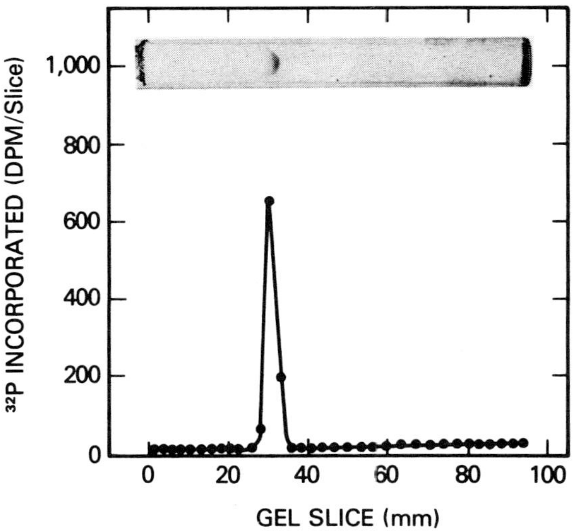

Figure 3 SDS gel electrophoresis of HMG-CoA reductase phosphorylated *in vivo*. Light–dark cycled rats ($n=4$) were injected intraperitoneally with 1 mCi of ^{32}P at 8.45 am and 9.45 am. At 10.00 am rats were anaesthetized and livers removed at 10.15 am for purification of HMG-CoA reductase by the method outlined in Table 1. Purification was performed in the presence of 5 mM EDTA and 50 mM NaF. The electrophoretic band in the reference gel indicates the electrophoretic position of the 51 000 molecular weight subunit of HMG-CoA reductase

These data provide evidence that HMG-CoA reductase can undergo phosphorylation *in vivo* and that the degree of phosphorylation and enzymic activity may be modulated by polypeptide hormones.

CONCLUSION

Based on the results reviewed here and detailed in previous publications, we have proposed a conceptual scheme of the regulation of HMG-CoA reductase (Figure 4)[6–8]. The enzymically active form of HMG-CoA reductase

Table 2 Effect of glucagon on the enzymic activity and phosphorylation of HMG-CoA reductase

Group	*Cyclic AMP* (nmol/g liver)	*ATP specific activity* (dpm/pmol)	*Microsomal HMG-CoA reductase activity** (nmol min^{-1} mg^{-1})	[^{32}P]*HMG-CoA reductase* (dpm/mg)
Saline	0.59 ± 0.18	14.8 ± 1.3	0.132 ± 0.014	15,250 ± 2431
Glucagon	4.98 ± 0.85	13.9 ± 1.4	0.080 ± 0.009	31,675 ± 1890

* Representative data of eight separate experiments in which a total of 32 rats were used to determine the effect of glucagon on the enzymic activity of HMG-CoA reductase. Light-dark cycled rats were injected with ^{32}P (intraperitoneally 1 mCi at 8.45 am and 9.45 am; 9.15 am saline (control) or glucagon 400 μg was injected subcutaneously; 10.00 am glucagon (200 μg) or saline injection was repeated and livers removed at 10.15 am for assay and purification of HMG-CoA reductase). Liver microsomes were prepared in buffer containing 5 mM EDTA and 50 mM NaF.

is regulated by a bicyclic cascade system. The enzymically active form of HMG-CoA reductase is dephosphorylated, whereas the active form of reductase kinase is phosphorylated. Increase in intracellular cAMP concentration would be expected to modulate the bicyclic cascade system by increasing the activity of the cAMP-dependent reductase kinase and to inhibit reductase kinase and HMG-CoA reductase phosphatases by increasing the activity of the phosphatase inhibitor protein, thereby influencing the dephosphorylation of both reductase kinase and the HMG-CoA reductase. The phosphoprotein phosphatase inhibitory protein is activated by a reversible phosphorylation reaction mediated by a cyclic AMP-dependent kinase[9–11].

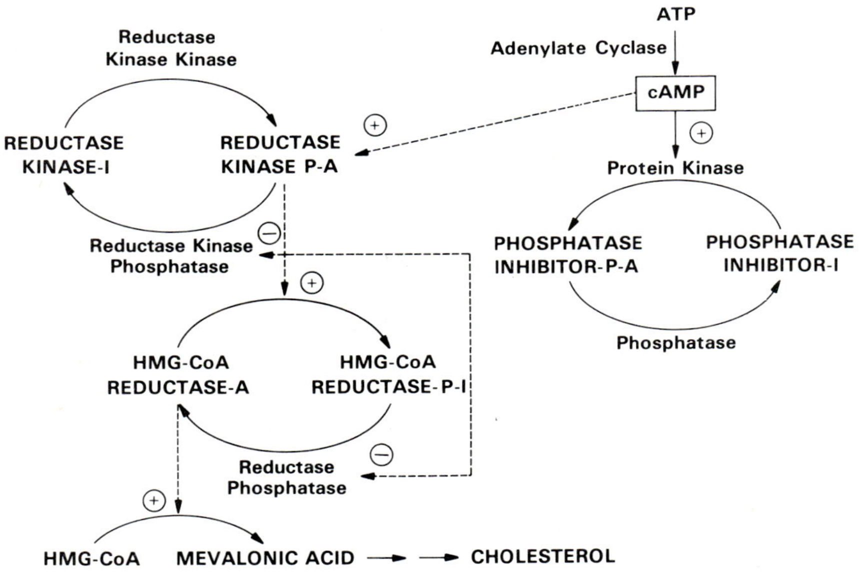

Figure 4 Schematic representation of the modulation of enzymic activity of hepatic reductase kinase and HMG-CoA reductase. The active, inactive, and phosphorylated forms of the enzymes are designated A, I, and P, respectively. The enzymically active form of HMG-CoA reductase is dephosphorylated, whereas the active form of reductase kinase and phosphatase inhibitor protein is phosphorylated. cAMP would be expected to modulate the bicyclic cascade system by increasing the activity of the cAMP-dependent reductase kinase and to inhibit reductase kinase and HMG-CoA reductase phosphatases by increasing the activity of the phosphatase inhibitor protein

This overall scheme for the regulation of the enzymic activity of HMG-CoA reductase involving reversible covalent modifications may represent an important short-term mechanism for the regulation of mevalonate formation and cholesterol biosynthesis.

Acknowledgments

We would like to thank Ms Barbara Ziarnik for typing the manuscript and John Stonik for expert technical assistance.

References

1. Siperstein, M. D. (1970). Regulation of cholesterol biosynthesis in normal and malignant tissue. In Horecker, B. L. and Stadtman, E. R. (eds.). *Current Topics in Cellular Regulation*, pp. 65–80. (New York: Academic Press)
2. Beytia, E. D. and Porter, J. W. (1976). Biochemistry of polyisoprenoid biosynthesis. *Ann. Rev. Biochem.*, **45,** 113
3. Rodwell, V. W., Nordstrum, J. L. and Mitschelen, J. J. (1976). Regulation of HMG-CoA reductase. In Paoletti, R. and Kretchevsky, D. (eds.) *Advances in Lipid Research*, pp. 2–42. (New York: Academic Press)
4. Beg, Z. H., Stonik, J. A. and Brewer, H. B. Jr. (1979). 3-hydroxy-3-methylglutaryl coenzyme A reductase from avian liver: catalytic properties. *Biochim. Biophys. Acta*, **572,** 93
5. Ingebritsen, T. S., Lee, H. S., Parker, R. A. and Gibson, D. M. (1978). Reversible modulation of the activities of both liver microsomal hydroxymethyl coenzyme A reductase and its activating enzyme: evidence for regulation of phosphorylation. *Biochem. Biophys. Res. Commun.*, **81,** 1268
6. Beg, Z. H., Stonik, J. A. and Brewer, H. B. Jr. (1978). 3-hydroxy-3-methylglutaryl coenzyme A reductase: regulation of enzymic activity by phosphorylation and dephosphorylation. *Proc. Natl. Acad. Sci.* (*USA*), **75,** 3678
7. Beg, Z. H., Stonik, J. A. and Brewer, H. B. Jr. (1979). Characterization and regulation of reductase kinase, a protein kinase that modulates the enzymic activity of 3-hyroxy-3-methylglutaryl-coenzyme A reductase. *Proc. Natl. Acad. Sci.* (*USA*), **76,** 4375
8. Beg, Z. H., Stonik, J. A. and Brewer, H. B. Jr. (1980). *In vitro* and *in vivo* phosphorylation of rat liver 3-hydroxy-3-methylglutaryl coenzyme A reductase and its modulation by glucagon. *J. Biol. Chem.*, **255,** 8541
9. Huang, F. L. and Glinsmann, W. H. (1975). Inactivation of rabbit muscle phosphorylase phosphatase by cyclic AMP-dependent kinase. *Proc. Natl. Acad. Sci.* (*USA*), **72,** 3004
10. Nimmo, H. G. and Cohen, P. (1977). Hormonal control of protein phosphorylation. *Advances in Cyclic Nucleotide Research*, vol. 8, pp. 145–192. (New York: Raven Press)
11. Goris, J., Defreyn, G., Vandeeheede, J. R. and Merlevede, W. (1978). Protein inhibitors of dog liver phosphorylase phosphatase dependent or independent of protein kinase. *Eur. J. Biochem.*, **91,** 457

5
Studies on properties of purified cholesterol 7α-hydroxylase from rabbit and rat liver microsomes

K. WIKVALL, H. BOSTRÖM, H. DANIELSSON,
R. HANSSON, I. KALLES AND B. LIDSTRÖM

INTRODUCTION

The introduction of a 7α-hydroxyl group is the first and rate-limiting step in the conversion of cholesterol into bile acids[1-4]. The cholesterol 7α-hydroxylase activity is regulated by the concentrations of bile acids in portal blood but also by nutritional and hormonal factors[3,4]. The reaction is catalysed by a mixed function oxidase system of liver microsomes and involves the participation of at least two components, a cytochrome P-450 and NADPH-cytochrome P-450 reductase[5-8].

There are several reports on the involvement of cytosolic proteins in the regulation of enzyme activities in cholesterol biosynthesis[9-12]. There is much less information concerning the role of cytosol in regulation of cholesterol 7α-hydroxylation. Early work showed that the 20,000 × *g* supernatant catalyses 7α-hydroxylation of cholesterol more efficiently than microsomal fraction fortified with NADPH[13]. Recently, Spence and Gaylor[12] have reported on the stimulatory effect of cytosol and ammonium sulphate-fractionated cytosol on cholesterol 7α-hydroxylation catalysed by whole microsomes. The stimulatory activity was found to be heat-labile. In a preliminary communication Craig *et al.*[14] have confirmed and extended the results of Spence and Gaylor[12].

It is now established that several species of cytochrome P-450 with differing, although overlapping, substrate specificities exist in liver microsomes[15,16]. At least six different cytochromes P-450 have been purified to apparent homogeneity on gel electrophoresis[15-19]. Recently, in this laboratory, cytochrome P-450 fractions from liver microsomes of cholestyramine-treated rats and rabbits have been purified which catalyse cholesterol 7α-hydroxylation when combined with homogeneous NADPH-cytochrome P-450 reductase[8,20]. The present work concerns attempts to identify and isolate the species of cytochrome P-450 involved in 7α-hydroxylation of cholesterol as well as studies on the properties of purified reconstituted 7α-hydroxylase system from liver microsomes. These studies include experiments on the effects of cytosolic protein fractions on reconstituted cholesterol 7α-hydroxylase activity.

MATERIALS AND METHODS

Materials

[4-^{14}C]Cholesterol (61 μCi/μmol) was obtained from the Radiochemical Centre, Amersham, England. The labelled cholesterol was purified by chromatography on a column of aluminium oxide, grade III. Octylamine-Sepharose 4B was prepared as described previously[20,21]. DEAE-Sepharose CL-6B and, CM-Sephadex C-50 were obtained from Pharmacia. Bio-Gel HTP and Cellex-P were from Bio-Rad and DEAE-cellulose (DE-52) from Whatman. Bio-Gel hydroxylapatite was mixed with an equal weight of Whatman CF1 cellulose powder. DEAE-cellulose, Triton X-100, Tween-80, sodium cholate, dilauroylglycero-3-phosphorylcholine and cofactors were from Sigma Chemical Co. Renex 690 was from Atlas Chemical Co., Emulgen 911 and 913 from Kao-Atlas, Tokyo, cholestyramine from Merck, Sharp & Dohme, and Amberlite XAD-2 from Rohm & Haas.

Male rabbits of the New Zealand strain, weighing 2–2.5 kg, and male rats of the Sprague-Dawley strain, weighing about 200 g, were used. The animals were treated with cholestyramine, 3% (w/v) in the diet for 5 days or with phenobarbital, 1 mg/ml of drinking water, for 1 week.

METHODS

Preparation of cytochromes P-450 and NADPH-cytochrome P-450 reductase

Rabbit and rat liver microsomes were prepared as described previously[8] and treated with sodium pyrophosphate buffer[22]. Liver microsomes from cholestyramine-treated rabbits and rats used for preparation of cytochromes P-450 A, I and II were subjected to the slow freezing and thawing procedure described by Heller and Gould[20,23].

Cytochromes P-450 LM_2, LM_{3b} and LM_4 were prepared from phenobarbital-treated, untreated and cholestyramine-treated rabbits as described by Coon and associates[18,22]. Cytochrome P-450 LM_4 was also prepared from phenobarbital-treated rabbits as described by Hansson and Wikvall[20]. Cytochromes P-450 I and II were prepared from liver microsomes of cholestyramine-treated rabbits by modifications of the procedures described by Imai and Sato[24,25,20]. The hydroxylapatite column was washed with 35 mM and 80 mM phosphate buffer before the cytochrome P-450 was eluted with 300 mM phosphate in the buffer. In the CM-Sephadex chromatography the column was first washed with 50 mM phosphate. Cytochrome P-450 I was then eluted with 100 mM phosphate and cytochrome P-450 II with 300 mM phosphate in the buffer.

Cytochromes P-450 B and D were prepared from phenobarbital-treated rats as described by Guengerich[26] with the exception that DEAE-Sepharose was used instead of DEAE-cellulose. A major phenobarbital-inducible form of cytochrome P-450, cytochrome P-450 'Fraction C' ,was isolated as described by West *et al.*[27]. Cytochromes P-450 I and II were prepared from liver microsomes of cholestyramine-treated rats as described above for the rabbit liver cytochromes. Cytochrome P-450 A was isolated from the 80 mM phosphate eluate in hydroxylapatite chromatography as described by Guengerich[26]. The cytochrome P-450, which eluted with 5 mM phosphate in DEAE-Sepharose chromatography, was further purified in room temperature on a DEAE-cellulose column as described by Ryan *et al.*[28]. Cytochrome P-450 A was eluted with the equilibration buffer.

Cytochrome P-450 was determined according to Omura and Sato[29] and protein as described by Lowry *et al.*[30].

NADPH-cytochrome P-450 reductase was prepared from liver microsomes of phenobarbital-treated rabbits and rats as described by Yasukochi and Masters[31] and contained 50 and 55 units/mg of protein respectively.

Preparation of protein fractions from rabbit and rat liver cytosol

The 100 000 × *g* supernatant obtained after the ultracentrifugation step in the preparation of microsomal fraction was used as starting material for the purification of cytosolic protein fractions. Ammonium sulphate (saturated solution adjusted to pH 7.5) was added to the 100 000 × *g* supernatant fraction to 60% of saturation. The resulting precipitate was collected by centrifugation, dissolved in 40 mM Tris-HCl buffer, pH 7.5, containing 0.25 M sucrose and 70 mM KCl and subjected to fractionation with acetone. The 35–60% acetone precipitate was further purified by ammonium sulphate fractionation and DEAE-cellulose chromatography. The acetone fractionation procedure and the following purification procedures were essentially those described by Nordstrom *et al.*[9] for the preparation of cytosolic activator and inactivator fractions involved in the HMG-CoA reductase reaction. The following modifications were made: dithiothreitol and EDTA were excluded from the buffers, ammonium sulphate fractionation from 0 to 60% was used instead of 0 to 40%, and the final Sephadex G-150 chromatography was omitted. The initial ammonium sulphate fractionation could be replaced by fractionation with polyethylene glycol 6000[22]. The fraction precipitating between 6 and 12% (w/v) of polyethylene glycol was further purified as described above. The final cytosolic subfractions (DEAE-cellulose fractions A and B) were concentrated in a Diaflo ultrafiltration cell using Amicon PM-10 filter and dialysed against 50 mM potassium phosphate buffer, pH 7.5 containing 0.25 M sucrose.

Incubation procedures and analyses of incubation mixtures

Incubations were performed at 37 °C for 20 min with 0.1–0.5 nmol of cytochrome P-450, 1–3 units of NADPH-cytochrome P-450 reductase, 25 μg of dilauroylglycero-3-phosphorylcholine, 1–2 μmol of NADPH in a total amount of 1–2 ml of 50 mM Tris-acetate buffer, pH 7.4, containing 20% glycerol and 0.1 mM EDTA. Cholesterol, 25–150 nmol, in 25 μl of acetone was added to the incubation mixture together with 0.6 mg of Triton X-100 in 20 μl of water. The incubations were performed, terminated and analysed as as described previously[28,8].

RESULTS

Attempts to identify the cytochrome P-450 component of the cholesterol 7α-hydroxylase system

Table 1 shows the catalytic properties of cytochromes P-450 LM_2, LM_{3b} and LM_4 from rabbit liver microsomes with respect to 7α-hydroxylation of cholesterol. The preparations of cytochromes P-450 LM_2 and LM_4 from phenobarbital-treated and cytochrome P-450 LM_{3b} from untreated rabbits were apparently homogeneous upon SDS-polyacrylamide gel electrophoresis and contained 19–20 nmol of cytochrome P-450/mg of protein. Preparations of cytochrome P-450 LM_4 from cholestyramine-treated rabbits were apparently homogeneous on gel electrophoresis and contained 10 nmol of cytochrome P-450/mg of protein. In addition, two fractions of cytochrome P-450 (I and II) were prepared from cholestyramine-treated rabbits by modifications of the procedures described by Imai and Sato[24]. These fractions had specific cytochrome P-450 contents of 6.1 nmol and 11.4 nmol/mg of protein respectively (Table 1).

Table 1 Cholesterol 7α-hydroxylase activity in preparations of rabbit liver microsomal cytochrome P-450

Fraction	*Cytochrome P-450* (nmol/mg protein)	*Cholesterol 7α-hydroxylation* (pmol nmol cytochrome P-450^{-1} min^{-1})
Microsomes phenobarbital)	3.0	1
Microsomes (untreated)	1.5	4
Microsomes (cholestyramine)	1.0	8
P-450 LM_2 (phenobarbital)	19.5	<0.5
P-450 LM_{3b} (untreated)	19.3	<0.5
P-450 LM_4 (phenobarbital)	19.0	<0.5
P-450 LM_4 (cholestyramine)	10.0	6
P-450 I (cholestyramine)	6.1	24
P-450 II (cholestyramine)	11.4	17

Cholesterol was incubated under standard conditions at 37 °C for 20 min with 0.5–1.0 nmol of cytochrome P-450, 1–3 units of NADPH-cytochrome P-450 reductase, 25 μg of dilauroyl-glycero-3-phosphorylcholine, 0.6 mg of Triton X-100 and 2 μmol of NADPH in a total volume of 1–2 nmol of 50 mM Tris-acetate buffer, pH 7.4, containing 20% glycerol and 0.1 mM EDTA

Liver microsomes from cholestyramine-fed rabbits were more active in cholesterol 7α-hydroxylation than microsomes from phenobarbital-treated or untreated animals. Cytochrome P-450 LM_2 showed no detectable 7α-hydroxylase activity, nor did cytochrome P-450 LM_{3b} and cytochrome P-450 LM_4 from phenobarbital-treated animals. These preparations catalysed hydroxylations of other substrates, such as ethylmorphine, testosterone and 5β-cholestane-3α,7α,12α-triol. It may be added that also cytochrome P-450 LM_4 preparations from β-naphthoflavone-treated and untreated rabbits were apparently inactive in 7α-hydroxylation of cholesterol. However, cytochrome

P-450 LM_4 preparations from cholestyramine-treated rabbits, as well as cytochromes P-450 I and II, catalysed 7α-hydroxylation of cholesterol. The rate of hydroxylation was comparable to or higher than that in microsomes.

Table 2 Cholesterol 7α-hydroxylase activity in preparations of rat liver microsomal cytochrome P-450

Fraction	*Cytochrome P-450* (nmol/mg protein)	*Cholesterol 7α-hydroxylation* (pmol nmol cytochrome P-450^{-1} min^{-1})
Microsomes (phenobarbital)	1.5	8
Microsomes (cholestyramine)	0.7	40
P-450 B (phenobarbital)	18.9	<0.5
P-450 D (phenobarbital)	15.9	<0.5
P-450 'Fraction C' (phenobarbital)	18.3	<0.5
P-450 A (cholestyramine)	18.5	<0.5
P-450 I (cholestyramine)	13.2	145
P-450 II (cholestyramine)	6.5	142

Cholesterol was incubated under the same conditions as in Table 1

Table 2 shows the catalytic properties of cytochromes P-450 B, D and 'Fraction C' from liver microsomes of phenobarbital-treated rats. The preparations were apparently homogeneous on gel electrophoresis and contained 15–19 nmol of cytochrome P-450/mg of protein. In addition, three heterogeneous fractions of cytochrome P-450 (A, I and II) were prepared from liver microsomes of cholestyramine-treated rats. Cytochrome P-450 fraction A contained 18.5 nmol of cytochrome P-450/mg of protein. This fraction showed two protein bands on gel electrophoresis. Cytochrome P-450 I contained 13.2 nmol of cytochrome P-450/mg of protein and cytochrome P-450 II 6.5 nmol/mg of protein.

Rat liver microsomes showed generally higher cholesterol 7α-hydroxylase activity than rabbit liver microsomes. Cholestyramine treatment stimulated the reaction. None of the cytochrome P-450 fractions obtained from phenobarbital-treated rats, cytochromes P-450 B, P-450 D and P-450 'Fraction C', showed cholesterol 7α-hydroxylase activity, nor did cytochrome P-450 A. These fractions catalysed hydroxylations of other substrates, e.g. 25-hydroxylation of 5β-cholestane-3α,7α-12α-triol. On the other hand, cytochrome P-450 I and cytochrome P-450 II catalysed 7α-hydroxylation of cholesterol more efficiently than the microsomes.

Some properties of purified cholesterol 7α-hydroxylase system

Cytochrome P-450 fractions I and II from liver microsomes of cholestyramine-treated rats and cytochrome P-450 fractions I, II and LM_4 from liver microsomes of cholestyramine-treated rabbits were used for further studies.

The purified cytochrome P-450 preparations were completely dependent on NADPH-cytochrome P-450 reductase to catalyse cholesterol 7α-hydroxylation. The rate of hydroxylation was linear with the amount of cytochrome P-450 up to approximately 1 nmol in the presence of a fixed amount of NADPH-cytochrome P-450 reductase (Figure 1). No saturation of cholesterol was obtained with the microsomal fraction but with purified cytochrome P-450 I from cholestyramine-treated rats the system was saturated with about 100 μM of cholesterol added (Figure 2). Substrate saturation was

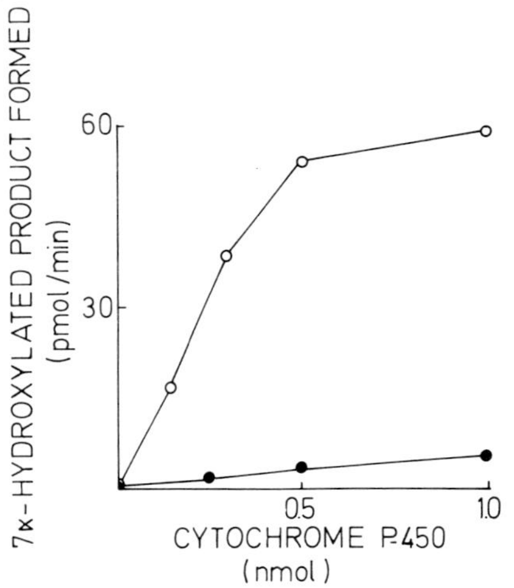

Figure 1 Effect of cytochrome P-450 concentration on the rate of 7α-hydroxylation of cholesterol. Cholesterol, 25 nmol, was incubated under standard conditions at 37 °C for 20 min with varying amounts of cytochrome P-450, 3 units of NADPH-cytochrome P-450 reductase, 25 μg dilauroylglyco-3-phosphorylcholine, 0.6 mg of Triton X-100 and 2 μmol of NADPH in a total volume of 1.5 ml of 50 mM Tris-acetate buffer, pH 7.4, containing 20% glycerol and 0.1mM EDTA. Cytochrome P-450 I (rat), ○——○; cytochrome P-450 LM_4 (rabbit), ●——●

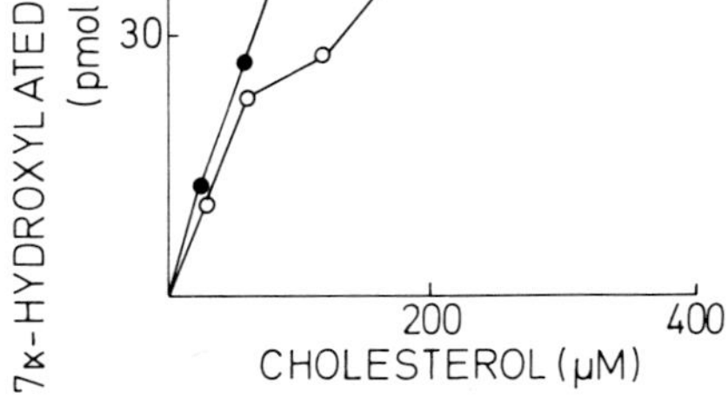

Figure 2 Effect of substrate concentration on the rate of 7α-hydroxylation of cholesterol. Incubation conditions were as in Figure 1 except for the varying concentrations of substrate. The amount of cytochrome P-450 I (rat) was 0.5 nmol. Cholesterol was added in a suspension of Tween 80 to incubations with microsomes, ○——○, and together with Triton X-100 to incubations with purified system, ●——●

Table 3 Effects of detergents used for solubilization of substrate on reconstituted cholesterol 7α-hydroxylase activity

Addition of substrate to incubation	*Cholesterol 7α-hydroxylation* (pmol nmol cytochrome P-450^{-1} min^{-1})
Cholesterol	
in Tween 80[a]	7
in Triton X-100[a]	48
in acetone	28
in acetone + Triton X-100[b]	56

[a] Final concentration of detergent in the incubation was 0.2% (w/v)
[b] Final concentration of Triton X-100 was 0.05% (w/v)
Cholesterol was added to incubation mixtures containing 0.5 nmol of cytochrome P-450, 2 units of NADPH-cytochrome P-450 reductase, 25 μg of dilauroylglycero-3-phosphorylcholine and 2 μmol of NADPH in a final volume of 1.5 ml of 50 mM Tris-acetate buffer, pH 7.4, containing 20% glycerol and 0.1 mM EDTA. Standard incubation conditions were used. A preparation of cytochrome P-450 I from rat liver microsomes containing 10 nmol of cytochrome P-450/mg of protein was used.

also obtained with cytochrome P-450 LM_4 from cholestyramine-treated rabbits. Addition of phospholipid was not obligatory to reconstitute 7α-hydroxylase activity.

Addition of cholesterol in a suspension of Triton X-100 to incubations with reconstituted system resulted in higher conversion of cholesterol into 7α-hydroxycholesterol than addition of the substrate in a suspension of Tween-80. Addition of cholesterol in acetone with separate addition of Triton X-100 was equally efficient (Table 3). A final concentration of Triton X-100 of 0.05% (w/v) was found to be optimal (Figure 3). Similar results

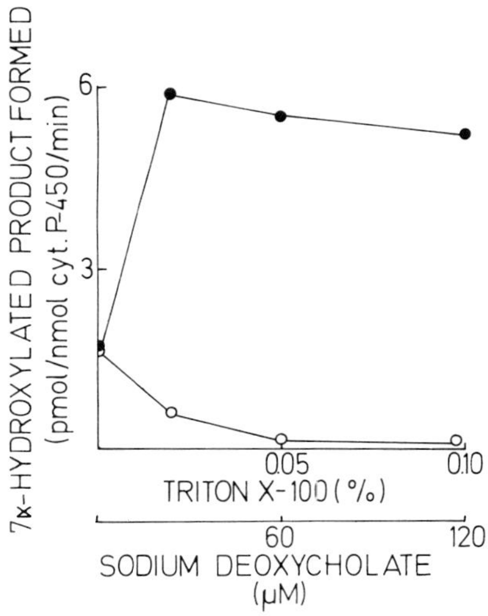

Figure 3 Effect of Triton X-100 and sodium deoxycholate on the rate of 7α-hydroxylation of cholesterol. Incubation conditions were as in Figure 1 except for the varying concentrations of detergent. Cytochrome P-450 LM_4, 0.5 nmol, from rabbit liver microsomes was used. Triton X-100, ● —— ●, sodium deoxycholate, ○ —— ○

were observed with all cytochrome P-450 fractions active in cholesterol 7α-hydroxylation. Sodium deoxycholate, on the other hand, had a marked inhibitory effect (Figure 3).

Modulation of reconstituted cholesterol 7α-hydroxylase activity with protein fractions from liver cytosol

Protein fractions from rat and rabbit liver cytosol which had stimulatory effect on reconstituted cholesterol 7α-hydroxylase activity were prepared by initial fractionation with ammonium sulphate or polyethylene glycol 6000 followed by acetone precipitation and DEAE-cellulose chromatography. The stimulatory activity was eluted with the equilibration buffer in DEAE-cellulose chromatography of the 35–60% acetone precipitate ('DEAE-cellulose fraction A'). Such fractions stimulated cholesterol 7α-hydroxylation, catalysed by cytochrome P-450 I and II from rat liver microsomes as well as from rabbit liver microsomes (Table 4). Figure 4A shows that the stimulatory activity from rat liver cytosol was approximately linear with the amount of protein up to a certain level and then remained constant. The stimulatory activity was destroyed upon heat treatment at 80 °C for 5 min.

Table 4 Effect of protein fractions from liver cytosol on reconstituted cholesterol 7α-hydroxylase activity

System	*Cholesterol 7α-hydroxylation* (pmol nmol cytochrome P-450^{-1} min^{-1})	
	Rat	*Rabbit*
Control	60	20
Control + DEAE-cellulose fraction A	128	37
Control + DEAE-cellulose fraction B	11	10

The control system contained 0.25 nmol of cytochrome P-450 I (rat) or 0.5 nmol of cytochrome P-450 II (rabbit), 2 units of NADPH-cytochrome P-450 reductase, 25 μg of dilauroylglycero-3-phosphorylcholine, 2 μmol NADPH, 0.6 mg Triton X-100 and 25 nmol of cholesterol. Cytochrome P-450, NADPH-cytochrome P-450 reductase and phospholipid were preincubated for 10 min before addition of cofactor and substrate. Incubations were then performed at 37 °C for 20 min. In experiments on the effects of DEAE-cellulose fractions A (0.5 mg) and B (0.1 mg) these fractions were included in the preincubation mixture

Fractions from rat and rabbit liver cytosol which had inhibitory effect on reconstituted cholesterol 7α-hydroxylase activity were obtained after DEAE-cellulose chromatography of the 35–60% acetone precipitate. The inhibitory activity was eluted from the DEAE-cellulose column with KCl-gradient and appeared after a protein peak eluting at a conductivity of 17 000–29 000 μmho ('DEAE-cellulose fraction B'). This fraction inhibited cholesterol 7α-hydroxylase activity catalysed by cytochrome P-450 fractions I and II from rat liver microsomes as well as from rabbit liver microsomes (Table 4). Figure 4B shows that the inhibitory activity from rat liver cytosol was dependent on the amount of protein. The inhibitory activity was stable to heat treatment at 80 °C for 5 min.

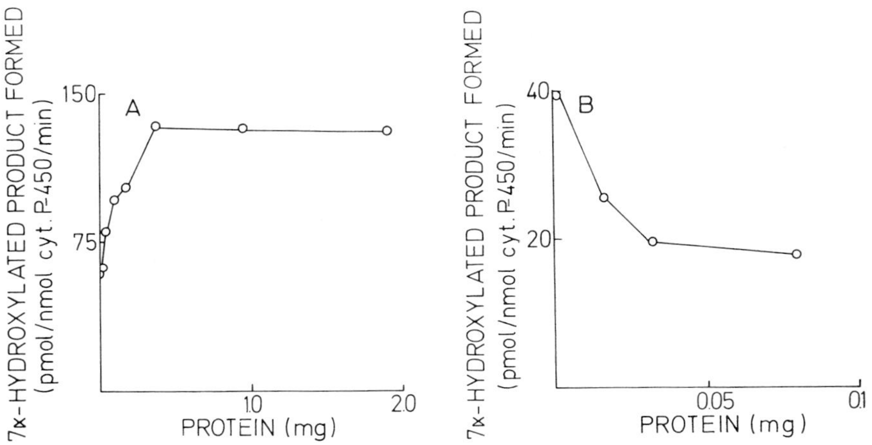

Figure 4 Effect of DEAE-cellulose fraction A (A) and DEAE-cellulose fraction B (B) from rat liver cytosol on reconstituted cholesterol 7α-hydroxylase activity. Incubation conditions were as in Table 4 except for the varying concentrations of cytosolic protein fractions. Cytochrome P-450 I, 0.25 nmol, from rat liver microsomes was used

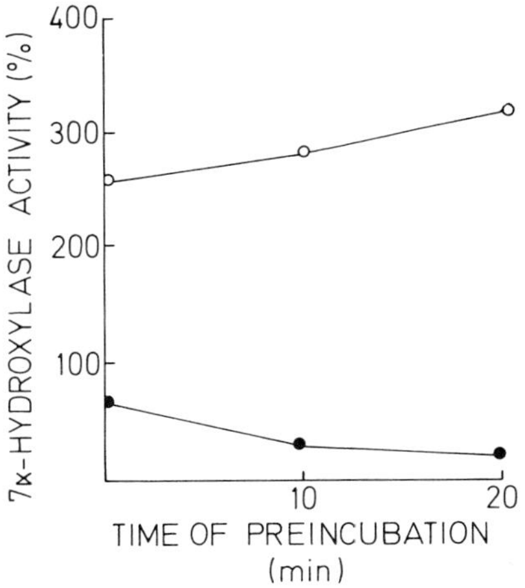

Figure 5 Effect of preincubation time on stimulation and inhibition of reconstituted cholesterol 7α-hydroxylase activity by cytosolic protein fractions. Incubation conditions were as in Figure 4 except for the varying preincubation time. DEAE-cellulose fraction A, ○——○; DEAE-cellulose fraction B, ●——●. Cholesterol 7α-hydroxylase activity is expressed as percentage of control values

Neither the stimulatory nor the inhibitory activity was dependent on ATP and $MgCl_2$. The activities were not affected by NaF. Figure 5 shows that preincubation of the cytosolic fractions from rat liver with reconstituted cholesterol 7α-hydroxylase system before assay of hydroxylase activity increased the effects of the stimulatory and inhibitory protein fractions. It should be noted that the 7α-hydroxylase activity in the control incubation decreased with increasing preincubation time.

DISCUSSION

Cholesterol 7α-hydroxylase activity is not stimulated by phenobarbital treatment nor by any other known mixed-function oxidase inducer[3]. The results of the present investigation also show that phenobarbital-induced species of cytochrome P-450, cytochromes P-450 B and 'Fraction C' from rat liver microsomes and cytochrome P-450 LM_2 from rabbit liver microsomes, are apparently inactive in 7α-hydroxylation of cholesterol. It is therefore likely that the cholesterol 7α-hydroxylase activity is associated with some constitutive species of cytochrome P-450. Such enzymes are difficult to isolate since they are present in rather low concentrations in liver microsomes.

Most information concerning the purification of cytochromes P-450 present in untreated animals has been obtained with rabbit liver. Koop and Coon[18] and Johnson[19] have recently described procedures for the isolation of cytochrome P-450 LM_{3b}. However, it seems less likely that this species is involved in cholesterol 7α-hydroxylation since the preparations used in the present study were not able to catalyse 7α-hydroxylation of cholesterol. Cytochrome P-450 LM_4 is one of the major forms present in rabbit liver microsomes. This species is induced by several xenobiotics such as β-naphthoflavone and methylcholantrene[15]. Cytochrome P-450 LM_4 is present also in liver microsomes of untreated rabbits[32]. We reported previously that cytochrome P-450 LM_4 isolated from phenobarbital-treated rabbits showed no cholesterol 7α-hydroxylase activity[20]. However, the rate of 7α-hydroxylation was very low also in the microsomal fraction from phenobarbital-treated rabbits. In the present work cholestyramine-fed rabbits have also been used. Liver microsomes from rabbits treated in this way catalysed 7α-hydroxylation of cholesterol considerably more efficiently than microsomes from phenobarbital-treated, β-naphthoflavone-treated as well as untreated rabbits. Cytochrome P-450 LM_4 preparations from cholestyramine-treated animals showed cholesterol 7α-hydroxylase activity when combined with NADPH-cytochrome P-450 reductase. Although the preparations were apparently homogeneous upon gel electrophoresis, the specific cytochrome P-450 content was not higher than about 10 nmol/mg of protein. Similar specific contents have been reported by Haugen and Coon[32] for cytochrome P-450 LM_4 prepared from untreated rabbits. These authors suggested that the cytochrome in microsomes from untreated animals might be deficient in haem or that the haem is lost more readily upon purification. Employing another purification procedure[20,24,25] two fractions of cytochrome P-450 (I and II) were obtained which were active in cholesterol 7α-hydroxylation. Cytochrome P-450 fraction II had similar cytochrome P-450 content as cytochrome P-450 LM_4 and showed a major protein band with similar mobility as cytochrome P-450 LM_4 on gel electrophoresis. From the present results it can not be definitely concluded whether cholesterol 7α-hydroxylation is catalysed by the major protein in the cytochrome P-450 LM_4 fraction or whether this fraction contains a species specific for cholesterol 7α-hydroxylation. Cytochrome P-450 LM_4 also catalyses 25-hydroxylation of 5β-cholestane-3α,7α,12α-triol[20]. This hydroxylase activity is not increased in cytochrome P-450 LM_4 preparations from cholestyramine-treated rabbits and seems to be more stable to storage at −20 °C than the cholesterol 7α-hydroxylase activity.

Cytochrome P-450 fractions I and II could be prepared from liver microsomes of cholestyramine-treated rats using the same procedure as that employed for rabbit liver microsomes. None of the fractions was homogeneous on gel electrophoresis but cytochrome P-450 fraction I had a specific cytochrome P-450 content of 13 nmol/mg of protein. Both fractions catalysed 7α-hydroxylation of cholesterol more efficiently than the corresponding microsomes and considerably more efficiently than any of the rabbit liver cytochromes P-450. In addition, a major fraction of cytochrome P-450 (A) was isolated with a specific cytochrome P-450 content of 18 nmol/mg of protein. This fraction was inactive in cholesterol 7α-hydroxylation but catalysed efficient 25-hydroxylation of 5β-cholestane-3α,7α,12α-triol.

The cytochrome P-450 preparations which were enriched in both 7α-hydroxylase activity and cytochrome P-450 were suitable for studies on the properties of cholesterol 7α-hydroxylase system. In contrast to cholesterol 7α-hydroxylation catalysed by rat and rabbit liver microsomes, the purified system was linear with the amount of cytochrome P-450 and could be saturated with cholesterol as substrate. This indicates that primarily exogenous cholesterol is 7α-hydroxylated by purified cytochromes P-450. It was observed that different types of detergents had different effects on the purified cholesterol 7α-hydroxylase system. The use of Tween-80 as solubilizing agent for the substrate was found to be less suitable since this detergent had an inhibitory effect on the purified cholesterol 7α-hydroxylase system. Sodium deoxycholate, which has a stimulatory effect on several reconstituted hydroxylase activities[15,27], was also inhibitory. Triton X-100, on the other hand, was found to stimulate reconstituted cholesterol 7α-hydroxylase activity. Similar stimulatory effects of Triton X-100 have been reported for the cholesterol side-chain cleavage activity catalysed by purified cytochrome P-450_{scc} from bovine adrenal mitochondria[33].

The results of the present communication also show that the activity of a purified, reconstituted cholesterol 7α-hydroxylase system from liver microsomes of rats and rabbits can be modulated by protein fractions from liver cytosol. It was possible to isolate stimulatory and inhibitory fractions from liver cytosol employing essentially the procedures described by Nordstrom *et al.*[9] for studies on regulation of HMG-CoA reductase. The use of purified cholesterol 7α-hydroxylase system to study the effects of cytosol on 7α-hydroxylase activity was found to be preferable to the use of whole microsomes. The effects obtained with the purified system were more reproducible, and the system seems to be suitable for studies on the mechanism of the stimulatory and inhibitory effects. It might be mentioned that a cholesterol-binding protein from rat liver cytosol prepared as described by Erickson *et al.*[34] stimulated cholesterol 7α-hydroxylase activity in whole microsomes but not in the purified system. It can be concluded that the function of this cholesterol-binding protein is probably not of a catalytic nature. The heat-labile stimulatory activity in DEAE-cellulose fraction A and the heat-stable inhibitory activity in DEAE-cellulose fraction B were not dependent on ATP and $MgCl_2$ and were not affected by NaF. This is in contrast to the protein fractions modulating HMG-CoA reductase activity described by Nordstrom *et al.*[9]. The stimulatory and inhibitory effects of DEAE-cellulose fractions A and B, respectively, were dependent on the amount of protein and time of preincubation with the cholesterol 7α-hydroxylase system. These findings indicate that the mode of action of these protein fractions does not involve carrier effects or substrate solubilization.

Acknowledgments

The skilful technical assistance of Miss Ann-Charlotte Dahlqvist, Mrs Britt-Marie Johansson and Mrs Anne Legnehed is gratefully acknowledged. This work was supported by the Swedish Medical Research Council (project 03X-218) and by the Loo and Hans Ostermans Foundation.

References

1. Danielsson, H., Einarsson, K. and Johansson, G. (1967). Effect of biliary drainage on individual reactions in the conversion of cholesterol to taurocholic acid. *Eur. J. Biochem.*, **2,** 44
2. Shefer, S., Hauser, S. and Mosbach, E. H. (1968). 7α-Hydroxylation of cholestanol by rat liver microsomes. *J. Lipid Res.*, **9,** 328
3. Danielsson, H. and Sjövall, J. (1975). Bile acid metabolism. *Ann. Rev. Biochem.*, **44,** 233
4. Myant, N. B. and Mitropoulos, K. A. (1977). Cholesterol 7α-hydroxylase. *J. Lipid Res.*, **18,** 135
5. Johansson, G. (1971). Oxidation of cholesterol, 3β-hydroxy-5-pregnen-20-one and 3β-hydroxy-5-androsten-17-one by rat liver microsomes. *Eur. J. Biochem.*, **21,** 68
6. Boyd, G. S., Grimwade, A. M. and Lawson, M. E. (1973). Studies on rat liver microsomal cholesterol 7α-hydroxylase. *Eur. J. Biochem.*, **37,** 334
7. Björkhem, I., Danielsson, H. and Wikvall, K. (1974). 7α-Hydroxylation of cholesterol by reconstituted systems from rat liver microsomes. *Biochem. Biophys. Res. Commun.*, **61,** 934
8. Hansson, R. and Wikvall, K. (1979). Properties of reconstituted cholesterol 7α-hydroxylase system from rat and rabbit liver microsomes. *Eur. J. Biochem.*, **93,** 419
9. Nordstrom, J. L., Rodwell, V. W. and Mitschelen, J. J. (1977). Interconversion of active and inactive forms of rat liver hydroxymethylglutaryl-CoA reductase. *J. Biol. Chem.*, **252,** 8924
10. Beg, Z. H., Stonik, J. A. and Brewer, H. B. (1979). Characterization and regulation of reductase kinase, a protein kinase that modulates the enzymic activity of 3-hydroxy-3-methylglutaryl-coenzyme A reductase. *Proc. Natl. Acad. Sci. USA*, **76,** 4375
11. Gibson, D. M. and Ingebritsen, T. S. (1978). Reversible modulation of liver hydroxymethylglutaryl-CoA reductase. *Life Sciences*, **23,** 2649
12. Spence, J. T. and Gaylor, J. L. (1977). Investigation of regulation of microsomal hydroxymethylglutaryl coenzyme A reductase and methyl sterol oxidase of cholesterol biosynthesis. *J. Biol. Chem.*, **252,** 5852
13. Danielsson, H. and Einarsson, K. (1964). The enzymic formation of 7α-hydroxycholesterol from cholesterol in rat liver homogenates. *Acta Chem. Scand.*, **18,** 831
14. Craig, J. F., Boyd, G. S., McLeod, R. J. and Suckling, K. E. (1979). Partial characterization of a protein from rat liver 100,000 *g* supernatant which stimulates cholesterol 7α-hydroxylase. *Biochem. Soc. Trans.*, **7,** 967
15. Coon, M. J., Vermilion, J. L., Vatsis, K. P., French, J. S., Dean, W. L. and Haugen, D. A. (1977). Biochemical studies on drug metabolism: isolation of multiple forms of liver microsomal cytochrome P-450. In Jerina, D. M. (ed.). *Drug Metabolism Concepts*, No. 44, pp. 46–71. Washington DC: American Chemical Society

16. Guerengrich, F. P. (1979). Isolation and purification of cytochrome P-450, and the existence of multiple forms. *Pharmacol. Ther.*, **6,** 99
17. Ryan, D. E., Thomas, P. E. and Levin, W. (1980). Hepatic microsomal cytochrome P-450 from rats treated with isosfarole: Purification and characterization of four enzymic forms. *J. Biol. Chem.*, **255,** 7941
18. Koop, D. R. and Coon, M. J. (1979). Purification and properties of P-450 LM_{3b}, a constitutive form of cytochrome P-450, from rabbit liver microsomes. *Biochem. Biophys. Res. Commun.*, **91,** 1075
19. Johnson, E. F. (1980). Isolation and characterization of a constitutive form of rabbit liver microsomal cytochrome P-450. *J. Biol. Chem.*, **255,** 304
20. Hansson, R. and Wikvall, K. (1980). Hydroxylations in biosynthesis and metabolism of bile acids: catalytic properties of different forms of cytochrome P-450. *J. Biol. Chem.*, **255,** 1643
21. Cuatrecasas, P. (1970). Protein purification by affinity chromatography: derivatizations of agarose and polyacrylamide beads. *J. Biol. Chem.*, **245,** 3059
22. Coon, M. J., van der Hoeven, T. A., Dahl, S. B. and Haugen, D. A. (1978). Two forms of liver microsomal cytochrome P-450, P-450 LM_2 and P-450 LM_4 (rabbit liver). *Methods Enzymol.*, **52C,** 109
23. Heller, A. R. and Gould, R. G. (1974). Reversible cold inactivation of microsomal 3-hydroxy-3-methylugltaryl coenzyme A reductase from rat liver. *J. Biol. Chem.*, **249,** 5254
24. Imai, Y. and Sato, R. (1974). A gel-electrophoretically homogeneous preparation of cytochrome P-450 from liver microsomes of phenobarbital-pretreated rabbits. *Biochem. Biophys. Res. Commun.*, **60,** 8
25. Negishi, M. and Kreibich, G. (1978). Coordinated polypeptide synthesis and insertion of protoheme in cytochrome P-450 during development of endoplasmic reticulum membranes. *J. Biol. Chem.*, **253,** 4791
26. Guengerich, F. P. (1978). Separation and purification of multiple forms of microsomal cytochrome P-450: partial characterization of three apparently homogeneous cytochromes P-450 prepared from livers of phenobarbital- and 3-methylcholantrene-treated rats. *J. Biol. Chem.*, **253,** 7931
27. West, S. B., Huang, M.-T., Miwa, G. and Lu, A. Y. M. (1979). A simple and rapid procedure for the purification of phenobarbital-inducible cytochrome P-450 from rat liver microsomes. *Arch. Biochem. Biophys.*, **193,** 42
28. Ryan, D. E., Thomas, P. E., Korzeniowski, D. and Levin, W. (1979). Separation and characterization of highly purified forms of liver microsomal cytochrome P-450 from rats treated with polychlorinated biphenyls, phenobarbital, and 3-methylcholantrene. *J. Biol. Chem.*, **254,** 1365
29. Omura, T. and Sato, R. (1964). The carbon monoxide-binding pigment of liver microsomes. *J. Biol. Chem.*, **239,** 2379
30. Lowry, O. H., Rosebrough, N. J., Farr, A. L. and Randall, R. J. (1951). Protein measurement with the Folin phenol reagent. *J. Biol. Chem.*, **193,** 265
31. Yasukochi, Y. and Masters, B. S. S. (1976). Some properties of a detergent-solubilized NADPH-cytochrome c (cytochrome P-450) reductase purified by biospecific affinity chromatography. *J. Biol. Chem.*, **251,** 5337
32. Haugen, D. A. and Coon, M. J. (1967). Properties of electrophoretically homogeneous phenobarbital-inducible and β-naphthoflavone inducible forms of liver microsomal cytochrome P-450. *J. Biol. Chem.*, **251,** 7929
33. Nakajin, S., Ishii, Y., Shinoda, M. and Shikita, M. (1979). Binding of Triton X-100 to purified cytochrome $P\text{-}450_{scc}$ and enchancement of the cholesterol side chain cleavage activity. *Biochem. Biophys. Res. Commun.*, **87,** 524
34. Erickson, S. K., Meyer, D. J. and Gould, R. G. (1978). Purification and characterization of a new cholesterol-binding protein from rat liver cytosol. *J. Biol. Chem.*, **253,** 1817

6
Effect of taurocholic acid on cholesterol synthesis in the cultured hepatocyte

C. A. BARTH, I. HILLMAR AND E. E. WEIS

INTRODUCTION

In the early 1950s it became clear that hepatic cholesterol synthesis is a regulated metabolic pathway[1]. At the end of the same decade Beher and Baker[2] proposed that bile salts might be one of the regulators; they showed that a 0.5% cholic acid diet supressed liver cholesterogenesis. Subsequently, a number of investigators[3–9] demonstrated a general inverse relationship between bile acid flux through the liver and rate of cholesterol synthesis.

Then it became doubtful whether bile acids regulate *directly* cholesterol synthesis in the liver cell. Weis and Dietschy[10], and Nervi and Dietschy[11] concluded from their experiments that the above findings are due to an enhanced absorption of cholesterol in the intestine. This would lead to a rise of the hepatic cholesterol concentration and hence cause an indirect inhibition of cholesterol synthesis.

During the following years several groups have tried to prove the original concept by Beher and Baker by using either animal models with diversion of absorbed cholesterol or *in vitro* preparations. Hamprecht and co-workers[12] observed an inhibitory effect of cholic acid on liver 3-hydroxy-3-methyl-glutaryl coenzyme-A reductase (E.C.1.1.1.34) in animals carrying a lymph fistula. Other investigators, including ourselves, did not observe this effect in the isolated perfused liver[13,14].

In this contribution a *direct* effect is defined in a strictly operational sense denoting an inhibition exerted within the liver cell irrespective of the underlying biochemical mechanism.

RESULTS

Experiments *in vivo*

According to Table 1 any proof of a direct effect necessitates an experimental model where cholesterol absorbed from the intestine is either diverted or, where the intestine cannot be the target for the bile salt, administered. We chose the latter way by infusing taurocholate to rats that simultaneously had a bile fistula.

Table 1 Criteria for a *direct* vs. *indirect* inhibition of hepatic cholesterol synthesis by bile salts

	Direct	*Indirect*
Flux of cholesterol, intestine→liver enhanced	No	Yes
Rise of hepatic cholesterol concentration	No*	Yes (obligatory)
Response to i.v. bile salt	Yes	No
Response in case of lymph diversion	Yes	No

* Only in case of primary action via inhibition of cholesterol 7-α mono-oxygenase a rise might be anticipated

As can be seen from Table 2, a 6 h intravenous (i.v.) infusion of taurocholate suppressed the rise of cholesterol synthesis which was observed in animals with the bile fistula alone. Because of the bile diversion in all experimental animals, taurocholate could not influence intestinal cholesterol absorption. Accordingly, no rise of hepatic cholesterol concentration was observed (Figure 1).

Table 2 Influence of sodium taurocholate on lipid synthesis of the liver (10.00 h) (dpm g wet weight^{-1} h^{-1})

Experimental details		[1-^{14}C]acetate incorporation → *Cholesterol*	→ *Fatty acids*	*n*
Intact controls		5.973 ± 1462	6.107 ± 557	11
Bile fistula, saline Mock infusion, albumin i.v.		22.747 ± 3775	12.116 ± 1895	5
Bile fistula,	taurocholate i.v. (33.4 μmol × 100g rat^{-1}h^{-1})	6.544 ± 801	7.548 ± 1279	6
Bile fistula,	taurocholate i.d. (33.4 μmol × 100g rat^{-1}h^{-1})	6.390 ± 1059	6.639 ± 1161	6

i.d. = intraduodenal
Data from Ref. 19
$\bar{x}$ ± SEM

The above findings were corroborated in another series of experiments which showed that also the activity of the cholesterogenic enzyme 3-hydroxy-3-methylglutaryl coenzyme-A (HMG-CoA) reductase of liver was lowered by i.v. taurocholate (Figure 1).

One reason why we obtained a positive result may be that a higher dose of taurocholate was infused as compared to previous investigators; the dose was chosen in agreement with earlier findings from this laboratory showing a surprisingly high flux of bile salts through the enterohepatic circulation of the intact rat[15].

Furthermore a more extensive inhibition of cholesterol synthesis by taurocholate during the light–dark transition of the diurnal cycle was observed (data not shown). This finding, which confirms earlier investigations[11,12], points to a greater sensitivity of cholesterogenic enzymes during phases of their most active synthesis.

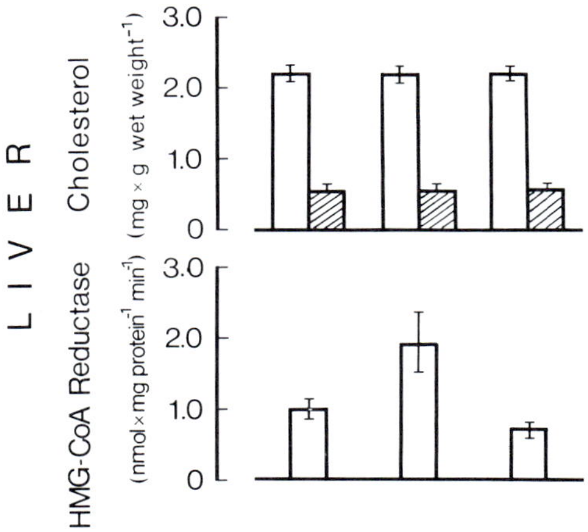

Figure 1 Hepatic cholesterol concentration and HMG-CoA reductase activity. Left: intact control rats; centre: bile fistula for 6 h; right: bile fistula plus i.v. infusion of 33.4 μmol taurocholate $\times$ 100 g body-weight^{-1} h^{-1}. For cholesterol levels either total hepatic cholesterol concentrations (white columns) or esterified cholesterol (hatched columns) are given

In conclusion, the route of application, the dose of the bile salt and the dynamics of the synthesis of cholesterogenic enzymes have to be considered when the regulation of cholesterol synthesis by bile salts is studied and discussed.

Experiments *in vitro*

The cultured hepatocyte is an ideal model in cases where the study of the parenchymal liver cell in the isolated state is a *sine qua non*. Monolayer cultures of rat hepatocytes show the full complement of regulatory responses including induction of enzymes by hormones[16]. Moreover, the active transport system for bile salts is preserved in the cultured cell[17]. Therefore, we have studied the influence of taurocholic acid on the activity of HMG-CoA reductase in this model. As can be seen, no influence of taurocholate on the basal activity of the enzyme was observed (Figure 2). On the contrary, in case of a simultaneous addition of glucocorticoid which causes a 2-fold rise of the enzyme activity (probably via a stimulation of protein synthesis[18]) a dose-dependent inhibition of enzyme activity was observed (Table 3).

Two features of this observation deserve a comment. First, the effective concentration of taurocholate was surprisingly low: it ranged between 0.01 and 10 μmol/l and was well below bile salt concentrations in the portal blood. Secondly, an 'induction' of the enzyme by glucocorticoid seems to be obligatory. This finding, again, indicates that the dynamics of enzyme synthesis are important for this regulatory phenomenon and that taurocholate may inhibit the synthesis of HMG-CoA reductase.

Table 3 Effect of taurocholate on HMG-CoA reductase activity of monolayer cultures of rat hepatocytes.

Addition Dexamethasone (10^{-5}M)	Taurocholate (M)	*n*	*HMG-CoA reductase activity* (pmol mg protein^{-1} min^{-1})
–	–	8	6.46 ± 1.12*
+	–	8	15.70 ± 2.92
+	10^{-9}	8	10.33 ± 2.26
+	10^{-7}	10	9.50 ± 1.98
+	10^{-5}	8	7.53 ± 1.24
+	5×10^{-4}	7	6.8 ± 0.8

* $\bar{x}$ ± SEM
Data from Ref. 20

CONCLUSIONS

In two different experimental models data have been obtained which contribute evidence for a direct inhibition of cholesterol synthesis by taurocholate. The bile acid inhibited both [^{14}C]acetate incorporation into cholesterol and the activity of HMG-CoA reductase, the regulatory enzyme of this metabolic pathway. In both experimental models an interference of intestinal cholesterol absorption was impossible so that the conclusion is justified that bile acids control the synthesis of their precursor, cholesterol, via negative feedback within the liver cell.

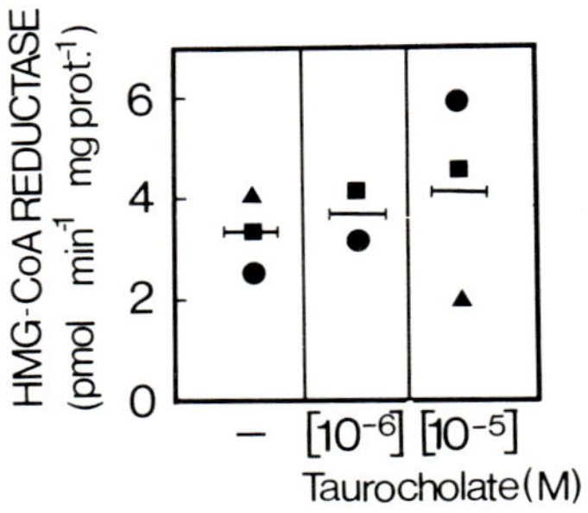

Figure 2 Effect of taurocholate on basal activity of HMG-CoA reductase in monolayer cultures of rat hepatocytes. Monolayers were incubated for 6 h with the concentration of taurocholate, as indicated on the abscissa. Horizontal bars show averages

No direct evidence is contributed in this study regarding the underlying biochemical mechanism. Nevertheless, a common characteristic emerges from studies both *in vivo* and *in vitro*: the sensitivity towards inhibition by taurocholate is greater when the rate of synthesis of HMG-CoA reductase is accelerated. This finding is compatible with a mechanism whereby the bile acid inhibits the rate of synthesis of the enzyme.

Finally, the data may contribute to our understanding of the metabolic defect of cholesterol gallstone disease and its successful therapy with oral bile acids. It has been proposed that the disease is due to an abnormal high rate of cholesterol synthesis in the liver and that chenodeoxycholic acid therapy acts by suppressing HMG-CoA reductase activity[21]. It is evident that any therapy can be successful only if it is not accompanied by a rise of liver cholesterol concentration which would cause a rise of biliary cholesterol secretion. As stated in Table 1, this is the case only if bile acids *directly* influence hepatic cholesterol synthesis. Hence, no beneficial effect on biliary cholesterol secretion can be expected unless a *direct* effect of the bile acid administered is operative.

Acknowledgments

This work has been supported by the Deutsche Forschungsgemeinschaft. We thank Mrs Brigitte Weber for excellent technical assistance and Ms Uta Rasche for typing the manuscript.

References

1. Gould, R. G. and Taylor, C. B. (1950). Effect of dietary cholesterol on hepatic cholesterol synthesis. *Fed. Proc.*, **9**, 179
2. Beher, T. and Baker, C. (1959). Build-up and regression of inhibitory effects of cholic acid on *in vivo* liver cholesterol synthesis. *Proc. Soc. Exp. Biol. Med.*, **101**, 214
3. Seitz, W. and v. Brand, V. (1961). Der Einfluß von gekoppelten Gallensäuren auf die Synthese von Fettsäuren und Cholesterin in der Leber. *Klin. Wochenschr.*, **39**, 891
4. Myant, N. B. and Eder, H. A. (1961). The effect of biliary drainage upon the synthesis of cholesterol in the liver. *J. Lipid Res.*, **2**, 363
5. Fimognari, G. M. and Rodwell, V. W. (1965). Cholesterol biosynthesis: mevalonate synthesis inhibited by bile salts. *Science (Wash.)*, **147**, 1038
6. Grundy, S. M., Hofmann, A. F., Davignon, J. and Ahrens, E. H. (1966). Human cholesterol synthesis is regulated by bile acids. *J. Clin. Invest.*, **45**, 1018
7. Danielsson, H., Einarsson, K. and Johansson, G. (1967). Effect of biliary drainage on individual reactions from cholesterol to taurocholic acid. *Eur. J. Biochem.*, **2**, 44
8. Back, P., Hamprecht, B. and Lynen, F. (1969). Regulation of cholesterol biosynthesis in rat liver: diurnal changes of activity and influence of bile acids. *Arch. Biochem. Biophys.*, **133**, 11
9. Shefer, S., Hauser, S., Lapar, V. and Mosbach, E. H. (1973). Regulatory effects of sterols and bile acids on hepatic 3-hydroxy-3-methylglutaryl CoA reductase and cholesterol 7x-hydroxylase in the rat. *J. Lipid Res.*, **14**, 573
10. Weis, H. J., and Dietschy, J. M. (1969). Failure of bile acids to control hepatic cholesterogenesis: evidence for endogenous cholesterol feedback. *J. Clin. Invest.*, **48**, 2398
11. Nervi, F. C. and Dietschy, J. M. (1978). The mechanism of and the interrelationship between bile acid and chylomicron-mediated regulation of hepatic cholesterol synthesis in the liver of the rat. *J. Clin. Invest.*, **61**, 895
12. Hamprecht, B., Roscher, R., Waltinger, G. and Nüssler, C. (1971). Influence of bile acids on the activity of rat liver 3-hydroxy-3-methylglutaryl CoA reductase. *Eur. J. Biochem.*, **18**, 15
13. Liersch, M. E. A., Barth, C. A., Hackenschmidt, H. J., Ullman, H. L. and Decker, K. F. A. (1973). Influence of bile salts on cholesterol synthesis in the isolated perfused rat liver. *Eur. J. Biochem.*, **32**, 365
14. Cooper, A. D. (1976). The regulation of 3-hydroxy-3-methylglutaryl CoA reductase in the isolated perfused rat liver. *J. Clin. Invest.*, **57**, 1461
15. Weis, E. E. and Barth, C. A. (1978). The extracorporeal bile duct: a new model for determination of bile flow and bile composition in the intact rat. *J. Lipid Res.*, **19**, 856
16. Wanson, J. C., Bernaert, D. and May, C. (1979). Morphology and functional proper-

ties of isolated and cultured hepatocytes. In Popper, H. and Schaffner, F. (eds.). *Progress in Liver Disease*, vol. VI, pp. 1–22

17. Schwarz, L. R. and Barth, C. A. (1979). Taurocholate uptake by adult rat hepatocytes in primary culture. *Z. Physiol. Chem.*, **360,** 1117
18. Lin, R. C. and Snodgrass, P. J. (1977). A steady state of 3-hydroxy-3-methylglutaryl coenzyme A reductase activity in cultured rat liver cells and the increase of its activity by dexamethasone. *FEBS Lett.*, **83,** 89
19. Weis, E. E. and Barth, C. A. (1980). Inhibition of cholesterol synthesis in rat liver by physiological doses of taurocholate. *Eur. J. Biochem.*, **111,** 479
20. Barth, C. A. and Hillmar, I. (1980). Taurocholate inhibits the glucocorticoid-induced rise of 3-hydroxy-3-methylglutaryl CoA reductase in primary culture of hepatocytes. *Eur. J. Biochem.*, **110,** 237
21. Salen, G., Nicolau, G., Shefer, S. and Mosbach, E. H. (1975). Hepatic metabolism in patients with gallstones. *Gastroenterology*, **69,** 676

7
Filter trapping of $^{14}CO_2$: a new approach to the study of cholesterol metabolism in hepatocyte monolayers

H. WIETHOLTZ, S. HOTTINGER AND R. PREISIG

INTRODUCTION

In recent years much effort has been devoted to a better understanding of the pathways involved in bile acid synthesis. It is now established that the two major steps of the biosynthetic pathway are the ring hydroxylation – especially at the 7α-position – and the side-chain oxidation of the cholesterol molecule. The 7α-hydroxylation is considered to be a microsomal process, exhibiting feedback inhibition by primary bile acids. In contrast, the subcellular localization of the side-chain oxidation has not been definitely resolved and potential feedback regulations of bile acids upon this special step are largely unknown[1].

Since the study of hepatic regulatory mechanism of cholesterol in the intact animal is complicated by factors such as the amount of cholesterol in diet, the caloric intake of the animal and the functional integrity of the enterohepatic circulation, our studies took advantage of hepatocyte monolayers. Hepatocyte monolayers are particularly suited for studying cellular function, since investigations may be performed under precisely defined conditions, without the potential influences of blood flow, hormonal or neural factors.

MATERIAL AND METHODS

All studies were performed in male Sprague-Dawley rats (Deutsche Versuchstierfarm, Tuttlingen, Germany). The animals were kept in individual cages in the same room under constant temperature (22 °C) and humidity (48 $\pm$ 2%), the circadian rhythm being governed by daylight. Free access to standard rat diet (Altromin R 300, Altromin GmbH, Lage, Germany) and water was allowed.

Preparation of monolayers

The animals were subjected to a standard *in situ* collagenase perfusion via the portal vein. Prior to infusing collagenase solution the liver was flushed for 3 min with a Ca^{2+}-free Krebs–Ringer–bicarbonate solution. Thereafter, to the same solution 50 mg/100 ml collagenase (CLS II, Worthington, Biochem., New Jersey, USA) was added, and the liver perfused for 30 min. During the perfusion, flow rate (10 ml/min), gassing (with 95% O_2 and 5% CO_2), pH (7.45) and temperature (37 °C) were kept constant.

After termination of the perfusion, the liver was flushed with 20 ml ice-cold (4 °C) Ca^{2+}-free Krebs–Ringer–bicarbonate and removed to a Petri dish on ice. The liver was weighed and the capsule gently removed with scissors and forceps. Following incubation at room temperature in 20 ml Ca^{2+}-free Krebs–Ringer–bicarbonate containing 50 mg/100 ml collagenase, the liver cells were dispersed with a 10 ml wide-bore sterile pipette and gently filtered through a 100 μm screen in a 25 mm Swinnex holder using a 50 ml syringe. Subsequently, the cell suspension was centrifuged at 50 *g* for 2 min, resuspended in 40 ml Ca^{2+} and Mg^{2+}-free Hanks solution (Gibco, Glasgow, Scotland) and again centrifuged at 70 *g* for 3 min. The pellet was resuspended in 10 ml Leibovitz L-15 medium (Gibco, Glasgow, Scotland) at pH 7.5 with 50 μg/ml Gentamicin (Seromed GmbH, Munich, Germany), 10 mU/ml Insulin (Sigma Chem. Comp., St Louis, USA) and 15% fetal calf serum added. Cell count and viability were determined in a haemocytometer chamber after mixing 0.2 ml (1:5) diluted cell suspension with 0.05 ml 0.4% Trypan Blue. Viability, as judged by the Trypan Blue test, was approximately 90%. The suspension volume was adjusted with medium to 2×10^6 cells/ml cell suspension, plated in a 25 cm^2 Falcon tissue flask (6×10^6 cells) and placed in an incubator at 37 °C using 5% CO_2 and air. The duration of the procedure from the end of perfusion until plating was about 50 min. The first medium exchange was performed 5 h after plating, with serum-free Leibowitz L-15 medium containing insulin (10 mU/ml), Gentamicin (50 μg/ml) and Hepes buffer (20 mM) pH 7.3 (Hepes p.A., MW-238; Fluka AG, Buchs SG, Switzerland). Afterwards, the medium was changed every 24 h. From each rat a batch of 30–50 monolayers was obtained, corresponding to $190–300 \times 10^6$ cells per liver.

Metabolic studies

All metabolic studies were performed in confluent monolayers, 48 h after plating. Prior to addition of the various substrates, the culture medium was replaced with 3 ml Hanks' BSS solution containing Ca^{2+} and Mg^{2+}. To capture the $^{14}CO_2$ derived from side-chain oxidation, a Whatman GFA filter, soaked with 200 μl 0.5 N NaOH was suspended with a plastic dipper above the medium in the closed culture flasks. 8, 10 or 12 h after addition of the tracer and the different cold bile acids, respectively, the filters were removed and transferred to counting vials. The test system is depicted in Figure 1.

Cholesterol side-chain oxidation was studied using [26-^{14}C]cholesterol (52.5 mCi/mmol, New England Nuclear, Boston, Mass., USA). Radiochemical purity was greater than 99% as determined by paper chromatography, thin-layer chromatography and isotopic dilution analysis. An addition of 1 μCi [26-^{14}C]cholesterol was made to a single culture flask. In

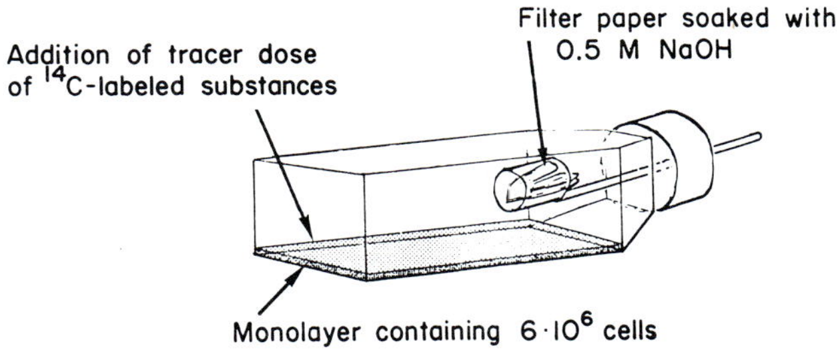

Figure 1 After addition of the [26-^{14}C]cholesterol to the monolayer, the culture flask was temporarily sealed and $^{14}CO_2$ resulting from cellular metabolism quantitatively captured on a filter paper soaked with NaOH. Thereafter the filter paper was removed and ^{14}C radioactivity counted in a liquid scintillation counter

order to facilitate hepatocellular uptake of the tracer, bovine serum (50 μl/ 1 μCi XOL) was used in the initial studies. Since this procedure did not allow precise quantification of the amounts of lipoproteins added, in subsequent investigations we used 50 μg/1 μCi XOL purified human low-density lipoprotein (kindly supplied by Professor S. Seiler, Innsbruck, Austria). In some investigations different bile acids of A grade were mixed with the cholesterol tracer/LDL solution to explore potential alterations of side-chain oxidation. These bile acids were cholic, chenodeoxycholic and ursodeoxycholic acid (Calbiochem., San Diego, Calif., USA).

Protein was analysed according to the modified method of Lowry *et al.* as described by Oyama and Eagle, using bovine serum albumine as standard[2].

^{14}C *radioactivity* was counted in a Packard-Tri-Carb 2660 liquid scintillation counter using 5 ml Lumagel as scintillator.

Statistical calculations

Where appropriate, regression analysis was performed; other results are given as means and standard deviations. Differences were calculated with the Student *t*-test. Because of the relatively small sample size, only error possibilities of $p < 0.01$ were regarded as statistically significant.

RESULTS

To establish the feasibility of the procedure in hepatocyte monolayers, in initial experiments we measured $^{14}CO_2$ yield resulting from side-chain oxidation up to 12 h after addition of labelled cholesterol. As shown in Figure 2, it became evident that after an incubation period of 6–8 h $^{14}CO_2$ yield rose linearly, exhibiting a small intraculture variation of $^{14}CO_2$ production. The slope of the regressive lines was $y = 409\,x–1720$, the coefficient of correlation being $r = 0.97$.

Based on this observation we proceeded to explore potential alterations of side-chain oxidation due to exogenous substances. Since bile acids are the end-products of this metabolism, we focused on the effects of cholic and chenodeoxycholic acid. In this study these primary bile acids in concentrations

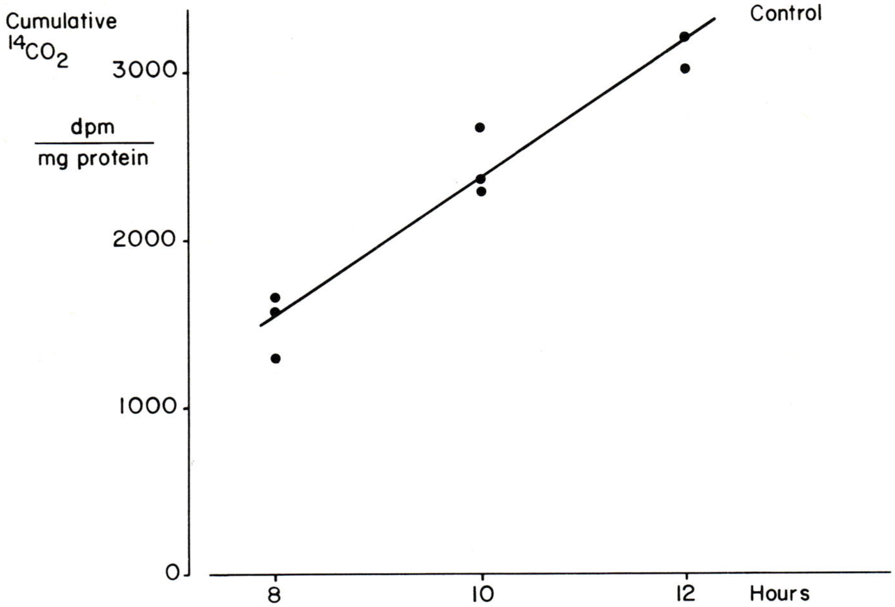

Figure 2 Side-chain oxidation of cholesterol. After addition of 1 μCi [26-^{14}C] cholesterol (together with LDL) to each hepatocyte monolayer, $^{14}CO_2$ yield rose linearly during the time of observation. Note the small variation in $^{14}CO_2$ yield between cultures

between 0 and 100 μmol/l were added to three cultures each, together with the labelled cholesterol and incubated for 12 h. The resultant $^{14}CO_2$ yield was compared to that of control cultures (without addition of bile acids). Cholic acid appeared to have little if any effect, since there was no significant difference of $^{14}CO_2$ yield at concentrations of 0 and 100 μmol/l cholic acid. In contrast, chenodeoxycholic acid clearly reduced side-chain oxidation of cholesterol. This was most pronounced at 100 μmol/l concentration, where $^{14}CO_2$ yield was decreased to 58%, a statistically significant difference from the control value ($p < 0.01$) (Table 1).

To confirm and expand this finding a further study was performed where in addition to cholic and chenodeoxycholic acid, ursodeoxycholic acid was used.

Table 1 Effect of cholic and chenodeoxycholic acid on side-chain oxidation of [26-^{14}C]cholesterol

Bile acid concentration (μmol/l)	$^{14}CO_2$ *yield* (dpm mg prot.$^{-1}$); $\bar{x} \pm$ SD; $n = 3$ *after addition of*	
	Cholic acid	*Chenodeoxycholic acid*
0	439 ± 134	427 ± 40
30	410 ± 103	433 ± 21
50	412 ± 87	341 ± 52
100	369 ± 52	248 ± 34*

* $p = 0.01$ significantly different from control

Figure 3 shows the effects of the three bile acids on the metabolic rate of cholesterol (calculated from $^{14}CO_2$ yield). Each point represents the mean of two cultures. It can be seen that the previous observations were confirmed. Once again, the suppressive effect of chenodeoxycholic acid was superior to that of cholic acid. In addition, the inhibition of side-chain oxidation using ursodeoxycholic acid was even more pronounced and evident at concentrations as low as 25 μmol/l.

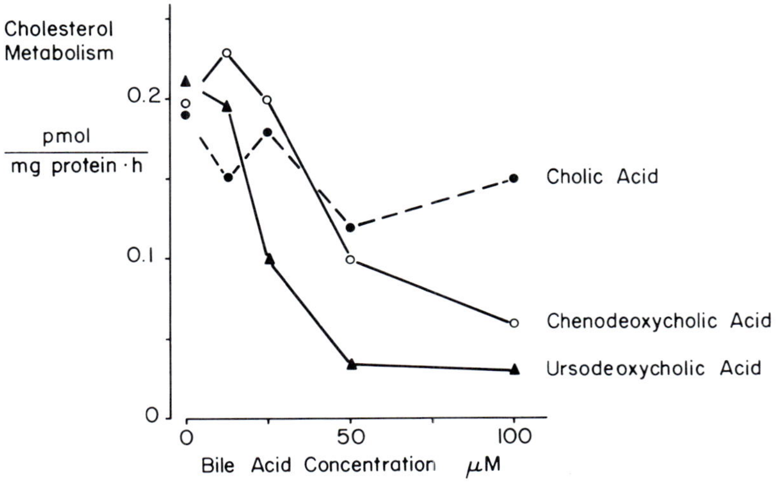

Figure 3 Effect of different concentrations of cholic, chenodeoxycholic and ursodeoxycholic acid on cholesterol side-chain oxidation (calculated from $^{14}CO_2$ yield). Whereas cholic acid does not appear to affect cholesterol metabolism, ursodeoxycholic acid produces a marked inhibition of side-chain oxidation. The inhibitory effects of chenodeoxycholic acid seem less pronounced

DISCUSSION

Previous investigations in the intact animal using cholesterol labelled with ^{14}C in position 26 have demonstrated that expired $^{14}CO_2$ yields an adequate estimate of bile acid synthesis[3,4]. Based on these observations it was reasonable to consider a similar approach for studies in hepatocyte monolayers. However, two conditions had to be fulfilled for obtaining valid measurements: it was necessary to assure uptake of cholesterol into the hepatocytes, and to ascertain quantitative collection of $^{14}CO_2$ in the culture flask.

Although bovine serum provided a suitable carrier system for cholesterol uptake, its lipoprotein content was not established. We therefore turned to low-density lipoprotein, extracted from human plasma by rate-zonal ultracentrifugation[5]. Using ring-labelled cholesterol [1a, 2a(n)-^{3}H]cholesterol, uptake into cells was shown to be 16.8 ± 6% of the dose added per mg protein within the incubation period of 12 h.

Quantitative collection of $^{14}CO_2$ was achieved with the previously described filter trapping system[6]. In this system recovery of $^{14}CO_2$ following addition of labelled bicarbonate amounts to 94 ± 4%.

As is evident from Figure 2, after 6–8 h of incubation cumulative $^{14}CO_2$ yield from side-chain oxidation of cholesterol achieves levels sufficient for precise measurement. Furthermore, during the ensuing hours, the metabolic rate is constant, as judged from the linear ^{14}CO production over time. Presumably, therefore, the system appeared sufficiently controlled for investigating the effects of exogenous compounds on cholesterol oxidation.

In a first set of experiments monolayers were exposed to different concentrations of cholic and chenodeoxycholic acid. Whereas cholic acid, even at concentrations of 100 μmol/l did not appear to affect $^{14}CO_2$ yield, side-chain oxidation of cholesterol was clearly affected by chenodeoxycholic acid. Thus, $^{14}CO_2$ yield tended to fall at concentrations of 50 μmol/l and was clearly suppressed at 100 μmol/l.

Encouraged by these results we undertook a second set of investigations, where the effects of ursodeoxycholic acid were also studied. In addition to confirming the previous results with primary bile acids, ursodeoxycholic acid proved to be the most potent inhibitor of side-chain oxidation. At concentrations as low as 25 μmol/l, cholesterol metabolism was already markedly depressed.

These results are obviously preliminary. Future studies will have to demonstrate, whether the observed phenomena represent substrate inhibition and if so, at what level of the bile acid pathways[1,7]. Nevertheless, our investigations point to the feasibility of studying regulation of cholesterol metabolism in hepatocyte monolayers without disturbing the integrity of the cells.

Acknowledgment

This work was supplied by the Swiss National Science Foundation.

References

1. Björkhem, J. and Danielsson, H. (1976). Biosynthesis and metabolism of bile acids in man. In Popper, H. and Schaffner, F. (eds.), *Progress in Liver Diseases*, vol. V, p. 215 (New York, San Francisco, London: Grune Stratton)
2. Oyama, V. J. and Eagle, H. (1956). Measurement of cell growth in tissue culture with a phenol reagent. *Proc. Soc. Exp. Biol. Med.*, **91,** 305
3. Chevallier, F. and Lufton, C. (1966). Cinétiques journalière et horaire de la transformation du cholésterol-26-^{14}C en acides biliaires. *Bull. Soc. Chem. Biol.*, **48,** 295
4. Davis, R. A. and Kern, F. (1976). Effects of ethinyl estradiol and phenobarbital on bile acid synthesis and biliary bile acid and cholesterol excretion. *Gastroenterology*, **70,** 1130
5. Patsch, J. R., Sailer, S., Kestner, G., Sandhofer, F., Holasek, A. and Braunsteiner, H. (1974). Separation of the main lipoprotein density classes from human plasma by rate-zonal ultracentrifugation. *J. Lipid Res.*, **15,** 356
6. Hottinger, S., Röllinghoff, W., Wietholtz, H. and Preisig, R. (1980). Filter trapping of $^{14}CO_2$: a simple and quantitative method for studying cell metabolism and assessing cell damage in hepatocyte monolayers. (Submitted for publication in *Exp. Cell Res.*)
7. Danielsson, H. and Johansson, G. (1974). Effects of long term feeding of chenodeoxycholic acid on biosynthesis and metabolism of bile acids in the rat. *Gastroenterology*, **67,** 126

8
Effects of cholesterol and bile acids on HMG-CoA reductase and brush border enzymes in organ-cultured intestine

E. F. STANGE, A. SCHNEIDER, M. ALAVI, H. DITSCHUNEIT AND J. R. POLEY

INTRODUCTION

Intestinal cholesterol synthesis contributes approximately 20% to the circulating cholesterol pool in animals fed a low cholesterol diet[1]. Increasing dietary cholesterol abolishes cholesterol synthesis in the liver[2], but has little[3,4] or no[5] effect on cholesterol production in rat and dog intestine. Consequently, in these species, the main site of endogenous cholesterol synthesis is shifted to the small intestine. This occurs also in the guinea pig[6,7] and the rabbit[8], although their intestinal cholesterogenesis seems more sensitive to exogenous cholesterol.

In liver and intestine, the key enzyme of cholesterol synthesis is 3-hydroxy-3-methylglutaryl coenzyme-A reductase[9] (HMG-CoA reductase; E.C.1.1.1.34).

The regulator of the enzyme in hepatocytes is probably cholesterol, rather than bile acids; the possible role of bile acids is controversial[10–13]. With regard to cholesterol synthesis in enterocytes, the issue has remained controversial as to whether cholesterol or bile acids, or both, control HMG-CoA reductase activity.

In vivo studies in the rat by Shefer *et al.*[5] demonstrated that cholesterol and bile acids lowered intestinal reductase during the basal period of the circadian rhythm. Bile acids alone only suppressed peak activity. In a similar study in the guinea pig, cholesterol alone decreased intestinal reductase activity. However, the rise of bile acid synthesis, which occurs in this species after cholesterol feeding[14], did not permit determination which of the two, cholesterol or bile acids, had a greater influence on reductase. On the other hand, the regulatory effects of bile acids on enteric reductase could be secondary, since they enhance absorption by its micellar dispersion[15]. Gebhard and Cooper[16] presented the first report on the *in vitro* regulation of intestinal cholesterol synthesis, using short-term (6 h) organ cultures of canine intestine. They have shown that cholesterol or bile acids alone considerably inhibited HMG-CoA reductase. However, the effect of both was not additive in near-physiological concentrations. Therefore, it is unlikely that cholesterol and bile acids as mixed micelles exert a suppressive effect of their own; at least not in a species which responds sluggishly to dietary cholesterol[4].

To further elucidate the role of cholesterol, and bile acids, alone or in combination, on the regulation of enteric cholesterol synthesis, we continued to use the rabbit as a more ideal animal species, for several reasons:

(1) the rabbit cannot expand its bile acid pool (cholesterol escape) in response to exogenous cholesterol[17];
(2) rabbit intestine is very sensitive to dietary cholesterol[8];
(3) in contrast to the rat[18], there is no circadian rhythm of intestinal reductase activity[8].

Finally, we have utilized organ cultures of rabbit ileum, since it can be preserved about 4 times longer than canine intestinal mucosa[19].

METHODS

Organ culture technique

In white New Zealand rabbits the ileum was excised, and full-thickness (including submucosa) biopsies were taken with a sterile scalpel blade 10–15 cm proximal to the caecal valve. Mucosal specimens were processed as follows: one portion was transferred into ice-cold homogenization medium (0.1 M sucrose, 0.5 M KCl, 0.04 M KH_2PO_4, 0.03 M EDTA and 0.25% Kyro EOB (kindly supplied by Procter and Gamble, Cincinatti) adjusted to pH 7.2) for enzyme determinations; the other portion was immediately cultured.

Organ culture was performed with 1–2 mm tissue fragments after thorough rinsing in Trowel's T8 medium (Gibco Biocult, Karlsruhe, GFR) as previously described[19]. Control medium consisted of 90% Trowel's T8, 10% lipo-protein-free fetal calf serum, pencillin 100 U/ml, streptomycin 100 μg/ml, neomycin 100 μg/ml. To obtain lipoprotein-free fetal calf serum, fresh serum was ultracentrifuged for 24 h at 105,000 $\times$ *g* with a density adjusted to 1.25 g/ml[20].

Histologic examination was carried out routinely on cultured tissue, and its good preservation after 24 h of culture was always evident.

Enzyme and chemical determinations

Alkaline phosphatase was assayed with the Merckotest enzyme kit according to the method of Bessey *et al.*[21]. Sucrase was determined using the glucose dehydrogenase kit (E. Merck, Darmstadt, GFR) as described by Dahlqvist[22]. Cholesterol was measured by the Boehringer Mannheim cholesterol oxidase kit; for tissue extraction methanol/chloroform was used.

Incorporation studies

[6-^{3}H]thymidine (28.5 Ci/mmol, NEN Chemicals, Dreieichenhain, GFR) incorporation into acid-precipitable DNA was measured, using ice-cold 10% trichloroacetic acid[23]. Medium radioactivity was 1 μCi/ml.

[4,5-^{3}H]L-leucine (5 Ci/mmol, NEN Chemicals) was diluted to 5 μCi/ml medium and incorporated into tissue protein. Protein was precipitated by 10% trichloroacetic acid and 1% phosphotungstic acid[24].

HMG-CoA reductase assay

HMG-CoA reductase was determined according to Shapiro *et al.*[25], with minor modifications[26]. The incubation solution contained 1.0 M potassium phosphate buffer, 1.0 M EDTA, 0.5 M glucose-6-phosphate, 0.1 M NADP, 0.24 dithiothreitol, 10 mg/ml serum albumin, 1 mg/ml glucose-6-phosphate dehydrogenase (Boehringer, Mannheim, GFR) in a total volume of 0.18 ml (pH 7.4), to which 0.07 ml of tissue homogenate were added. After a preincubation period of 15 min the reaction was started by the addition of 24 nmol D,L-[3-^{14}C]HMG-CoA (10 m Ci/nmol, NEN Chemicals) in 0.05 ml.

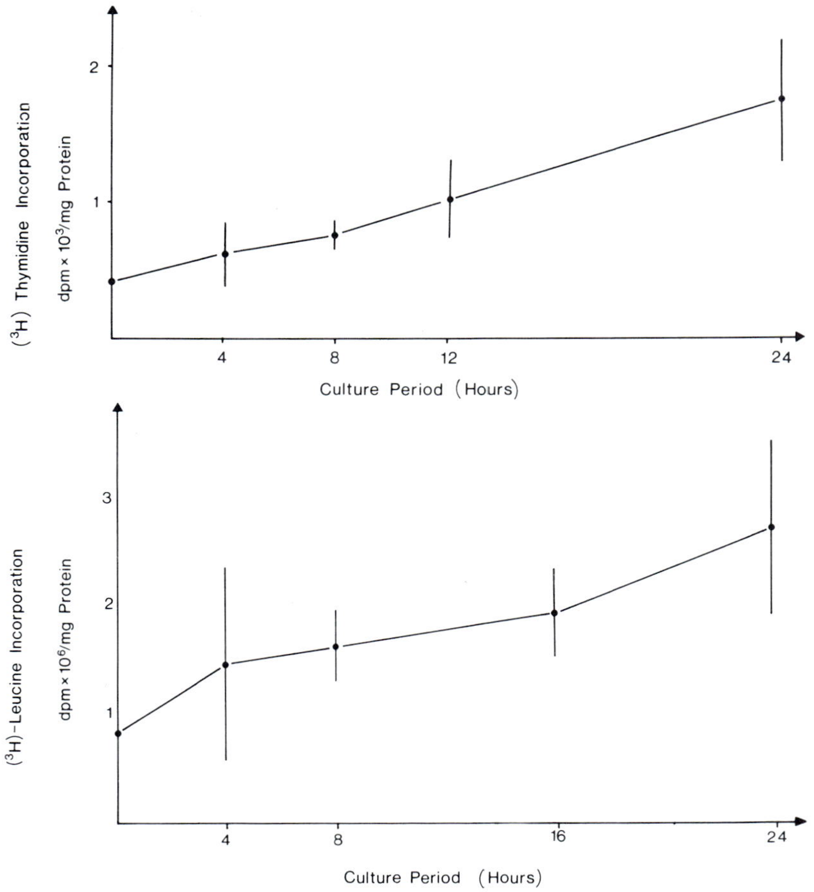

Figure 1 Viability test (±1SD). Incorporation of (a) [^{3}H]thymidine into DNA (n=8); and (b)[^{3}H]leucine into protein (n=10), of organ-cultured rabbit ileum over 24 h. Boiled biopsies were used for 0 h values. Culture was stopped at times indicated

RESULTS

Viability of cultured mucosa (Figure 1)

The mucosal specimens were kept viable in the organ culture system for 24 h. Inclusion of 0.2 and 1.0 mmol/l cycloheximide into the culture medium suppressed [^{3}H]leucine labelling of protein by at least 98% in comparison with controls ($n=4$).

Effects of various compounds on HMG-CoA reductase and brush border enzymes

Ethanol and cholesterol (Figure 2)
Reductase activity in ileal biopsies prior to culture averaged 0.042 ± 0.015 nmol mg^{-1} h^{-1}. After 12 h of culture it increased to 0.096 ± 0.016 ($p < 0.001$), whereafter it remained unchanged for the remaining 12 h.

The addition of 1% ethanol and of 0.05 mmol/l cholesterol to the culture medium had no effect on reductase. However, addition of cholesterol in higher concentrations clearly suppressed the increase in reductase activity

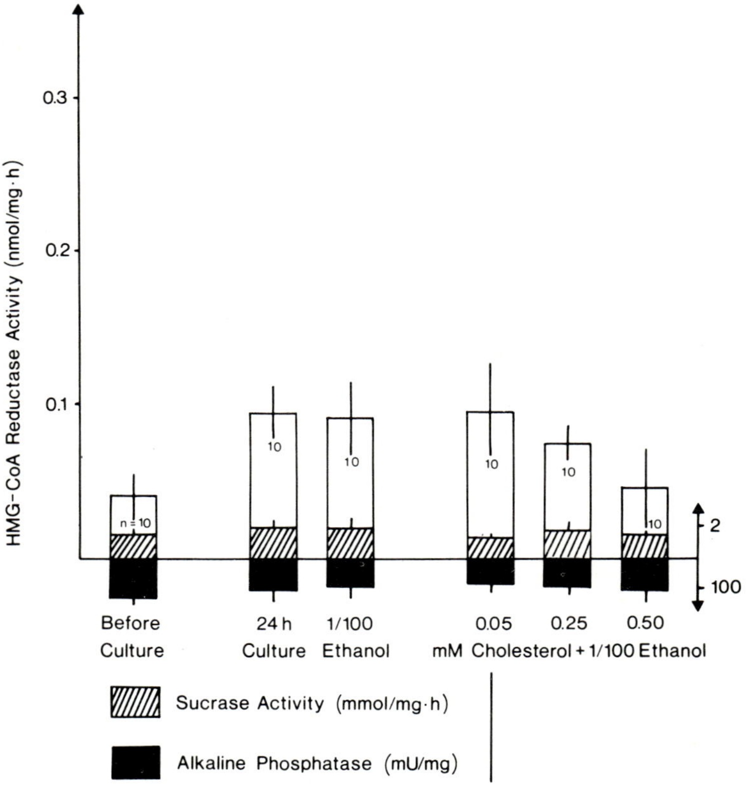

Figure 2 Effect of cholesterol and ethanol on HMG-CoA reductase, sucrase and alkaline phosphatase in cultured rabbit ileum after 24 h. Horizontal bars: mean values of n animals; vertical lines: SD (n = number or rabbits)

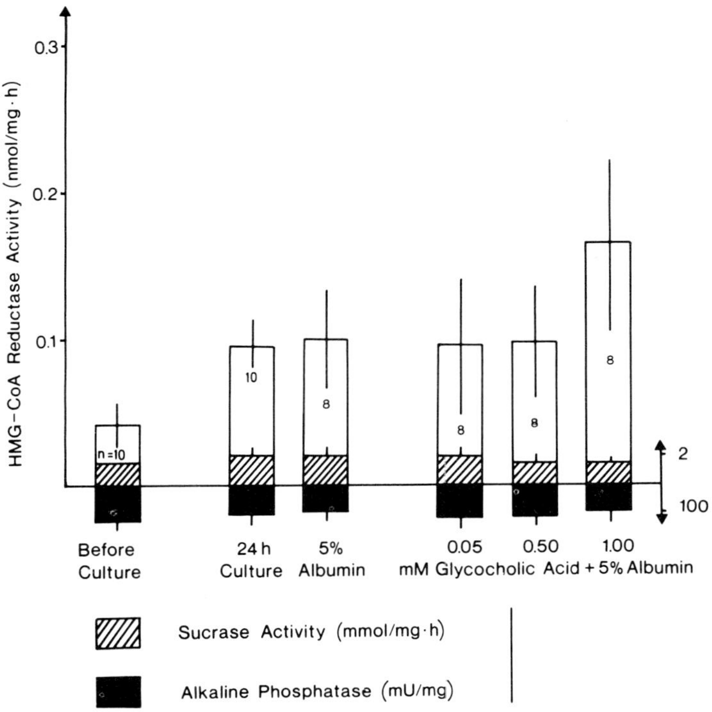

Figure 3 Effect of glycocholic acid and albumin on HMG-CoA reductase, sucrase and alkaline phosphatase in cultured rabbit ileum after 24 h. Horizontal bars: mean values of *n* animals; vertical lines: SD (*n* = number of rabbits)

($p < 0.05$). Both ethanol and cholesterol had no influence on the activity of sucrase and alkaline phosphatase for the entire duration of the organ culture.

Albumin and glycocholic acid (Figure 3)
The addition of 5% bovine serum albumin or glycocholic acid in concentrations of 0.05 and 0.5 mmol/l respectively, failed to influence reductase activity. However, 1.0 mmol/l glycocholic acid produced a significant ($p < 0.01$) stimulation of HMG-CoA reductase. On the other hand, sucrase and alkaline phosphatase remained essentially unchanged by albumin and, following the addition of bile acid, only a slight decrease in their activity was observed.

Glycodeoxycholic acid (Figure 4; Table 1)
The effect of the main bile acid of the rabbit, glycodeoxycholic acid, was more pronounced than that of glycocholic acid. When added in concentrations of 1.0 mmol/l, reductase activity doubled ($p < 0.001$) and it tripled ($p < 0.001$) over control values after the addition of 5.0 mmol/l glycodeoxycholate. At the same time, there was a slight tendency for sucrase and alkaline phosphatase activities to decline. However, when glycodeoxycholic acid was presented in concentrations exceeding 10 mmol/l, there was a notable decrease of reductase activity, as well as that of alkaline phosphatase (Table 1).

Table 1 Influence of glycodeoxycoholic acid on HMG-CoA reductase and alkaline phosphatase of ileum organ culture I means, $n = 3$

Glycodeoxycholic acid (mM)	*HMG-CoA reductase* (%)	*Alkaline phosphatase* (%)
5	100	100
10	14	50
50	0	0
5 + 0.2 mM cycloheximide	3	65

The addition of 0.2 mmol/l cycloheximide to 5 mmol/l glycodeoxycholate, almost completely abolishes reductase activity, whereas alkaline phosphatase was still about 65% active (Table 1).

To exclude a direct action of bile acid on preformed enzymes, ileal mucosal homogenates were incubated with varying concentrations (1.0–5.0 mmol/l) of glycodeoxycholate. After 1 h of incubation, a decrease of reductase activity of 66 and 77%, respectively, was observed in comparison with studies when bile acids were not included into the medium during the hour of incubation.

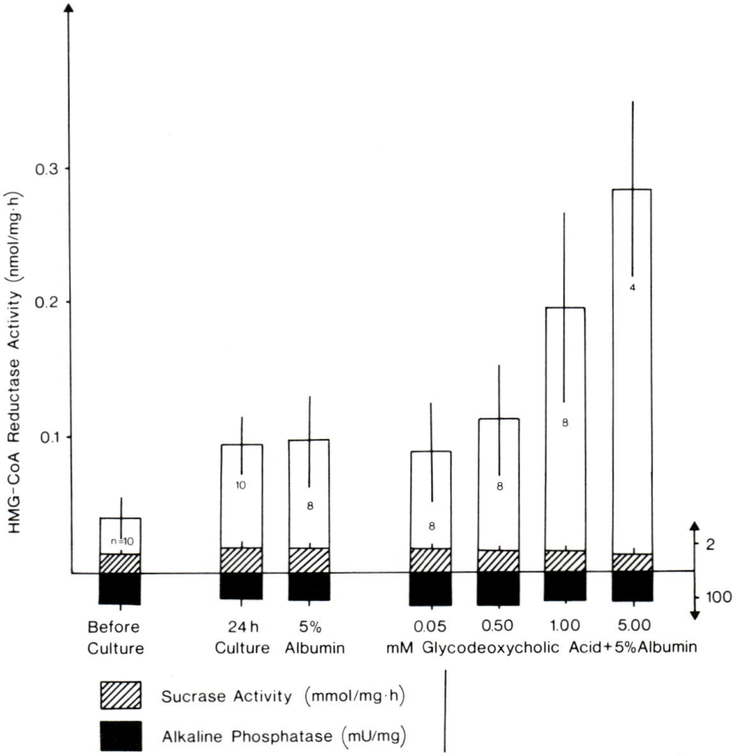

Figure 4 Influence of glycodeoxycholic acid on HMG-CoA reductase, sucrase and alkaline phosphatase in cultured rabbit ileum after 24 h. Horizontal bars: mean values of *n* animals; vertical lines: SD (*n* = number of rabbits)

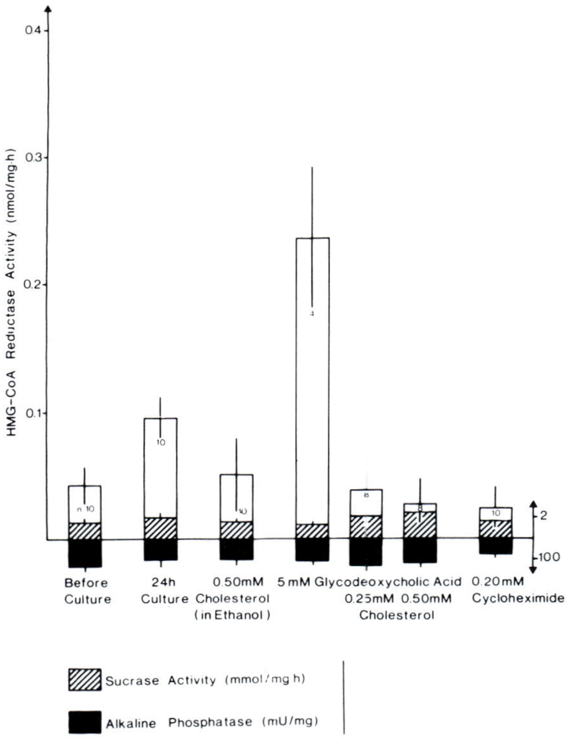

Figure 5 Influence of cholesterol/bile acid micelles and cycloheximide on HMG-CoA reductase, sucrase and alkaline phosphatase in cultured rabbit ileum after 24 h. Horizontal bars: mean values of *n* animals; vertical lines: SD (*n* = number of rabbits)

Cholesterol and bile acid micelles (Figure 5)

As demonstrated in Figures 3 and 4, cholesterol in 0.5 mmol/l solution decreased, and 5.0 mmol/l glycodeoxycholic acid markedly increased reductase activity. However, when cholesterol was presented to the culture medium in a mixed micellar solution, a drastic decrease of reductase activity was noted ($p < 0.001$).

The decrease of reductase activity using 0.5 mmol/l micellar cholesterol was of similar magnitude to that of 0.2 mmol/l cycloheximide, which blocks protein synthesis in the mucosa, resulting in a marked decrease of sucrase and alkaline phosphatase activities. Cholesterol in micellar form had no influence on these marker enzymes.

Bile acids and mucosal cholesterol contents (Table 2)

During the 24 h culture period the cholesterol contents of the biopsies increased relative both to wet weight and protein. In the presence of bile acids a pronounced cholesterol depletion occurred in the cultured tissue, if compared to controls. Therefore, the increased HMG-CoA reductase did not fully compensate for this loss.

Table 2 Effect of glycodeoxycholate on tissue cholesterol contents (means ± SD); $n = 5$

Culture period (h)	*Glycodeoxycholate* (mM)	*Tissue cholesterol* (mg/g wet weight)	*Cholesterol protein ratio* (weight/weight)
0	0	0.87 ± 0.19	0.047 ± 0.016
24	0	1.87 ± 0.28	0.093 ± 0.030
24	2	1.35 ± 0.28	0.086 ± 0.025
24	5	1.43 ± 0.70	0.075 ± 0.033

DISCUSSION

Results of available *in vivo* studies suggest that three regulator candidates for intestinal HMG-CoA reductase may exist: (1) luminal cholesterol; (2) luminal bile acids, absorbed in micellar form; (3) plasma lipoprotein cholesterol. Lipoprotein regulation is supported by work from our laboratory[26] and by Andersen and Dietschy[27], who stimulated intestinal reductase in rats made hypolipoproteinaemic by 4-aminopyrazol-(3,4D)-pyrimidine. This decrease was reversible after the infusion of plasma lipoprotein. These experiments lend continued support to the view that cholesterol biosynthesis in enterocytes and other cell systems is under constant surveillance and control by cholesterol itself.

Our investigations in cultured rabbit ileal mucosa (in a lipoprotein-free system) have demonstrated that cholesterol exerted a marked suppressor effect on enteric HMG-CoA reductase, when present in concentrations greater than 0.25 mmol/l, either as 1% ethanolic solution, or in mixed micellar solution. These findings support data obtained previously by *in vivo* studies in the rabbit[8]. Cholesterol by itself had no effect on membrane-associated enzymes, such as sucrase and alkaline phosphatase.

Both glycocholic and glycodeoxycholic acid were strong stimulators of HMG-CoA reductase, the latter bile acid in particular. The range of concentrations at which bile acids were most effective, was between 1.0 and 5.0 mmol/l. Higher concentrations were probably toxic, as indicated by a marked decline of sucrase and alkaline phosphatase activities. By contrast, these membrane-bound enzymes were not affected by the culture procedure, rendering unlikely a change in the proportion of villous to crypt cells. Bile acids also stimulate reductase activity of cultured fibroblasts[28] and hepatocytes[29].

The suppressor effect of cholesterol on HMG-CoA reductase is likely to be mediated directly by cholesterol itself, which probably inhibits enzyme synthesis. The action of bile acids on the stimulation of reductase is less well understood, but may proceed directly by influencing physicochemical properties of membranes. Hepatic reductase activity is increased after bile duct ligation[11], resulting in a rise of bile acid concentration in tissue. This increase of tissue bile acids is followed by an increase in membrane fluidity[30], a function of membrane cholesterol content. The detergent effect of bile acids leads to a depletion of cholesterol in plasma membranes and in microsomes in the environment of reductase, so that enzyme activity is stimulated or new enzyme synthesized. Although we did not measure membrane fluidity, the conclusion may be valid that the action of bile acids does influence membrane behaviour and integrity, as judged by a decrease of membrane-bound enzymes, sucrase and alkaline phosphatase. Feeding of deoxycholic acid resulted in a loss of sucrase activity, as shown in another study[31], suggesting a 'damaging' effect on enterocyte membranes.

In our organ-culture model we could not demonstrate a suppressive effect on intestinal reductase when low concentrations of bile acids (1.0 mmol/l) were used, as had been proposed[16]. However, we could not rule out a slight temporary decrease of reductase activity after 6 h of culture, a time used for culture of canine mucosa for reasons of limited viability.

In summary, the data obtained in this study tend to support the following:

(1) It is cholesterol itself which regulates its own synthesis in cultured rabbit ileum. A negative feedback mechanism is likely.
(2) When cholesterol is presented in micellar form, a greater inhibitory capacity is demonstrated as compared to cholesterol dissolved in ethanol. Micellar cholesterol probably has a higher tissue-uptake rate.
(3) The stimulatory effect of bile acids is probably secondary, due to their detergent action, by depleting membrane and tissue cholesterol, inducing new synthesis of HMG-CoA reductase.
(4) That new enzyme synthesis is involved as demonstrated by two lines of evidence: (a) the stimulatory effect of bile acids is blocked completely by cycloheximide; (b) bile acids in concentrations of 1.0 and 5.0 mmol/l decrease, rather than increase, the activity of the preformed enzyme.

Acknowledgments

This study was supported by a grant from the Deutsche Forschungsgemeinschaft, SFB 112 (D3). The excellent and skilful technical assistance of Mrs B. Jansohn and Mrs M. Lauster, and the typing of the manuscript by Mrs D. Moser, are gratefully acknowledged.

References

1. Dietschy, J. M. and Wilson, J. D. (1969). Regulation of cholesterol metabolism. *N. Engl. J. Med.*, **282,** 1128
2. Shapiro, D. J. and Rodwell, V. W. (1971). Regulation of hepatic HMG-CoA reductase and cholesterol synthesis. *J. Biol. Chem.*, **246,** 3210
3. Dietschy, J. M. (1968). The role of bile salts in controlling the rate of intestinal cholesterogenesis. *J. Clin. Invest.*, **47,** 286
4. Gould, G., Taylor, C. G., Hagermann, J. S., Warner, I. and Campbell, J. D. (1953). Effect of dietary cholesterol on the synthesis of cholesterol in dog tissue *in vitro*. *J. Biol. Chem.*, **201,** 519
5. Shefer, S., Hauser, S., Lapar, V. and Mosbach, E. H. (1973). Regulatory effects of dietary sterols and bile acids on rat intestinal HMG-CoA-reductase. *J. Lipid Res.*, **14,** 400
6. Turley, S. D. and West, C. E. (1976). Effect of cholesterol and cholestyramine feeding and of fasting on sterol synthesis in the liver, ileum and lung of the guinea pig. *Lipids*, **11,** 571
7. Swann, A., Wiley, M. H. and Siperstein, M. D. (1975). Tissue distribution of cholesterol feedback control in the guinea pig. *J. Lipid Res.*, **16,** 360
8. Stange, E. F., Alavi, M., Schneider, A., Ditschuneit, H. and Poley, J. R. (1981). Influence of dietary cholesterol, saturated and unsaturated lipid on 3-hydroxy-3-methylglutaryl CoA reductase in rabbit intestine and liver. *J. Lipid Res.* **22,** 47

9. Shefer, S., Hauser, S., Lapar, V. and Mosbach, E. H. (1972). HMG-CoA reductase of intestinal mucosa and liver of the rat. *J. Lipid Res.*, **13**, 402
10. Nervi, F. O. and Dietschy, J. M. (1975). Ability of six different lipoprotein fractions to regulate the rate of hepatic cholesterogenesis in vivo. *J. Biol. Chem.*, **250**, 8704
11. Weis, H. J. and Dietschy, J. M. (1969). Failure of bile acids to control hepatic cholesterogenesis: evidence for endogenous cholesterol feedback. *J. Clin. Invest.*, **48**, 2398
12. Cooper, A. D. and Ockner, R. K. (1974). Studies of hepatic cholesterol synthesis in experimental acute biliary obstruction. *Gastroenterology*, **66**, 586
13. Hamprecht, B., Roscher, R., Waltinger, G. and Nüssler, C. (1971). Influence of bile acids on the activity of rat liver 3-hydroxy-3-methylglutaryl coenzyme A reductase, *Eur. J. Biochem.*, **18**, 15
14. Hansma, H. and Ostwald, R. (1974). Effects of dietary cholesterol upon bile acid metabolism in guinea pig. *Lipids*, **9**, 731
15. Poley, J. R. (1976). Fat digestion and absorption in lipase and bile acid deficiency. In Rommel, K. and Goebell, H. (eds.). *Lipid Absorption: Biochemical and Clinical Aspects*, pp. 151–202. (Lancaster: MTP Press)
16. Gebhard, R. L. and Cooper, A. D. (1978). Regulation of cholesterol synthesis in cultured canine intestinal mucosa. *J. Biol. Chem.*, **253**, 2790
17. Hellström, K. (1965). On the bile acid and neutral fecal steroid excretion in man and rabbits following cholesterol feeding. *Acta Physiol. Scand.*, **63**, 21
18. Shefer, S., Hauser, S., Lapar, V. and Mosbach, E. H. (1972). Diurnal variation of HMG-CoA reductase activity in rat intestine. *J. Lipid Res.*, **13**, 571
19. Kagnoff, M. F., Donaldson, R. M. and Trier, J. S. (1972). Organ culture of rabbit small intestine. Prolonged *in vitro* steady state protein synthesis and secretion and secretory IgA secretion. *Gastroenterology*, **63/4**, 541
20. Stange, E., Agostini, B. and Papenberg, J. (1975). Changes in rabbit lipoprotein properties by dietary cholesterol, and saturated and polyunsaturated fats. *Atherosclerosis*, **22**, 125
21. Bessey, O. A., Lowry, O. H. and Brock, M. J. (1946). A method for the rapid determination of alkaline phosphatase in five cubic milliliters of serum. *J. Biol. Chem.*, **164**, 321
22. Dahlqvist, A. (1968). Assay of intestinal disaccharidases. *Anal. Biochem.*, **22**, 99
23. Alpers, D. H. and Philpott, G. W. (1975). Control of deoxyribonucleic acid synthesis in normal rabbit colonic mucosa. *Gastroenterology*, **69**, 951
24. MacDermott, R. P., Donaldson, R. M. and Trier, J. S. (1974). Glycoprotein synthesis and secretion by mucosal biopsies of rabbit colon and human rectum. *J. Clin. Invest.*, **54**, 545
25. Shapiro, D. J., Nordstrom, J. L., Mitschelen, J. J., Rodwell, V. W. and Schimke, R. T. (1974). Micro assay for HMG-CoA-reductase in rat liver and in L-cell fibroblasts. *Biochim. Biophys. Acta*, **370**, 369
26. Stange, E. F., Alavi, M., Schneider, A., Preclik, G. and Ditschuneit, H. (1980). Lipoprotein regulation of 3-hydroxy-3-methylglutaryl CoA reductase in cultured intestinal mucosa. *Biochim. Biophys. Acta*, **620**, 520
27. Andersen, J. M., and Dietschy, J. M. (1977). Regulation of sterol synthesis in 15 tissues of the rat. *J. Biol. Chem.*, **252**, 3652
28. Brown, M. S. and Goldstein, J. L. (1974). Suppression of 3-hydroxy-3-methlyglutaryl coenzyme. A reductase activity and inhibition of growth of human fibroblasts by 7-keto-cholesterol *J. Biol. Chem.*, **249**, 7306
29. Kandutsch, A. A. and Chen, H. W. (1973). Inhibition of sterol synthesis in cultured mouse cells by 7a-hydroxycholesterol, 7b-hydroxycholesterol and 7-ketocholesterol. *J. Biol. Chem.*, **248**, 8408
30. Mitropoulos, K. A., Venkatesan, S. and Balasubramaniam, S. (1979). On the role of bile acids in the regulation of hepatic cholesterogenesis. In Paumgartner, G., Stiehl, A. and Gerok, W. (eds). *Biological Effects of Bile Acids*, p. 137. (Lancaster: MTP Press)
31. Gracey, M., Houghton, M. and Thomas, J. (1975). Deoxycholate depresses small-intestinal enzyme activity. *Gut*, **16**, 53

9
Bile acids and hepatic HMG-CoA reductase in man

K. EINARSSON, J. AHLBERG, B. ANGELIN AND S. EWERTH

INTRODUCTION

The liver is a key organ in the metabolism of cholesterol in man. Although most tissues are capable of synthesizing cholesterol, the liver supplies the major part of endogenously formed cholesterol. The rate-determining step in the biosynthesis of cholesterol is the conversion of 3-hydroxy,-3-methylglutaryl coenzyme A (HMG-CoA) to mevalonate, catalyzed by the microsomal enzyme HMG-CoA reductase (mevalonate: NADP oxido-reductase, EC 1.1.1.34). The activity of this enzyme is subject to a sensitive feedback control, still incompletely known in its details.

The aim of this presentation is to summarize some recent studies performed in our laboratory concerning HMG-CoA reductase in human liver with special reference to the effects of bile acid feeding.

MATERIAL AND METHODS

The following groups of patients were investigated:

(1) gallstone-free subjects undergoing cholecystectomy because of adeno-myoma or polyps of the gallbladder wall; these patients served as controls;

(2) normolipidaemic, normal-weight patients with uncomplicated cholesterol gallstone disease undergoing elective cholecystectomy; and

(3) patients with cholesterol gallstone disease pretreated with cholic acid (CA) or chenodeoxycholic acid (CDCA) at a daily dose of 15 mg/kg body weight for 4–8 weeks prior to operation.

All patients were hospitalized 2–3 days prior to operation. They were given the regular hospital diet. The operations were performed at 9 a.m. after a 12 h fast, and standardized anaesthesia was given. Directly after opening the abdomen, a biopsy was obtained from the left lobe of the liver, and the microsomal fraction was prepared immediately.

The activity of the microsomal HMG-CoA reductase was assayed essentially as described by Nicolau *et al.*[1]. The incubation system contained, in a total volume of 0.85 ml, 0.15–0.5 mg of microsomal protein, 100 mM phosphate buffer (pH 7.2), 3 mM $MgCl_2$, 3 mM NADP, 10 mM glucose-6-phosphate, 5 units of glucose-6-phosphate dehydrogenase, 20 mM mercaptoethanol, and 0.4 mM (0.5 μCi) of [3-^{14}C]HMG-CoA. Details of incubation conditions, analysis of mevalonate formation, and calculation of HMG-CoA reductase activity have been described recently[2,3].

RESULTS

The HMG-CoA reductase activity displayed a rather wide interindividual variation both in gallstone-free controls and in patients with cholesterol gallstones (Figure 1). In the series of patients investigated, we did not find any relationships between enzyme activity and factors such as age, sex, or absolute or relative body weight[2,3]. There was no difference in HMG-CoA reductase activity between patients with cholesterol gallstone disease and gallstone-free controls.

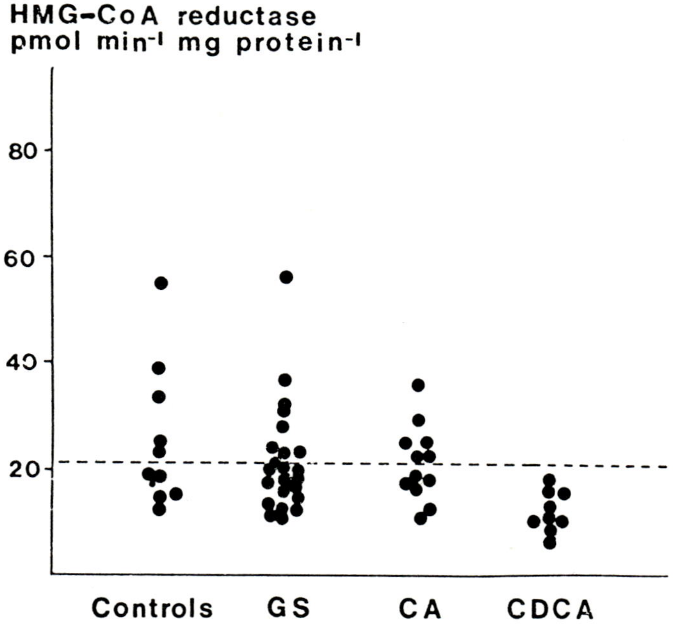

Figure 1. Hepatic microsomal HMG-CoA reductase activity in gallstone-free subjects (controls) and patients with cholesterol gallstones, untreated (GS), pretreated with cholic acid (CA), and chenodeoxycholic acid (CDCA). Data from ref. 3

Pretreatment with CA did not influence hepatic microsomal HMG-CoA reductase activity. Administration of CDCA, on the other hand, was associated with a 40% reduction of enzyme activity (Figure 1).

DISCUSSION

In the present work, microsomal HMG-CoA reductase was assayed in surgical liver biopsies obtained in the fasting state. The activity of this enzyme is known from animal studies to be influenced by several regulatory factors such as stress, caloric intake, hormonal activation, and diurnal variation. Great care was therefore taken to standardize preoperative conditions, timing of operation, and operative as well as anaesthetic procedures.

Studies in rat liver have furthermore shown that the activity of HMG-CoA reductase may be regulated by changes in the total amount of enzyme protein and by activation–inactivation due to the state of phosphorylation[4–6]. Recent data from our laboratory[7] have shown that the HMG-CoA reductase activity of human microsomes prepared in the presence of fluoride (which prevents dephosphorylation of the enzyme) was several-fold lower than in microsomes prepared in the absence of fluoride. Preincubation of microsomes with alkaline phosphatase, on the other hand, resulted in activation of enzyme activity. However, although there is at present some uncertainty as to which type of assay actually reflects true 'physiological' activity, measurements of maximally and minimally activated enzyme activity appear to parallel those obtained by the standard procedure used in the present work[6].

The 4–5-fold range of fasting HMG-CoA reductase activity seen in healthy controls is of similar magnitude to that seen for *in vivo* determinations of net steroid balance[8], reflecting whole-body cholesterol synthesis. Under the present conditions we did not observe any influence of sex or body weight on enzyme activity. However, grossly obese patients appear to have increased HMG-CoA reductase activity[9].

The gallbladder bile of patients with cholesterol gallstones is generally supersaturated with cholesterol. According to current views the liver is the source of this abnormal bile[10]. The results of the present work give no support to the concept that the formation of supersaturated bile in normal-weight, normolipidaemic patients with cholesterol gallstones is the result of an increased hepatic synthesis of cholesterol. Instead, the metabolic 'defect' in these patients appears to be a reduced bile acid pool size and a deficient secretion of bile acids into bile[11,12].

Treatment with CDCA but not with CA is associated with unsaturation of gallbladder bile. This difference is due to a reduced secretion of cholesterol during treatment with CDCA[13–15]. The exact mechanism(s) by which CDCA lowers cholesterol secretion have not been clarified. The present data support the concept that CDCA may reduce the hepatic secretion of cholesterol at least partly by suppressing hepatic cholesterogenesis.

Administration of ursodeoxycholic acid (UDCA) also makes gallbladder bile unsaturated with cholesterol by reducing hepatic secretion of cholesterol[16]. The mechanisms behind these effects of UDCA are not known. Given to patients with cholesterol gallstones under similar conditions as those described for CA and CDCA, UDCA did not significantly influence hepatic HMG-CoA reductase activity[17]. This would suggest that UDCA may suppress hepatic cholesterol secretion in other ways than by affecting hepatic cholesterol synthesis.

Thus treatment with CDCA but not with CA or UDCA seems to inhibit hepatic HMG-CoA reductase activity in man. Whether this effect is specific to the CDCA molecule or not cannot be decided from the present work. Preliminary results suggest that the fasting portal venous concentration of bile acids is higher during treatment with CDCA than during CA administration[18]. This higher inflow of bile acids to the liver may be of importance for the more efficient suppression of HMG-CoA reductase activity. Further work is needed to clarify whether the effect of CDCA treatment is exerted by influencing the amount of enzyme, the state of phosphorylation, or both.

Acknowledgments

The skilful technical assistance of Mrs Eija Varhenmaa, Mrs Margret Wahlström, Miss Gerd Ledin and Mrs Gunvor Alvelius is gratefully acknowledged. The work summarized here has been supported by grants from the Swedish Medical Research Council (19x–04793), from the Swedish National Association against Heart and Chest Diseases, and from the Tore Nilson Foundation. Dr Angelin is the recipient of a Fellowship from the Ernst Klenk Foundation.

References

1. Nicolau, G., Shefer, S., Salen, G. and Mosbach, E. H. (1974). Determination of hepatic 3-hydroxy-3-methylglutaryl CoA reductase activity in man. *J. Lipid Res.*, **15,** 94
2. Ahlberg, J., Angelin, B., Björkhem, I., Einarsson, K. and Leijd, B. (1979). Hepatic cholesterol metabolism in normo- and hyperlipidemic patients with cholesterol gallstones. *J. Lipid Res.*, **20,** 107
3. Ahlberg, J., Angelin, B. and Einarsson, K. (1981). Hepatic 3-hydroxy-3-methylglutaryl coenzyme A reductase activity and biliary lipid composition in man: relation to cholesterol gallstone disease and effects of cholic acid and chenodeoxycholic acid treatment. *J. Lipid Res.*, **21** (In press)
4. Nordstrom, J. L., Rodwell, V. W. and Mitschelen, J. J. (1977). Interconversion of active and inactive forms of rat liver hydroxymethylglutaryl-CoA reductase. *J. Biol. Chem.*, **252,** 8924
5. Beg, Z. H., Stonik, J. A. and Brewer, H. B. Jr (1978). 3-Hydroxy-3-methylglutaryl coenzyme A reductase: regulation of enzymatic activity by phosphorylation and dephosphorylation. *Proc. Natl. Acad. Sci. USA*, **75,** 3678
6. Brown, M. S., Goldstein, J. L. and Dietschy, J. M. (1979). Active and inactive form of 3-hydroxy-3-methylglutaryl coenzyme A reductase in the liver of the rat. *J. Biol. Chem.*, **254,** 5144
7. Angelin, B., Einarsson, K. and Ewerth, S. (1981). Active and inactive form of 3-hydroxy-3-methylglutaryl coenzyme A in human liver microsomes. (In preparation)
8. Angelin, B., Einarsson, K., Hellström, K. and Kallner, M. (1976). Elimination of cholesterol in hyperlipoproteinaemia. *Clin. Sci. Mol. Med.*, **51,** 393
9. Angelin, B., Backman, L., Einarsson, K. and Ewerth, S. (1981). Hepatic cholesterol metabolism in obesity. (In preparation)
10. Small, D. M. (1976). The etiology and pathogenesis of gallstones. *Adv. Surg.*, **10,** 63
11. Vlahcevic, Z. R., Bell, C. C. Jr, Buhac, I., Farrar, J. T. and Swell, L. (1970). Diminished bile acid pool size in patients with gallstones. *Gastroenterology*, **59,** 165
12. Shaffer, E. A. and Small, D. M. (1977). Biliary lipid secretion in cholesterol gallstone disease. The effect of cholecystectomy and obesity. *J. Clin. Invest.*, **59,** 828
13. Adler, R. D., Bennion, L. J., Duane, W. C. and Grundy, S. M. (1975). Effects of low dose chenodeoxycholic acid feeding on biliary lipid metabolism. *Gastroenterology*, **68,** 326
14. LaRusso, N. F., Hoffman, N. E., Hofmann, A. F., Northfield, T. C. and Thistle, J. L. (1975). Effect of primary bile acid ingestion on bile acid metabolism and biliary lipid secretion in gallstone patients. *Gastroenterology*, **68,** 1301
15. Einarsson, K. and Grundy, S. M. (1980). Effects of feeding cholic acid and chenodeoxy-

cholic acid on cholesterol absorption and hepatic secretion of biliary lipids in man. *J. Lipid Res.*, **21**, 23

16. Von Bergmann, K., Gutsfeld, M., Schulze-Hagen, K. and von Unruh, G. (1979). Effects of ursodeoxycholic acid on biliary lipid secretion in patients with radiolucent gallstones. In Paumgartner, G., Stiehl, A. and Gerok, W. (eds.). *Biological Effects of Bile Acids*, pp. 61–66. (Lancaster: MTP Press)
17. Angelin, B., Einarsson, K. and Ewerth, S. (1981). Effects of ursodeoxycholic acid on hepatic cholesterol metabolism and on biliary lipid composition in man. (In preparation)
18. Angelin, B., Ahlberg, J., Björkhem, I., Einarsson, K. and Ewerth, S. (1979). Serum levels of individual bile acids in portal venous and systemic circulation during treatment with chenodeoxycholic acid and cholic acid. In Paumgartner, G., Stiehl, A. and Gerok, W. (eds.). *Biological Effects of Bile Acids*, pp. 107–108. (Lancaster: MTP Press)

10

Effect of a bile alcohol and a bile acid analogue on sterol metabolism in the rat

E. H. MOSBACH, A. K. SINGHAL, N. K. N. AYENGAR, P. S. MAY AND C. K. McSHERRY

INTRODUCTION

The discovery of gallstone dissolution by bile acids raises the question whether specific molecular features are required to impart cholelitholytic properties to a drug or enhance such properties. Therefore, studies were initiated to find or develop substances which, like chenodeoxycholic acid (CDCA) and ursodeoxycholic acid (UDCA), produce changes in biliary lipid levels and cholesterol/bile acid metabolism. The present paper describes preliminary studies of the effect of two compounds, a bile alcohol and a synthetic bile acid analogue, on sterol metabolism in the rat.

METHODS

Sterol balance studies were carried out with male rats of the Wistar or Fischer strains weighing 250–350 g. The animals were kept in individual metabolism cages and received a semi-synthetic low cholesterol diet (Bio-Serv, Frenchtown, N.J., catalog no. 1441) to which 5% corn oil was added. The details of the balance method as applied to rats, the procedures for determining serum and tissue sterols, biliary and faecal steroids, hepatic HMG-CoA reductase and cholesterol 7α-hydroxylase activities have all been described previously[1–3]. Since the young rats used for the balance experiments gained weight during the period of the study they were, strictly speaking, not in a steady state (as required by the balance method). Consequently, the experimental drug-treated animals were always compared to a control group maintained simultaneously under identical conditions.

RESULTS AND DISCUSSION

Studies with 5β-cholestane-3α, 7α, 12α, 25-tetrol ('tetrol')

This tetrahydroxy C_{27}-steroid is the major biliary and faecal bile alcohol in patients with the rare inherited sterol storage disease cerebrotendinous xanthomatosis (CTX). Such patients exhibit striking peculiarities of sterol metabolism, for example, low serum cholesterol concentrations, elevated activities of the hepatic microsomal rate-limiting enzymes HMG-CoA reductase and cholesterol 7α-hydroxylase, preponderance of cholic acid (CA) in bile at the expense of the dihydroxycholanoic acids and low concentrations of secondary bile acids in bile and faeces[4]. It was postulated that some of the abnormalities of sterol metabolism in CTX were secondary to the presence of the tetrol and other bile alcohols in the enterohepatic circulation or in tissues. In a preliminary experiment, 20 mg of [7β-^{3}H]tetrol (specific radioactivity 6×10^4 dpm/mg), suspended in 1 ml of 20% ethanol by sonication, were administered to each of four rats by stomach tube. The animals were kept in restraining cages for 24 h to collect bile, urine and faeces. During the experimental period less than 0.5% of the administered label was excreted in bile or urine. On the average. about 4% of the radioactivity was detected in the liver, while 75% or more was recovered in the faeces. None of the faecal metabolites was identical with the starting material (tetrol). It was concluded that the tetrol was rather poorly absorbed, degraded extensively by the intestinal bacterial flora and would not be expected to exert significant effects on tissue sterol metabolism.

Table 1 Effect of 0.1% dietary tetrol[a] on serum and bile cholesterol and hepatic rate-limiting enzymes

				Hepatic enzyme activities	
Treatment	*Number of animals*	*Serum cholesterol* (mg/dl)	*Biliary cholesterol* (mg/ml)	*HMG-CoA reductase* (pmole min^{-1} mg^{-1})	*Cholesterol 7α-hydroxylase* (pmole min^{-1} mg^{-1})
Control	4	71.7 ±2.5	0.09±0.016	46.2±9.28	13.8±2.95
Tetrol	5	93.5[b]±8.6	0.12±0.031	45.9±4.08	16.0±4.70

[a] 5β-Cholestane-3α,7α,12α,25-tetrol was added to the semi-synthetic low cholesterol diet (Bio-Serv No.1441) and fed to male Fischer-344 rats for 2 weeks

[b] Differs from controls ($P < 0.01$)

In a balance study a group of five rats fed 0.1% tetrol for 2 weeks was compared with a control group of 5 animals (Table 1). Weight gain, food intake and faecal output of the groups were identical, and there was no evidence of hepatotoxicity. In the tetrol-treated group, serum cholesterol levels were 30% higher than in the controls; biliary cholesterol, hepatic HMG-CoA reductase and cholesterol 7α-hydroxylase activities were unchanged. As expected on the basis of the enzyme activities, faecal sterol and bile acid output were not affected by the administered bile alcohol (Table 2).

The tetrol or its bacterial metabolites had no effect on the composition of the faecal sterol fraction: The coprostanol/cholesterol ratio was similar in the two groups. In contrast, the faecal bile acid pattern was altered profoundly: in the control group, hyodeoxycholic acid was the major bile acid accounting for 53% of the total while ω-muricholic acid predominated in the tetrol-treated animals (31.6% of total bile acids). As a consequence the ratio of ω-muricholic acid to hyodeoxycholic acid changed from 0.02 to 2.20. Presumably the 7β-dehydroxylation of ω-muricholic acid was inhibited by the bile alcohol.

Table 2 Faecal steroids of rats fed 0.1% tetrol[a] for 2 weeks

Treatment	*Faecal steroid output* Neutral (mg/day)	Acidic (mg/day)	*Faecal steroid ratios*[b] Coprostanol / Cholesterol	ω-Muricholic acid / Hyodeoxycholic acid
Control ($n = 4$)	7.34 ± 0.96	8.84 ± 2.09	0.92	0.03
Tetrol ($n = 5$)	7.29 ± 0.31	7.01 ± 1.77	1.09	2.20[c]

[a] 5β-Cholestane-3α,7α,12α,25-tetrol
[b] Faecal sterols and bile acids were analysed by gas–liquid chromatography as described in references 1 and 3
[c] Differs from controls ($p < 0.01$)

It was concluded that the administered bile alcohol did not produce striking changes of sterol metabolism in the rat, but caused a decrease in the concentration of certain bacterial strains which normally convert ω-muricholic acid to hyodeoxycholic acid.

Studies with bile acid analogues

A few years ago A. F. Hofmann suggested that it might be advantageous to prepare new cholelitholytic drugs resistant to degradation by intestinal bacteria. Such agents, in order to be more useful than CDCA or UDCA, should give rise to less lithocholic acid than the naturally occurring bile acids. Ideally, they should not be convertible to lithocholic acid at all. If the bacterial degradation of these hypothetical drugs were abolished, they might participate in enterohepatic cycling for longer periods, thus making it possible theoretically to achieve gallstone dissolution with smaller dosages of the

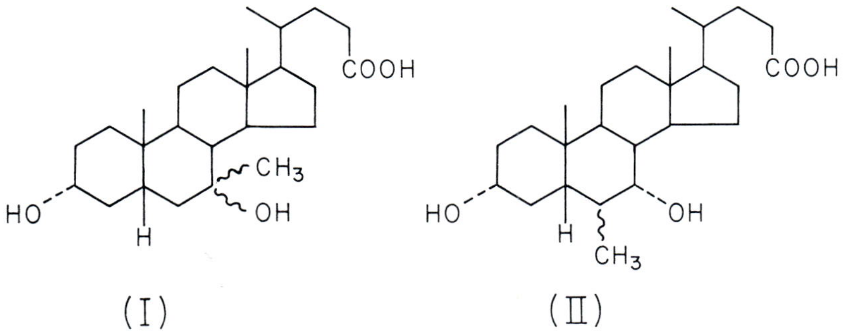

Figure 1 I = 3α,7ξ-dihydroxy-7ξ-methyl-5β-cholan-24-oic acid; II = 3α,7α-dihydroxy-6ξ-methyl-5β-cholan-24-oic acid

drugs. Prototypes of such compounds are 7-methyl- or 6-methyl-substituted 3,7-dihydroxy bile acids (Figure 1, I and II). We decided to attempt the synthesis of these compounds and, wherever feasible, to test each intermediate obtained during the synthesis for toxicity and effect on cholesterol/bile acid metabolism.

The first synthetic intermediate was the amide of 7-ketolithocholic acid with 2-amino-2-methyl-1-propanol (Figure 2). When fed to male Wistar rats at a level of 0.1% of the diet for 4 weeks the compound was well tolerated and caused no liver damage. Body weight, serum and biliary cholesterol concentrations, and bile acid pool size were unchanged from those of the control group, and the amide was therefore not studied further in this species.

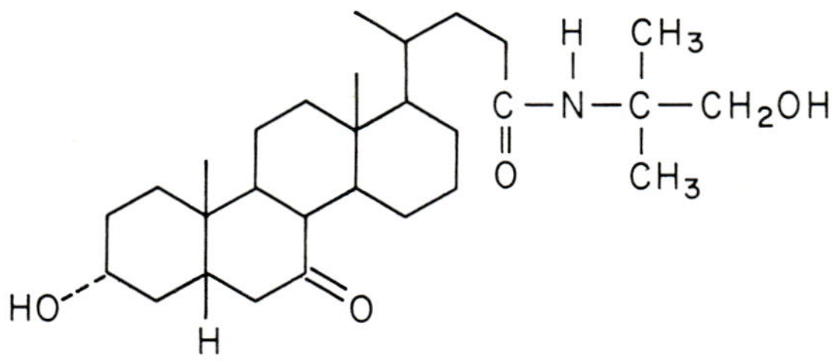

Figure 2 2-(3α-hydroxy-7-keto-5β-cholan-24-amido)-2-methyl-1-propanol ('amide')

When the amide was cyclized and treated with methyl magnesium iodide in a Grignard reaction we obtained a 4,4-dimethyl-2-oxazoline derivative of 3α-7ξ-dihydroxy-7ξ-methyl-24-nor-5β-cholane (Figure 3), referred to henceforth as 'oxazoline'.

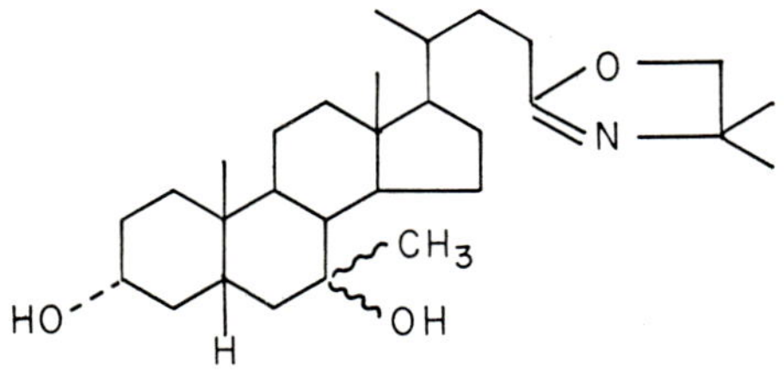

Figure 3 2-(3α-7ξ-dihydroxy-7ξ-methyl-24-nor-5β-cholanyl)-4,4-dimethyl-2-oxazoline ('oxazoline')

Because of the relatively poor yield this compound was fed to only two Fischer-344 rats at a level of 0.1% of the diet for 2 weeks and compared to a control group of three animals.

There was no hepatotoxicity, and the oxazoline was apparently absorbed for its administration did produce significant changes in cholesterol metabolism. In the experimental group, serum cholesterol but not biliary cholesterol concentrations were elevated and hepatic microsomal HMG-CoA reductase and cholesterol 7α-hydroxylase increased by 50 and 70%, respectively (Table 3). Surprisingly, these increases in the activities of the

Table 3 Effect of 0.1% dietary oxazoline[a] on serum and bile cholesterol and rate-limiting hepatic enzymes

Treatment	*Number of animals*	*Serum cholesterol* (mg/dl)	*Biliary cholesterol* (mg/ml)	*Hepatic enzyme activities* *HMG-CoA reductase* (pmole mg^{-1} min^{-1})	*Hepatic enzyme activities* *Cholesterol 7α-hydroxylase* (pmole mg^{-1} min^{-1})
Control	3	73	0.18	110	16
Oxazoline[a]	2	98	0.16	170	27

[a] 2-(3α,7ξ-dihydroxy-7ξ-methyl-24-nor-5β-cholanyl)-4,4-dimethyl-2-oxazoline was added to the stock diet (Bio-Serv No. 1441) and fed to male Fischer-344 rats for 2 weeks

rate-limiting enzymes were not associated with corresponding changes in sterol or bile acid output (Table 4).

Since the administered oxazoline was not isotopically labelled, detailed studies of its metabolic fate were not attempted. The following preliminary results seem pertinent, however:

(1) administration of oxazoline produced a 50% decrease of bile acid pool size;
(2) the oxazoline was metabolized to bile acid-like compounds which accounted for about 50% of this reduced bile acid pool;
(3) a major biliary metabolite was a monounsaturated 7-methylcholenoic acid, but at present it cannot be stated whether this compound was produced in the tissues, by intestinal bacteria, or by dehydration during the chemical work-up of the bile.

Table 4 Faecal steroids of rats fed 0.1% oxazoline[a] for 2 weeks

Treatment	*Number of animals*	*Faecal steroid output* *Neutral* (mg/day)	*Faecal steroid output* *Acidic* (mg/day)	*Faecal steroid ratios* *Coprostanol* / *Cholesterol*	*Faecal steroid ratios* *ω-Muricholic acid* / *Hyodeoxycholic acid*
Control	3	7.3	8.8	0.92	0.02
Oxazoline[a]	2	7.5	8.8	0.75	63.0

[a] 2-(3α,7ξ-dihydroxy-7ξ-methyl-24-nor-5β-cholanyl)-4,4-dimethyl-2-oxazoline was added to the stock diet (Bio-Serv No. 1441) and fed to male Fischer-344 rats for 2 weeks

The oxazoline had no effect on the composition of the faecal sterol fraction but profoundly altered the faecal bile acid pattern. At the end of the 2-week feeding period, hyodeoxycholic acid, the predominant faecal bile acid in the controls (53% of total bile acids), had been replaced almost completely by ω-muricholic acid (62% of total bile acids) thus producing a large change in the ω-muricholic acid to hyodeoxycholic acid ratio (Table 4).

Since this bile acid analogue was not hepatotoxic, and its administration produced an increase of the rate-limiting enzyme activities and a profound change in the faecal bile acid pattern, further studies of bile acid oxazolines may be useful.

Acknowledgment

This research was supported by US Public Health Service Grant HL 10894.

References

1. Cohen, B. I., Raicht, R. F. and Mosbach, E. H. (1974). Effect of dietary bile acids, cholesterol and β-sitosterol upon formation of coprostanol and 7-dehydroxylation of bile acids by rats. *Lipids*, **9**, 1024
2. Cohen, B. I., Raicht, R. F., Salen, G. and Mosbach, E. H. (1975). An improved method for the isolation, quantitation, and identification of bile acids in rat faeces. *Anal. Biochem.*, **64**, 567
3. Raicht, R. F., Cohen, B. I., Shefer, S. and Mosbach, E. H. (1975). Sterol balance studies in the rat. Effects of dietary cholesterol and β-sitosterol on sterol balance and rate-limiting enzymes of sterol metabolism. *Biochim. Biophys. Acta*, **388**, 374
4. Salen, G. and Mosbach, E. H. (1976). The metabolism of sterols and bile acids in cerebrotendinous xanthomatosis. In Nair, P. P. and Kritchevsky, D. (eds.). *The Bile Acids*, vol. 3, pp. 115–153. (New York: Plenum Press)

11
Pathways of cholesterol removal via bile acid synthesis and biliary cholesterol excretion in man

C. C. SCHWARTZ, Z. R. VLAHCEVIC AND L. SWELL

INTRODUCTION

The major pathway for excretion of cholesterol from the body takes place in the liver via formation of bile acids and via biliary cholesterol excretion. About 1 g of cholesterol is lost daily from the body, of which approximately 0.5 g is degraded to bile acids while biliary cholesterol secretion accounts for the remainder. Recent studies from our laboratories[1] have demonstrated that hepatic cholesterol destined for excretion in bile is compartmentalized, one compartment for bile acid synthesis and one for biliary cholesterol secretion. The specific activity time curves of bile acids and biliary cholesterol following injection of labelled mevalonate and cholesterol could only be simulated mathematically if plasma free cholesterol furnished 60–70% of cholesterol in these precursor compartments while newly synthesized cholesterol contributed 20–30% and plasma esterified cholesterol 5–10% (Figure 1).

In order to test the conclusions derived from these initial studies a series of experiments were designed to determine which lipoprotein fraction is a major contributor of free cholesterol to bile acid synthesis and biliary cholesterol excretion. High-density lipoprotein (HDL), and low-density lipoprotein (LDL) fractions, in which only free cholesterol was labelled, were administered to subjects with a bile fistula or intact enterohepatic circulation; the specific activities of bile acids and biliary cholesterol were determined at early and frequent intervals. The interpretation of data obtained in these experiments was based on the assumption that following the injection of autologous HDL and LDL labelled with ^{3}H and ^{14}C free cholesterol (or vice versa) human liver will preferentially and/or selectively utilize free cholesterol for bile acid synthesis and biliary cholesterol secretion from one of the administered lipoprotein fractions. The preferential (or selective) utilization of free cholesterol by the liver would result in differences in the specific activities of bile acid or biliary cholesterol prior to the equilibration of the labelled cholesterol between the various lipoprotein fractions. The data of these studies[2,3] demonstrated that free cholesterol from HDL was more rapidly incorporated into bile acids and biliary cholesterol than the

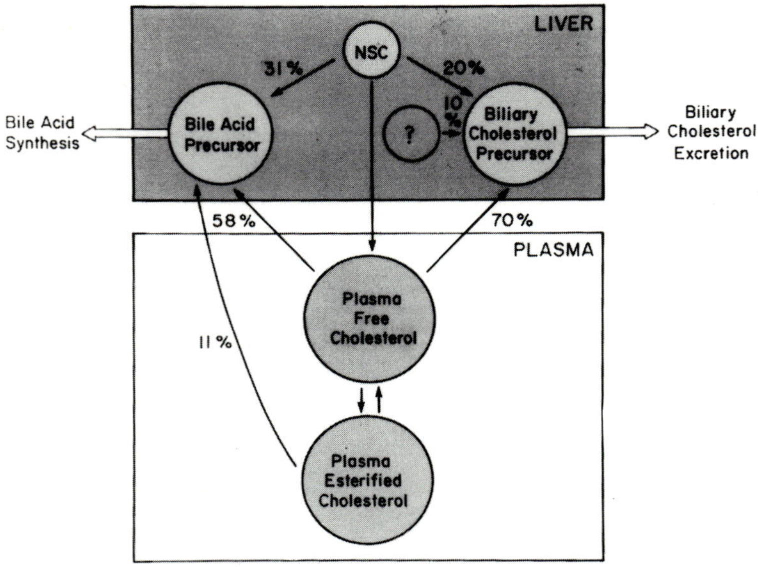

Figure 1 Schematic presentation of the percentage contribution of plasma free cholesterol, plasma esterified cholesterol and newly synthesized cholesterol (NSC) to the hepatic precursor compartments for bile acid synthesis and biliary cholesterol excretion[1]

free cholesterol from LDL. This observation suggested that HDL-free cholesterol may be a major substrate in man for bile acid synthesis and biliary cholesterol secretion (Figure 2). Simulation analysis and modelling of the ^3H and ^{14}C data have been carried out using the SAAM-27 computer program (unpublished). The best fits were obtained when the flux from the LDL free cholesterol to hepatic cholesterol precursor pools for bile acid synthesis and biliary cholesterol secretion was zero; HDL was the only source of plasma free cholesterol needed to fit the obtained specific activity curves (cholic acid (CA), chenodeoxycholic acid (CDCA), and biliary cholesterol). The precise mechanism by which HDL free cholesterol is preferentially selected by the liver for catabolism to bile acids or secretion as biliary cholesterol is not known but the most plausible hypothesis is that HDL, or a fraction thereof, shuttles free cholesterol to the liver where it may be removed from the surface of the HDL particle. Cholesterol can be exchanged by one-for-one molecular exchange (no net movement) or by transfer which implies net movement. Differentiation between the two types of movement in experiments in which radioactive cholesterol is used is sometimes difficult. The precursor compartments for bile acid synthesis and biliary cholesterol excretion have large fluxes to the outside (>1 g/day) and a compensatory net input is required to maintain steady state. The movement of cholesterol by exchange would be associated with a zero net flux. However, the design of the above studies[1–3] has not allowed us to resolve these possibilities.

The present report represents an extension of our efforts to ascertain the origin of cholesterol for bile acid synthesis and biliary cholesterol excretion. The specific aims of this study were:

(a) to determine whether lipoprotein cholesterol esters make a significant contribution to the pools of hepatocellular cholesterol destined for bile acid synthesis and biliary cholesterol excretion; and
(b) to provide some new information on the biochemical pathways of degradation of hepatic cholesterol into bile acids.

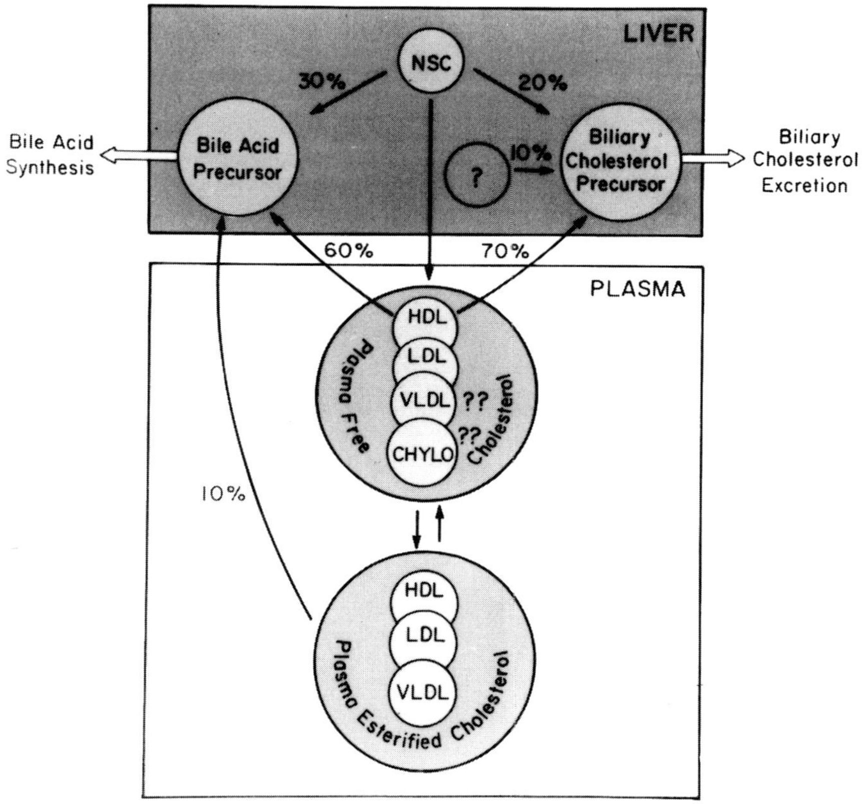

Figure 2 Contribution of free cholesterol from various lipoprotein fractions to bile acid synthesis and biliary cholesterol excretion. Recent studies[2,3] indicate that HDL free cholesterol is preferentially utilized

EXPERIMENTAL DESIGN AND DISCUSSION

Cholesterol sources for bile acid synthesis and biliary cholesterol excretion

Plasma was obtained from two patients (one with a bile fistula and one with an intact enterohepatic circulation) and incubated for 4 h with 75 μCi of

[1,2-^{3}H]cholesterol at 37 °C. At that temperature both free and esterified cholesterol were labelled with tritium. Following this procedure the same plasma was reincubated twice with 10 μCi [4-^{14}C]cholesterol at 4 °C at which temperature LCAT is inhibited. In one patient (patient A.V.) the plasma was then subjected to rapid lipoprotein separation using the heparin–manganese method[4] into α- and β-lipoprotein fractions. The α-lipoprotein fraction was dialyzed against 5% $BaCl_2$ (pH 7.7) overnight and the Ba–heparin complex was then removed by centrifugation. Addition of 7.5% $NaHCO_3$ resulted in formation of $BaCO_3$ and $MnCO_3$ which was also removed by centrifugation. After an overnight dialysis with saline the density of α-lipoprotein solution was adjusted to 1.21 g/ml with solid KBr and the solution was ultra-centrifuged. The 1.21 g/ml supernatant was dialyzed against saline with 0.01% EDTA (pH 7.4). In the second patient (patient S.W.) the same labelling procedure was followed with the exception that lipoproteins were separated by ultracentrifugation only. The autologous labelled lipoprotein fractions (HDL and LDL) were then administered to the patients via a 0.2 μm Millipore filter. Bile samples were obtained by the Grundy method in the first patient[5] and via a bile fistula in the second patient. Bile acids, biliary cholesterol, plasma lipoprotein free and esterified cholesterol were analyzed for mass and radioactivity[1–3]. Incubation of the plasma with [^{3}H]cholesterol at 37 °C resulted in the labelling of free and esterified cholesterol. The cholesterol esters in HDL were labelled by the action of LCAT. Subsequent incubation of plasma at 4 °C with [^{14}C]cholesterol achieved labelling of only the free cholesterol fraction since LCAT activity is inhibited at 4 °C. The final lipoprotein products administered to the patients contained free [^{3}H]cholesterol, esterified [^{3}H]cholesterol and free [^{14}C]cholesterol. The *in vivo* appearance of esterified [^{14}C]cholesterol affords a means of differentiating between the esterified [^{3}H]cholesterol derived *in vivo* from injected free [^{3}H]cholesterol and the administered esterified [^{3}H]cholesterol.

The administered lipoproteins were checked for homogeneity of mass and label by agarose gel electrophoresis[6] and immunoelectrophoresis. When recentrifuged the label floated in the appropriate lipoprotein density range. The ^{3}H activity was found in the free and esterified cholesterol while ^{14}C was only present in free cholesterol (by silicic acid column chromatography, thin-layer chromatography and by digitonide precipitation).

Figure 3 shows the data in A.V. with an intact enterohepatic circulation. The ^{3}H/^{14}C ratio is plotted against time in minutes. The *administered* total cholesterol ^{3}H/^{14}C ratio represents free [^{3}H]cholesterol plus esterified [^{3}H]cholesterol over free [^{14}C]cholesterol as administered to the patient. The *administered* free cholesterol ^{3}H/^{14}C ratio is the ratio of free [^{3}H]cholesterol over free [^{14}C]cholesterol. The ^{3}H/^{14}C ratios in α-lipoprotein-free cholesterol in α- and β-lipoprotein fractions of cholesterol esters and in CA and biliary cholesterol were used to interpret the data. CDCA ^{3}H/^{14}C ratio was identical to that of CA. The interpretation of the data was based on the assumption that *if* bile acids and biliary cholesterol derived most of their cholesterol from lipoprotein esterified cholesterol (after hydrolysis) they should have ^{3}H/^{14}C ratios similar to that in lipoprotein esterified cholesterol. Conversely, if bile acid and biliary cholesterol derived most of their cholesterol from plasma

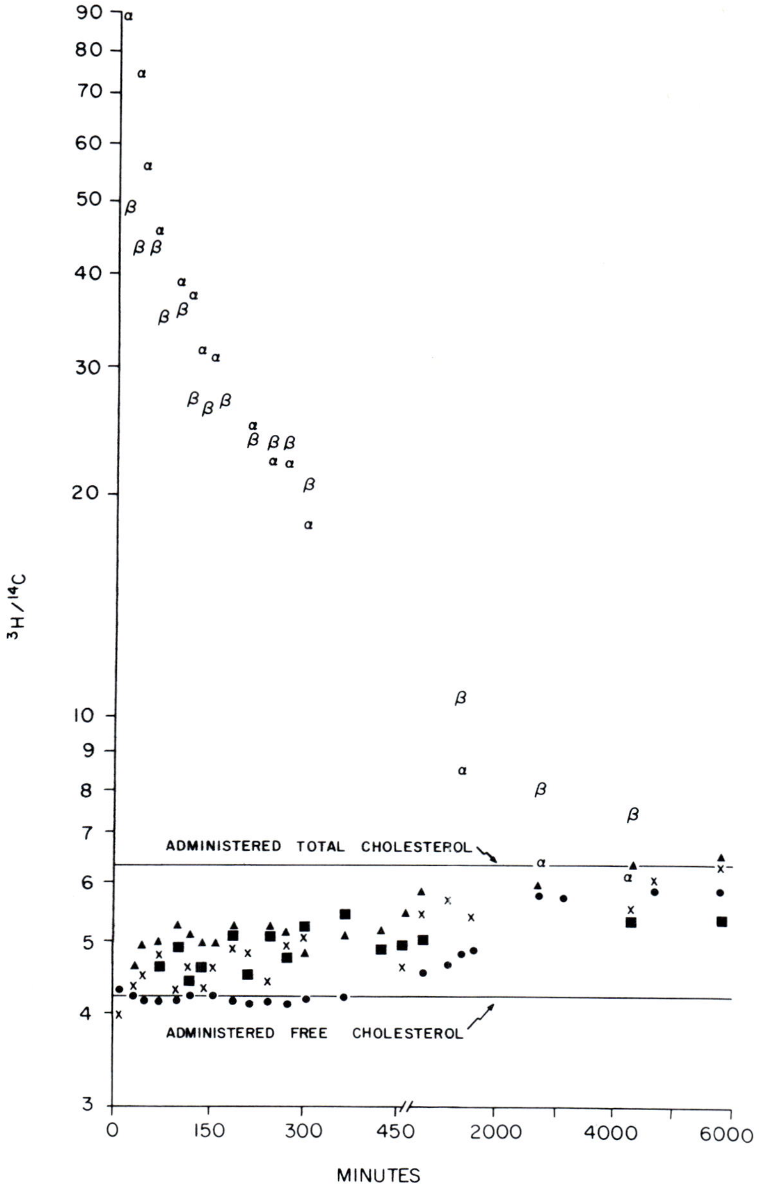

Figure 3 $^3H/^{14}C$ activity ratio *vs*. time in patient A.V. with intact enterohepatic circulation who received autologous labelled HDL (esterified [^3H]cholesterol and free [^3H] and [^{14}C]cholesterol). The administered total $^3H/^{14}C$ ratio and administered free $^3H/^{14}C$ ratio are denoted as horizontal lines. α(HDL) esterified cholesterol (α); β-lipoprotein esterified cholesterol (β); α(HDL) free cholesterol (×); biliary cholesterol (Δ); cholic acid (■): red blood cell cholesterol(●). (Reprinted from ref. 7 with publisher's permission)

free cholesterol (as postulated by our previous studies), the $^{3}H/^{14}C$ ratios of all three should be similar. Lastly, if plasma free cholesterol and esterified cholesterol both contributed cholesterol substrate to bile acid synthesis and biliary cholesterol excretion, the $^{3}H/^{14}C$ ratios in bile acids and biliary cholesterol should be intermediate.

The data in patient A.V. (Figure 3) clearly demonstrate that the $^{3}H/^{14}C$ ratios of CA, biliary cholesterol and α-lipoprotein free cholesterol were virtually identical to each other and only slightly higher than the administered free cholesterol $^{3}H/^{14}C$ ratio. This similarity strongly suggests that the bile acids (CA and CDCA) and biliary cholesterol originate from plasma free cholesterol. The gradual rise of the $^{3}H/^{14}C$ ratio (after 450 min) in α-lipoprotein free cholesterol in tandem with the rise of $^{3}H/^{14}C$ ratios in CA and biliary cholesterol suggest an input of free [^{3}H]cholesterol from hydrolysis of administered labelled cholesterol esters into the plasma free cholesterol pool (lipoprotein free cholesterol) which in turn serves as a substrate for bile acid synthesis and biliary cholesterol excretion.

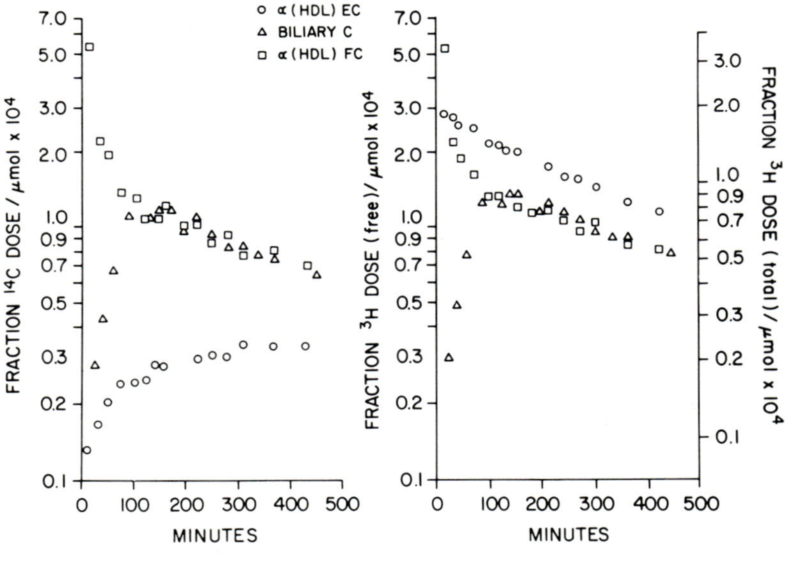

Figure 4 ^{3}H and ^{14}C specific activity time curves of α(HDL) esterified cholesterol (○); biliary cholesterol (△) and α(HDL) free cholesterol (□) expressed as fraction of ^{14}C and ^{3}H dose/μmol. (Reprinted from ref. 7 with publisher's permission)

By contrast, the $^{3}H/^{14}C$ ratios in α- and β-lipoprotein cholesterol ester fractions were initially very high and rapidly declined over the period of study and were clearly different from the $^{3}H/^{14}C$ ratios in bile acids and biliary cholesterol. It should be noted that during the early periods when the $^{3}H/^{14}C$ ratio in α-lipoprotein cholesterol esters was very high and rapidly declining no such trend was present in biliary sterols. The similarity of $^{3}H/^{14}C$ ratio

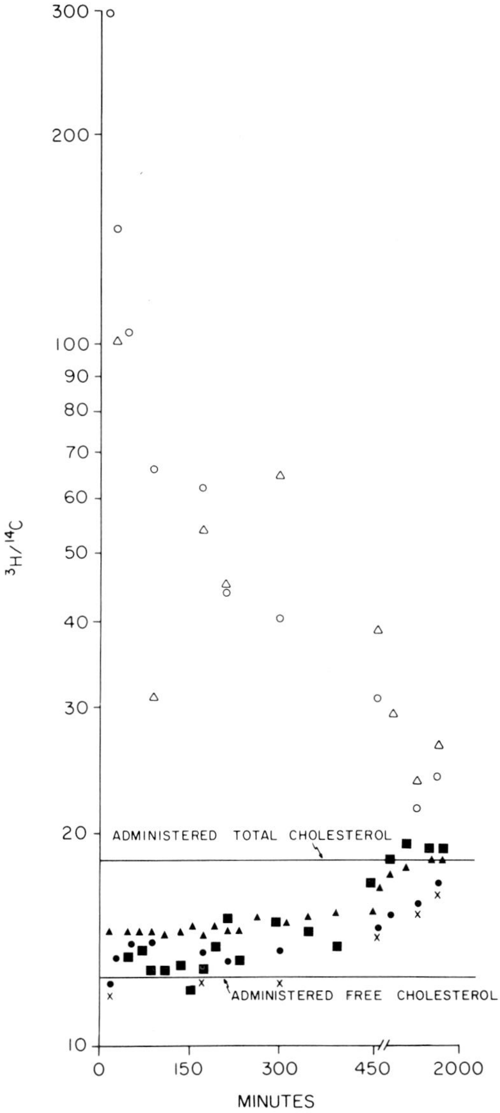

Figure 5 $^3H/^{14}C$ activity ratio *vs.* time in patient S.W. with bile fistula who received autologous labelled HDL ester [^{3}H], free [^{14}C] and free [^{3}H]cholesterol. HDL esterified cholesterol (○); LDL esterified cholesterol (△); lipoprotein free cholesterol (×); biliary cholesterol (▲); cholic acid (■); red blood cell cholesterol (●). (Reprinted from ref. 7 with publisher's permission)

of α- and β-lipoprotein cholesterol ester fractions suggest that β-lipoprotein cholesterol esters are probably derived in part from α-lipoprotein (HDL) esterified cholesterol possibly via cholesterol exchange protein.

Figure 4 shows the interrelationship between the ^{14}C and ^{3}H specific activities of α-lipoprotein free cholesterol, biliary cholesterol and α(HDL) esterified cholesterol. When the data are expressed as percentages of dose of administered free cholesterol the ^{3}H and ^{14}C specific activities of α-lipoprotein (HDL) free cholesterol and biliary cholesterol were virtually superimposable. Moreover, there is a classic precursor–product relationship between α-lipoprotein free cholesterol and biliary cholesterol, suggesting strongly that plasma free cholesterol is the major precursor for biliary cholesterol. The finding of a classical precursor–product relationship is present in A.V. because the contribution of the newly synthesized cholesterol in subjects with an intact enterohepatic circulation is very low (unpublished observations). The specific activity time curves for α-lipoprotein cholesterol esters (^{3}H and ^{14}C) were divergent and had no relationship to the biliary cholesterol specific activity time curves.

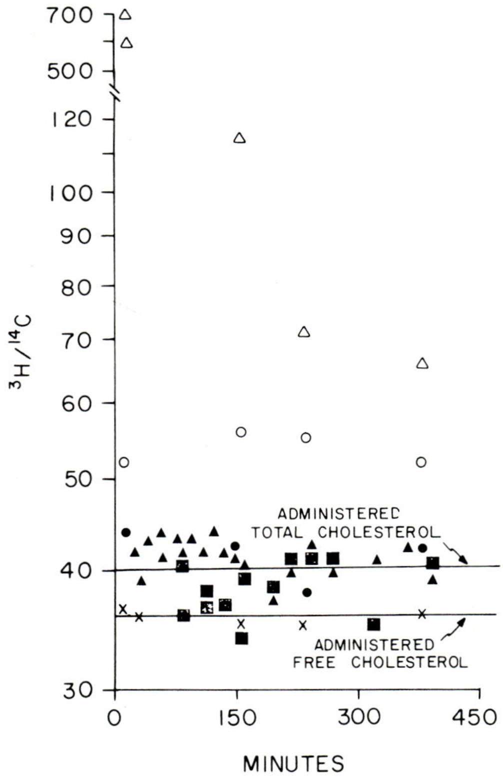

Figure 6 $^{3}H/^{14}C$ activity ratio in a patient with bile fistula who received autologous labelled LDL ester [^{3}H], free [^{14}C] and free [^{3}H]cholesterol. The symbols are identical with those in Figure 5. (Reprinted from ref. 7 with publisher's permission)

Figure 5 demonstrates the $^3H/^{14}C$ ratios in the patient with a bile fistula who received HDL free [^3H]cholesterol and esterified [^3H]cholesterol and free [^{14}C]cholesterol. As in the patient with an intact enterohepatic circulation there were marked similarities between $^3H/^{14}C$ ratios in plasma lipoprotein free cholesterol, CA and biliary cholesterol. By contrast, the $^3H/^{14}C$ ratios in HDL, VLDL and LDL cholesterol esters were high and rapidly declining as the administered cholesterol esters were replaced with cholesterol esters newly formed from free cholesterol with the lower $^3H/^{14}C$ ratio.

Figure 6 shows the data in a patient (patient S.W.) with a bile fistula who was administered LDL esterified [^3H]cholesterol and LDL free [^3H]cholesterol and free [^{14}C]cholesterol. As in the previous experiments the ratios of $^3H/^{14}C$ in lipoprotein free cholesterol, bile acids and biliary cholesterol were similar. By contrast, the $^3H/^{14}C$ ratios in LDL cholesterol esters were initially high and then gradually declined. It was of interest that the $^3H/^{14}C$ ratio of HDL cholesterol ester was intermediate between LDL esterified cholesterol and plasma lipoprotein free cholesterol, suggesting that some of the administered radioactivity in LDL cholesterol esters must have been transferred to HDL probably via the cholesterol ester transport protein.

The quantitation of plasma sources for bile sterol production was carried out as previously described[7]. The calculations assume that activity exiting bile acid and biliary cholesterol precursor pools is insignificant relative to activity entering (in early time periods) and that plasma free cholesterol and esterified cholesterol are the only plasma sources for hepatic precursor compartment of cholesterol destined for bile acid synthesis. According to these calculations the HDL lipoprotein cholesterol esters (after hydrolysis) contribute a very small amount (between 10 and 20%) of substrate in the hepatic precursor compartments for bile acid synthesis and biliary cholesterol excretion. LDL cholesterol ester also contributes less than 10% to bile acid synthesis but the contribution to biliary cholesterol excretion in one patient was about 40%. Thus the major contributor of cholesterol substrate for bile acid synthesis and biliary cholesterol secretion appears to be plasma free cholesterol. The data also suggest that cholesterol esters after hydrolysis return to the systemic circulation as free cholesterol rather than contributing to bile acid synthesis or biliary cholesterol excretion. It is unlikely that there is a large cholesterol ester pool in the liver which furnishes cholesterol for bile sterol formation as if this were the case one would not expect to observe precursor–product relationship between plasma free cholesterol (precursor) and biliary cholesterol (product). These data, therefore, qualitatively and quantitatively support our previous conclusions which were obtained using an entirely different experimental design that included simulation analysis and modelling of the data[1].

Cholesterol degradation to bile acids

Once the plasma free cholesterol enters the hepatic microsomal precursor compartment for bile acid synthesis it undergoes conversion to bile acids. This complex process involves the action of a variety of microsomal, cytosolic and mitochondrial enzymes resulting in a series of changes on the sterol nucleus and side-chain which eventually transform a water-insoluble molecule (cholesterol) into a water-soluble product (CA and CDCA)[8]. The key enzyme in this transformation is microsomal cholesterol 7α-hydroxylase which converts cholesterol into 7α-hydroxycholesterol. This enzyme is considered to be rate-limiting for bile acid synthesis and is subject to feedback regulation. 7α-hydroxycholesterol is further transformed to 7α-hydroxy-4-cholesten-3-one which is considered to be a branching point in the major bile acid synthetic pathway from which CA is formed via 12α-hydroxylation of this precursor while β-reduction results in eventual formation of CDCA[8]. These conventional concepts of the bile acid biosynthetic pathway and sequence of reactions were derived predominantly from *in vivo* and *in vitro* studies in rats. In light of the many differences in bile acid and cholesterol metabolism between the rat and man it was important to re-examine the bile acid biosynthetic pathways in man. A number of *in vivo* studies have been carried out in this laboratory in which a variety of labelled intermediates (7α-hydroxycholesterol; 7α-hydroxy-4-cholesten-3-one; 7α,26-dihydroxy-4-cholesten-3-one) were administered to patients with a bile fistula. The efficiency of their

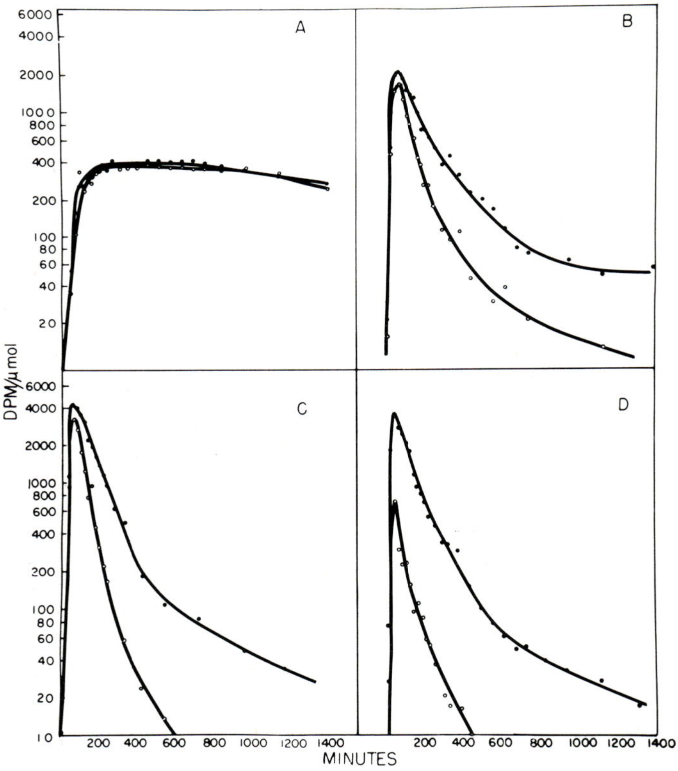

Figure 7 Specific activity time curves of cholic acid (○) and chenodeoxycholic acid (●) after administration of [4-^{14}C]cholesterol, 7α[7β-^{3}H]hydroxycholesterol, 7α[6β-^{3}H]-hydroxy-4-cholesten-3-one and 7α,26[6β-^{3}H]dihydroxycholest-4-ene-3-one

conversion to CA and CDCA were compared after administration to patients with bile fistulas.

The administration of labelled 7α-hydroxycholesterol (Figure 7B) and 7α-hydroxy-4-cholesten-3-one (Figure 7C) to a patient with a bile fistula demonstrated that the specific activities of CA were always lower than the specific activities of CDCA[9]. By contrast, the specific activities of CA and CDCA after administration of [4-^{14}C]cholesterol were identical (Figure 7A). The lower specific activities of CA after administration of labelled 7α-hydroxycholesterol and 7α-hydroxy-4-cholesten-3-one suggest that a portion of this bile acid must have been derived from a substrate proximal to the administered labelled 7α-hydroxycholesterol, i.e. from the cholesterol itself. This 'bypass' pathway from cholesterol to CA does not involve initial 7α-hydroxylation of cholesterol. It has been estimated that about 20–30% of CA

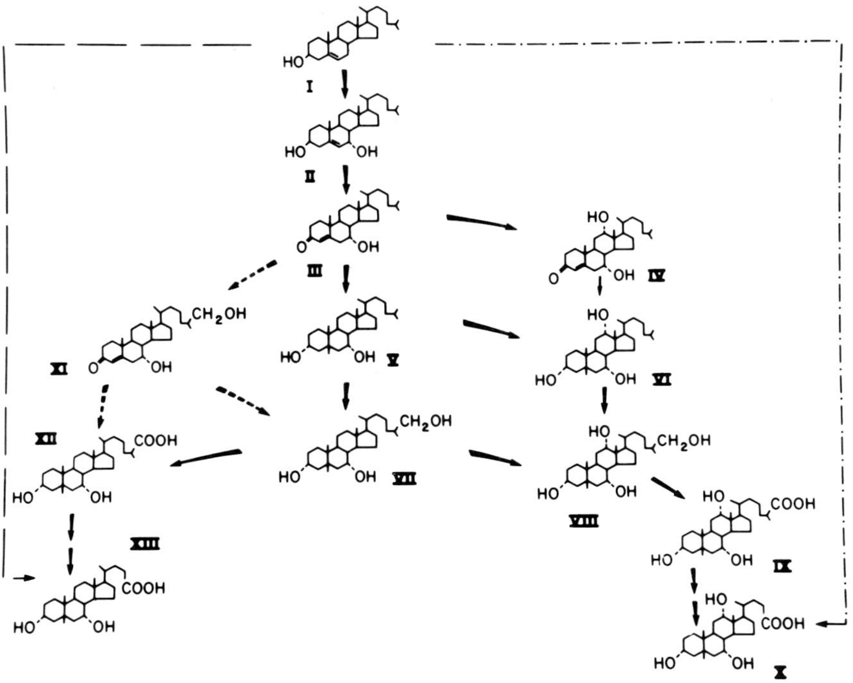

Figure 8 Present concept of bile acid pathways in man. I, cholesterol; II, 7α-hydroxycholesterol; III, 7α-hydroxy-4-cholesten-3-one; IV, 7α,12α-dihydroxy-4-cholesten-3-one; V, 5β-cholestane-3α,7α-diol; VI, 5β-cholestane-3α,7α,12α-triol; VII, 5β-cholestane-3α,7α,26-triol; VIII, 5β-cholestane-3α,7α,12α,26-tetrol; IX, 3α,7α,12α-trihydroxy-5β-cholestanoic acid; X, 3α,7α,12α-trihydroxy-5β-cholanoic acid (cholic); XI, 7α-26-dihydroxy-4-cholesten-3-one; XII, 3α,7α-dihydroxy-5β-cholestanoic acid; XIII, 3α,7α-dihydroxy-5β-cholanoic acid (chenodeoxycholic). Dotted arrows represent the hypothetical pathway to chenodeoxycholic acid and cholic acid via 26-hydroxylation of 7α-hydroxy-4-cholesten-3-one (III). –·–·–, bypass pathway to cholic acid; ——, bypass pathway to chenodeoxycholic acid (via 26-hydroxy-cholesterol)

in man is synthesized via this pathway. The sequence of reactions from cholesterol to CA via this pathway is not known. Additional studies, however, have excluded the likelihood that CA synthesized via this pathway is formed via the intermediate formation of 12α-hydroxycholesterol[10], 26-hydroxycholesterol[10,11] or 25-hydroxycholesterol[12]. In addition, these *in vivo* studies have demonstrated that 5β-cholestane-3α,7α,26-triol, a presumed sole precursor of CDCA, could also be 12α-hydroxylated and subsequently converted to cholic acid[10,13]. In the process of these *in vivo* studies it was also shown that CDCA may be synthesized via 26-hydroxylation of cholesterol[10,11] and 7α-hydroxy-4-cholesten-3-one via intermediate formation of 7α,26-dihydroxy-4-cholesten-3-one[10]. When administered intravenously to a patient with a bile fistula this latter compound (Figure 7D) was preferentially converted to CDCA in the ratio of 7 to 1 and may represent an important intermediate in the pathway of CDCA synthesis.

From these recent studies in man it appears that cholesterol degradation to bile acids probably occurs via multiple pathways. However, the contribution of these pathways to overall bile acid economy is not known. More detailed knowledge of the pathways by which bile acids are formed from cholesterol in normal subjects and in patients with hyperlipidaemia may be of importance, since the eventual disposition of cholesterol from the body takes place to a significant extent through its transformation to bile acids. These newer concepts of bile acid pathways originating from *in vivo* studies in man are shown in Figure 8.

References

1. Schwartz, C. C., Berman, M., Vlahcevic, Z. R., Halloran, L. G., Gregory, D. H. and Swell, L. (1978). Multicompartmental analysis of cholesterol metabolism in man. I. Characterization of the hepatic bile acid and biliary cholesterol precursor sites. *J. Clin. Invest.*, **61,** 408
2. Schwartz, C. C., Halloran, L. G., Vlahcevic, Z. R., Gregory, D. H. and Swell, L. (1978). Preferential utilization of free cholesterol from high-density lipoproteins for biliary cholesterol secretion in man. *Science*, **200,** 62
3. Halloran, L. G., Schwartz, C. C., Vlahcevic, Z. R., Nisman, R. M. and Swell, L. (1973). Evidence for high density lipoprotein-free cholesterol as the primary precursor for bile acid synthesis in man. *Surgery*, **84,** 1
4. Burstein, M. and Scholnick, H. R. (1973). Lipoprotein–polyanion–metal interactions. *Adv. Lipid Res.*, **11,** 67
5. Grundy, S. M. and Metzer, D. A. (1972). A physiological method for estimation of hepatic secretion of biliary lipids in man. *Gastroenterology*, **62,** 1200
6. Noble, R. P. (1968). Electrophoretic separation of plasma lipoproteins in agarose gel. *J. Lipid Res.*, **9,** 693
7. Schwartz, C. C., Vlahcevic, Z. R., Halloran, L. G. and Swell, L. (1981). An *in vivo* evaluation in man of the transfer of esterified cholesterol between lipoproteins and into the liver and bile. *Biochim. Biophys. Acta*, **663,** 143
8. Danielsson, H. and Sjovall, J. (1975). Bile acid metabolism. *Ann. Rev. Biochem.*, **44,** 233
9. Vlahcevic, Z. R., Schwartz, C. C., Gustafsson, J., Halloran, L. G., Danielsson, H. and Swell, L. (1980). Biosynthesis of bile acids in man: Multiple pathways to cholic and chenodeoxycholic acid. *J. Biol. Chem.*, **255,** 2925
10. Swell, L., Gustafsson, J., Schwartz, C. C., Halloran, L. G., Danielsson, H. and Vlahcevic, Z. R. (1980). An *in vivo* evaluation of the quantitative significance of several potential pathways to cholic and chenodeoxycholic acids from cholesterol in man. *J. Lipid Res.*, **21,** 455

11. Anderson, K. E., Kok, E. and Javitt, N. B. (1972). Bile acid synthesis in man: Metabolism of 7α-hydroxycholesterol-^{14}C and 26-hydroxycholesterol-^{3}H. *J. Clin. Invest.*, **51,** 112
12. Swell, L., Schwartz, C. C., Gustafsson, J., Danielsson, H. and Vlahcevic, Z. R. (1981). *In vivo* metabolism of 25-hydroxycholesterol in man. *Biochim. Biophys. Acta*, **663,** 163
13. Schwartz, C. C., Cohen, B. I., Vlahcevic, Z. R., Gregory, D. H., Halloran, L. G., Kuramoto, T., Mosbach, E. H. and Swell, Leon (1976). Quantitative aspects of the conversion of 5β-cholestane intermediates to bile acids in man. *J. Biol. Chem.*, **251,** 6308

12
Bile acid biosynthesis: metabolism of 3β-hydroxy-5-cholenoic acid

N. B. JAVITT, E. KOK, S. BURSTEIN, P. F. MISKOVITZ AND M. GUT

Studies from our laboratory have shown that cholesten-3β-26-diol (26-hydroxycholesterol) is metabolized to both chenodeoxycholic acid (CDCA) and cholic acid (CA) in the rat[1], hamster[2] and in man[3]. These findings challenged the traditional view that oxidation of the side-chain prior to transformation of the sterol ring to di- or tri-hydroxycoprostane does not lead to the formation of primary bile acids.

More recent studies in man[4] confirm the metabolic fate of 26-hydroxycholesterol and conclude that multiple pathways for bile acid synthesis may exist including the occurrence of side-chain oxidation products with cholesterol rather than coprostane-type sterol rings.

Although the occurrence of 26-hydroxylation as an initial step in bile acid synthesis is still not fully accepted by some investigators, the presence of 26-hydroxycholesterol in normal human meconium[5] together with 3β-hydroxy-5-cholenoic acid[6] which is also normally found in amniotic fluid[7] makes it most logical that a precursor–product relationship exists. In addition, in animals this monohydroxy bile acid has been demonstrated to be a metabolite of 26-hydroxycholesterol[1]. Thus, although further study would be useful, it does appear that at least in neonatal life a pathway exists in which cholesterol is metabolized to 26-hydroxycholesterol which is then either metabolized to (a) CDCA and CA, (b) 3β-hydroxy-5-cholenoic acid and (c) 26-hydroxycholesterol disulphate, all of which can be found in meconium.

We have succeeded recently in preparing a radioactive isotope of 3β-hydroxy-5-cholenoic acid and are studying its metabolic fate in the hamster Substitution of tritium into the 1, 2-position of the ring provides radioactivity at sites in the molecule that do not exchange or are biologically transformed. Synthesis was accomplished by Oppenauer oxidation followed by unsaturation of the 1–2 position and then tritiation by methods described previously in detail[8]. Following tritiation, the compound is reduced with sodium borohydride after formation of the acetate to yield both 3α- and 3β-hydroxy-5-cholenoic acids which can be separated by chromatographic methods. A previous study of the metabolism of 3β-hydroxy-5-cholenoic acid in the rat was done by Mitropolous and Myant using a tracer prepared by catalytic exchange using tritiated acetic acid in which the stability and location of the tritium was unknown and the material could not be purified to a known specific activity[9].

We administered the radioactive 3β-hydroxy-5-cholenoic acid together with [^{14}C]CDCA intravenously. More than 50% of the CDCA was recovered in bile within 4 h and more than 70% within 24 h. In contrast, only 40% of the 3β-hydroxy-5-cholenoate was recovered during this period of time.

Analysis of the bile for the distribution of the tritium indicated that it had been metabolized to other compounds. Following solvolysis and hydrolysis, the bile acids were fractionated on a column of glycophase G into mono, di and trihydroxy bile acids. All the tritium was found in either the mono or dihydroxy zones with none detected in the trihydroxy region. As expected all the ^{14}C derived from CDCA was found in the dihydroxy region.

The fractions obtained after separation on glycophase-G were then separated by HPLC using microporasil. Using these techniques we found that the monohydroxy region contained the infused 3β-hydroxy-5-cholenoic acid together with a new radioactive peak which we could confirm by chromatography as both the methyl ester, methyl ester acetate and by reverse isotope dilution to be 3α-hydroxy-5β-cholanoate (Lithocholic acid).

Using similar techniques we were also able to identify CDCA as a metabolite of 3β-hydroxy-5-cholenoic acid.

In summary, our recent studies now provide a more complete picture of the metabolic fate of the 26-hydroxycholesterol in man. Following oxidation of cholesterol to 26-hydroxycholesterol it may undergo 7α-hydroxylation and ultimately be metabolized to both CDCA and CA. Further oxidation of the side-chain to 3β-hydroxy-5-cholenoic acid can be followed either by excretion as the sulphate ester or further metabolism to lithocholic acid and CDCA. The pathway by which 3β-hydroxy-5-cholenoic acid is metabolized to CDCA is not specified at present. It also appears that oxidation of the side-chain beyond 26-hydroxycholesterol precludes 12α-hydroxylation to CA. Finally, 26-hydroxycholesterol can undergo esterification with sulphate and be excreted without further biotransformation.

References

1. Javitt, N. B. and Emerman, S. (1970). Metabolic pathways of bile acid formation in the rat. *Mt. Sinai J. Med.*, **37**, 977
2. Wachtel, N., Emerman, S. and Javitt, N. B. (1968). Metabolism of cholest-5-ene-3β, 26-diol in the rat and hamster. *J. Biol. Chem.*, **243**, 5207
3. Anderson, K., Kok, E. and Javitt, N. B. (1972). Bile acid synthesis in man. Metabolism of 7α-hydroxycholesterol-^{14}C and 26-hydroxy-cholesterol-^{3}H. *J. Clin. Invest.*, **51**, 112
4. Swell, L., Gustafsson, J., Schwartz, C., Halloran, L., Danielsson, H., and Vlahcevic, R. (1980). An *in vivo* evaluation of the quantitative significance of several potential pathways to cholic and chenodeoxycholic acids. *J. Lipid Res.*, **21**, 456
5. Lavy, U., Burstein, S., Gut, M. and Javitt, N. B. (1977). Bile acid synthesis in man. II. Determination of 7α-hydroxycholesterol, (22R)-22-hydroxycholesterol, and 26-hydroxy-cholesterol in human meconium. *J. Lipid Res.*, **18**, 232
6. Back, P. and Ross, K. (1973). Identification of 3β-hydroxy-5-cholenoic acid in human meconium. *Hoppe-Seyler's Z. Physiol. Chem.*, **354**, 83
7. Paumgartner, G., Deleze, G., Karlaganis, G., and Sidiropoulous, D. (1976). Bile acid pattern in human amniotic fluid: an index of fetal liver maturity. *Gastroenterology*, **71**, 923

8. Kok, E., Burstein, S., Javitt, N. B., Gut, M. and Byon, C. Y. (1981). Bile acid synthesis: Metabolism of 3β-hydroxy-5-cholenoic acid in the hamster. *J. Biol. Chem.* (In press)
9. Mitropoulos, K. A. and Myant, N. B. (1967). The formation of lithocholic acid and other bile acids from 3β-hydroxychol-5-enoic-acid *in vitro* and *in vivo*. *Biochim. Biophys. Acta*, **144**, 430

13
The metabolism of 7-ketolithocholic acid in man

G. SALEN, G. S. TINT, D. VERGA AND S. SHEFER

During the past few years, chenodeoxycholic acid (CDCA)[1] (Figure 1) and its 7β-hydroxy epimer ursodeoxycholic acid (UDCA)[2,3] have become established as gallstone-dissolving agents in man. In most subjects the administration of CDCA or UDCA reduces biliary cholesterol saturation and inhibits endogenous bile acid production[4]. As a result, the concentrations of biliary cholic acid (CA) and deoxycholic acid (DCA) decrease, and CDCA or UDCA, whichever was fed, becomes the predominant biliary bile acid. Lithocholic acid, which is produced from CDCA or UDCA through the action of intestinal bacteria, rises in the bile but less is found during

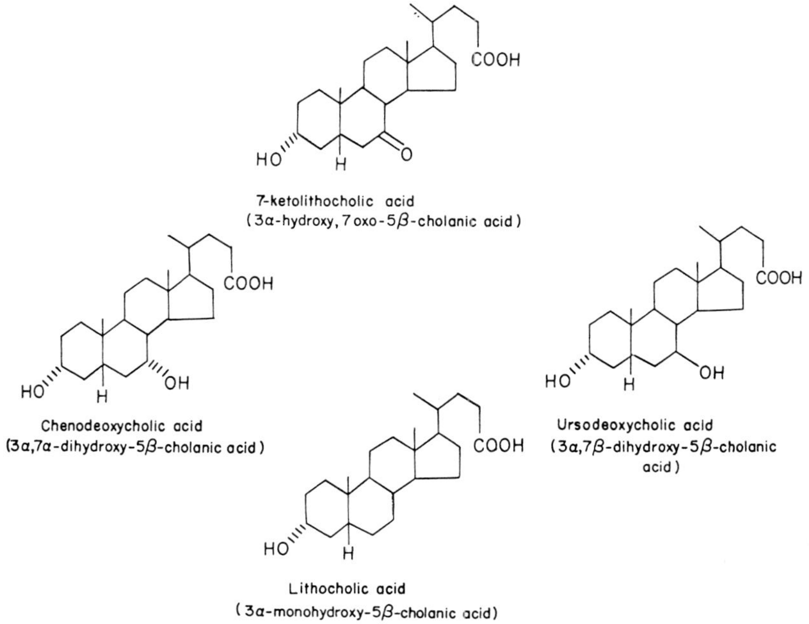

Figure 1 Structures of bile acids studied

UDCA treatment[2,4]. In some individuals 7-ketolithocholic acid (7KLCA), a putative bacterial metabolite of CDCA, was found in the bile and faeces[4]. This bile acid may also be a precursor of UDCA in the transformation of CDCA to UDCA in man[5]. To obtain additional information, the metabolism of 7KLCA was investigated under two different experimental conditions. Five subjects were fed 400 mg/day of 7KLCA for 2 weeks; a tracer dose of [24-^{14}C]CDCA was administered intravenously as a pulse-label and the transformation of CDCA to UDCA was examined. In another group of five subjects, 400 mg/day of uniformly labelled [24-^{14}C]7KLCA (specific activity, 1000 ± 10 dpm/mg) was fed for 2 weeks and the conversion of 7KLCA into CDCA and UDCA was tested. In both groups, biliary-free and conjugated bile acid composition was measured and biliary lithogenic index was determined.

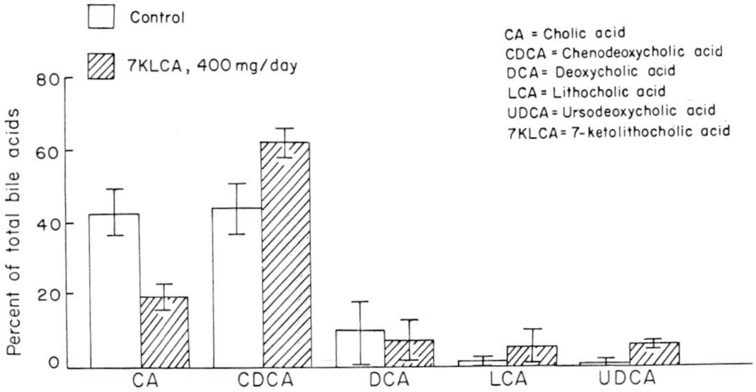

Figure 2 The effect of 7KLCA on biliary bile acid composition

Figure 2 lists the effects of feeding 400 mg/day of 7KLCA on biliary bile acid composition. After 2 weeks, the proportions of cholic acid and its bacterial metabolite, DCA, declined from 42 to 18% and from 12 to 8% of the total bile acids respectively, while the proportion of CDCA increased from 42 to 62% and UDCA from 1 to 8%. The differences in CA, CDCA and DCA composition were statistically significant. Free lithocholic acid rose in the bile from 2 to 5% (no sulphated lithocholic acid was detected) and trace amounts of 7KLCA were present also. These results indicate the 7KLCA was absorbed and converted predominantly to CDCA. The reductions in CA and DCA indicate that endogenous bile acid production during the administration of 7KLCA was inhibited. However, it is not clear whether the 7KLCA acted directly to suppress bile acid synthesis or alternatively whether CDCA, its major product, was responsible for hepatic suppression of synthesis. Table 1 shows the effect of 7KLCA on the conjugation pattern of biliary bile acids. Prior to treatment, 55% of the bile acids were excreted, conjugated with glycine and 45% conjugated with taurine. After 2 weeks of 7KLCA the proportion of glycine conjugates had risen to 73% and taurine conjugates declined to 27%. Thus, the administration of substantial quantities of free 7KLCA increases the requirement for hepatic conjugation and depletes the

Table 1 Effect of 7-ketolithocholic acid on bile acid conjugates

Treatment	*Glycine conjugates* (%)	*Taurine conjugates* (%)
Pre-7KLCA	55.1	44.9
7KLCA	72.9	27.1

hepatic pool of taurine. As a result, the bile becomes composed overwhelmingly of glycine conjugates.

Figure 3 illustrates the effects of 7KLCA on biliary cholesterol saturation. Prior to treatment the cholesterol saturation index in these subjects was clearly lithogenic (2.25) which was expected since all subjects had gallstones. After 2 weeks of 400 mg/day of 7KLCA, the cholesterol saturation index fell to 0.8. Thus, 7KLCA caused a substantial reduction in biliary cholesterol secretion. However, it is not clear whether this effect is related directly to 7KLCA or to the increased amounts of its major transformation product, CDCA.

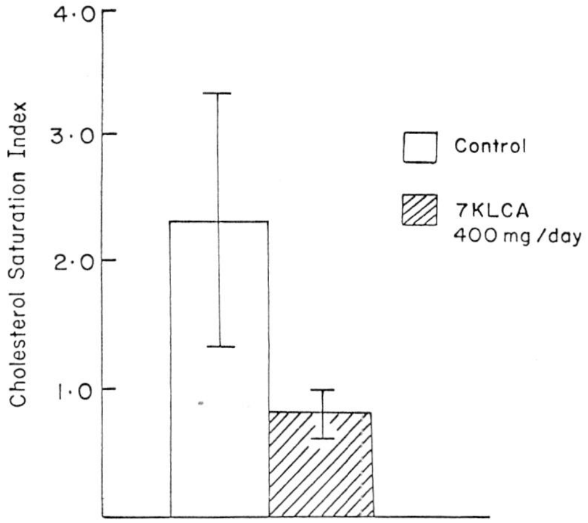

Figure 3 Effect of 7KLCA on the lithogenicity of bile

In order to study the transformation of CDCA to UDCA and identify intermediates in the pathway, [24-^{14}C]CDCA was administered intravenously as a pulse-label to five subjects during the feeding of unlabelled 7KLCA. Figure 4 shows the specific activity *versus* time curves for biliary CDCA, UDCA, and LCA. The specific activities of CDCA decayed linearly over the first 7 days after isotope injection, which indicated that a single pool of this bile acid existed. Further, both UDCA and LCA were labelled also and their respective specific activity curves intersected with the declining curve of CDCA and then continued to parallel the decay curve of CDCA forming a precursor–product relationship between CDCA and UDCA and LCA. No radioactive 7KLCA was detected. This experiment shows that UDCA was

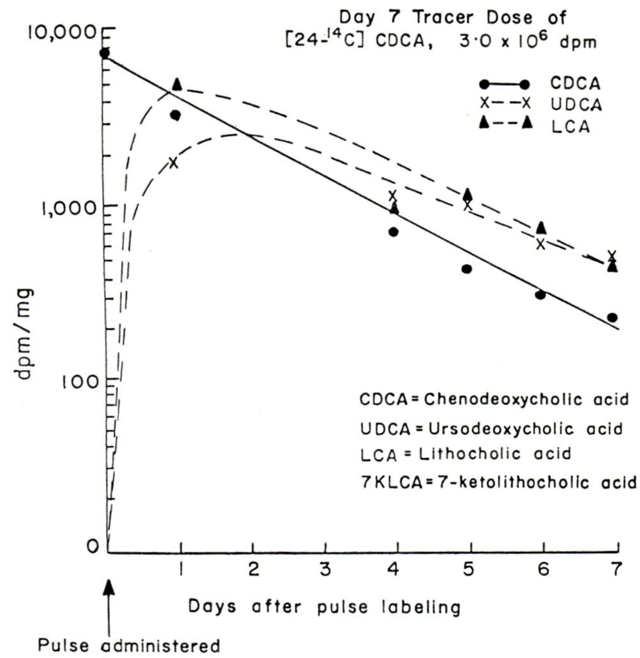

Figure 4 Specific activity decay curves of CDCA, UDCA and LCA after intravenous administration of tracer dose of [24-^{14}C]CDCA during 7KLCA feeding (400 mg/day for 14 days)

derived solely from CDCA and not from unlabelled 7KLCA, since the unlabelled 7KLCA – if converted into UDCA – would have diluted the specific activities of the UDCA and resulted in values that were less than CDCA. As expected, the precursor–product relationship between LCA and CDCA showed that lithocholic acid was produced predominantly from CDCA. Despite the modest increase in biliary-free lithocholic acid, the sulphate was not present (Figure 2).

In another experiment designed to study the formation of CDCA and UDCA from 7KLCA, uniformly labelled [24-^{14}C]7KLCA was fed for 2 weeks and biliary CDCA and UDCA specific activities were measured and are reported in Figure 5. Both UDCA and CDCA became radioactive and their respective specific activities increased over the first week to reach a plateau by day 8 when these values became constant. The mean specific activity for the final five determinations for CDCA was 761 $\pm$ 33 and for UDCA 720 $\pm$ 24. Both values are significantly lower than the specific activity of fed 7KLCA. Since CDCA is normally present in bile and is produced from cholesterol in the liver, the lower specific activity of biliary CDCA reflects dilution with endogenously synthesized CDCA. Since the specific activity of biliary CDCA was approximately 70% of the specific activity of fed 7KLCA, about 70% of the biliary CDCA was derived from this precursor. In contrast, only trace amounts of UDCA are usually present in the bile. Therefore the fact that the specific activity of UDCA equalled CDCA, and not 7KLCA, indicated that UDCA was derived directly from CDCA and not via 7KLCA. If 7KLCA was transformed into UDCA the specific activity of the UDCA should approximate that of the fed 7KLCA which was not the case.

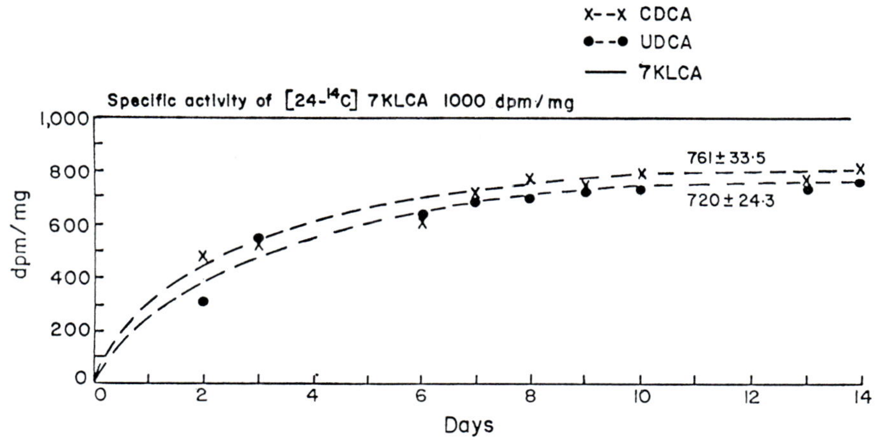

Figure 5 Specific activity curves of CDCA and UDCA during administration of uniformly labelled [24-^{14}C]7KLCA (specific activity 1000 dpm/mg), 400 mg/day

Acknowledgment

This work was supported by US Public Health Service Grants AM-18707, HL-17818, and AM-26756.

References

1. Danzinger, R. G., Hofmann, A. F., Schoenfeld, L. S. and Thistle, J. L. (1972). Dissolution of cholesterol gallstones by chenodeoxycholic acid. *N. Engl. J. Med.*, **286,** 1
2. Nakagawa, S., Makino, I. and Iskizaki, T. (1977). Dissolution of cholesterol gallstones by ursodeoxycholic acid. *Lancet*, **2,** 367
3. Salen, G., Colallilo, A., Verga, D., Bagan, E., Tint, G. S. and Shefer, S. (1980). Effect of high and low doses of ursodeoxycholic acid on gallstone dissolution in humans. *Gastroenterology*, **78,** 1412
4. Fedorowski, T., Salen, G., Colallilo, A. and Mosbach, E. H. (1977). Metabolism of ursodeoxycholic acid in man. *Gastroenterology*, **73,** 1131
5. Salen, G., Tint, G. S., Eliav, B. and Mosbach, E. H. (1974). Increased formation of ursodeoxycholic acid in patients treated with chenodeoxycholic acid. *J. Clin. Invest.*, **53,** 612

14
Hydroxylation of bile acids in man

A. BREMMELGAARD AND J. SJÖVALL

INTRODUCTION

Urine from humans contains bile acids which may be structurally regarded as 1- and 6-hydroxylation products of the common biliary bile acids[1,2]. Several of these acids are excreted in increased amounts in patients with cholestasis (Figure 1)[2–6]. This study was carried out in order to test the assumption that cholic acid (CA), chenodeoxycholic acid (CDCA) and deoxycholic acid (DCA) can be hydroxylated in patients with cholestasis.

MATERIALS AND METHODS

Bile acids

Bile acids labelled with ^{14}C in the carboxyl group and having specific activities of 50–55 mCi/mmol were from the Radiochemical Centre, Amersham, England, and NEN Chemicals, Dreieich, West Germany. Unlabelled bile acids were those used previously[2], except for 3α,6α,7α,12α-tetrahydroxy-5β-cholanoic acid which was prepared from 3α,6α-dihydroxy-12α-acetoxy-7-oxo-5β-cholanoic acid (kindly supplied by Dr K. Takeda, Shionogi Research Laboratory, Osaka, Japan) by $NaBH_4$ reduction followed by hydrolysis.

Patients

About 10 μCi of a labelled bile acid were given to a patient with primary biliary cirrhosis (E.H., [^{14}C]CA intravenously) and two patients with intermittent intrahepatic cholestasis of unknown aetiology in resolution phase (J.M.L., [^{14}C]DCA orally, and J.P.D., [^{14}C]CDCA intravenously). E.H. had severe itching and was treated with cholestyramine, J.M.L. and J.P.D. had moderate and no itching, respectively, and were not treated with bile acid binding resin. Urine was collected in 24 h portions and was stored at −20 °C until analysed.

Trivial names and abbreviations: cholic (CA), 3α,7α,12α-trihydroxy-5β-cholanoic; chenodeoxycholic (CDCA), 3α,7α-dihydroxy-5β-cholanoic; deoxycholic (DCA), 3α,12α-dihydroxy-5β-cholanoic; hyocholic, 3α, 6α,7α-trihydroxy-5β-cholanoic. TMS, trimethylsilyl; t_R, retention time relative to that of the TMS ether of methyl cholate; GC/MS, gas chromatography–mass spectrometry.

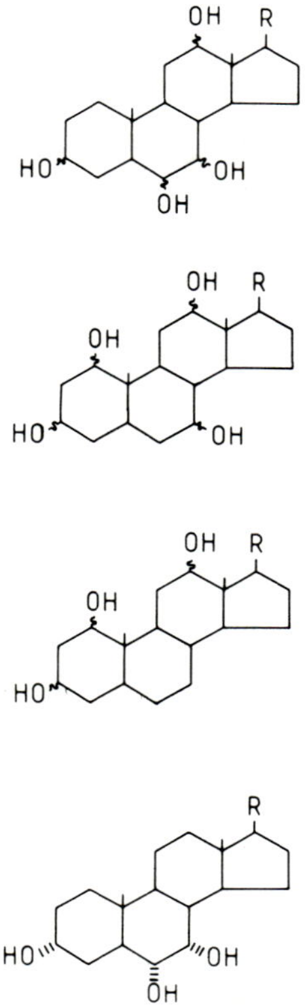

% of Total Urinary Bile Acids	
Healthy	Cholestasis
0	0 - 19
0	0 - 12
1 - 7	0 - 15
0 - 2	0 - 20

Figure 1 Structures and relative amounts of the most common 1- and 6-hydroxylated bile acids excreted in urine in healthy subjects and patients with cholestasis. Adapted from refs. 2 and 5

Bile acid analyses

Analyses of bile acids were carried out, using procedures described in Ref. 2. About 300–400 ml of urine was extracted, and bile acids were separated into groups according to mode of conjugation. The fractions containing glycine and taurine conjugates were combined and hydrolysed. The resulting unconjugated bile acids were extracted, purified on the lipophilic ion exchanger and methylated with diazomethane. The methyl esters were subfractionated according to number of hydroxyl groups on a 4 g column of Lipidex 5000, which was eluted with chloroform/hexane, 1 : 4, 3 : 7, 1 : 1 (v/v) in a stepwise manner to yield mono-, di- and trihydroxycholanoates, respectively. Tetrahydroxycholanoates were recovered by elution with methanol. The extraction and subfractionations were monitored by liquid scintillation counting of suitable aliquots of the fractions.

As an aid in the purification and identification of bile acids, acetonides were prepared in 1 ml dimethoxypropane and 50 μl 0.1 N hydrochloric acid for 30 min at 37 °C. The acid was then removed by filtration through a small column of DEAE Sephadex A-25 in OH^--form in 72% methanol. Following evaporation of solvents, compounds which yielded acetonides were separated from other components by a second chromatography on Lipidex 5000.

GC/MS analyses

These were performed as described previously, using the TMS ether derivatives and 1% SE-30 or 1.5% HiEff 8 BP as stationary phases. The bile acid derivatives were quantified by measurement of peak areas in selected fragment ion current chromatograms[2]. Thus, specific radioactivities of labelled bile acids in purified fractions could be calculated.

RESULTS

One urine sample from each patient was analysed in detail. The distribution of radioactivity between different fractions in the three experiments is shown in Figure 2.

In all three experiments a major part of the radioactivity was present in the sulphate fraction. Most of this activity is probably due to a sulphate of the administered compound and the sulphates were not further studied. Hydroxylated metabolites were expected to be found in the glycine and taurine conjugate fractions (see Ref. 2), and these fractions were hydrolysed and subfractionated. As seen in Figure 2, about 60% of the glycine- and taurine-conjugated metabolites of CDCA appeared in the trihydroxycholanoate fraction. All of this material reacted with dimethoxypropane (Figure 2). The mass spectra and retention times of the TMS derivatives of the radioactive compound and its acetonide were identical with those of the corresponding derivatives of methyl hyocholate. The specific activities of CDCA and hyocholic acid were essentially the same.

Most of the radioactivity in the glycine and taurine conjugated fraction from the CA experiment was due to CA. However, about 10% of the activity was eluted in the tetrahydroxycholanoate fraction and about half of this radioactive material reacted with dimethoxypropane (Figure 2). GC/MS analysis of the latter material revealed the presence of a compound which gave all the mass spectral peaks expected of the acetonide–TMS ether derivative of a tetrahydroxycholanoate (e.g. m/z 607 (M–15), 474 (M–90–58), 457 (M–90–75), 431 (M–90–101), 367 (base peak, M–2·90–75)). The spectrum showed several analogies with that of the acetonide–TMS ether derivative of methyl hyocholate. A comparison of GC/MS data was therefore made between the TMS ether and acetonide–TMS ether derivatives of methyl 3α,6α,7α,12α-tetrahydroxy-5β-cholanoate and the methyl ester of the CA metabolite. Identical retention times on SE-30 (t_R (TMS): 1.25; t_R (acetonide–TMS): 1.45) and HiEff 8 BP (t_R (TMS): 0.80) and identical mass spectra were obtained. The specific radioactivity was closely similar to that of CA.

The material not reacting with dimethoxypropane contained at least four tetrahydroxycholanoates. The TMS ether of the predominant component

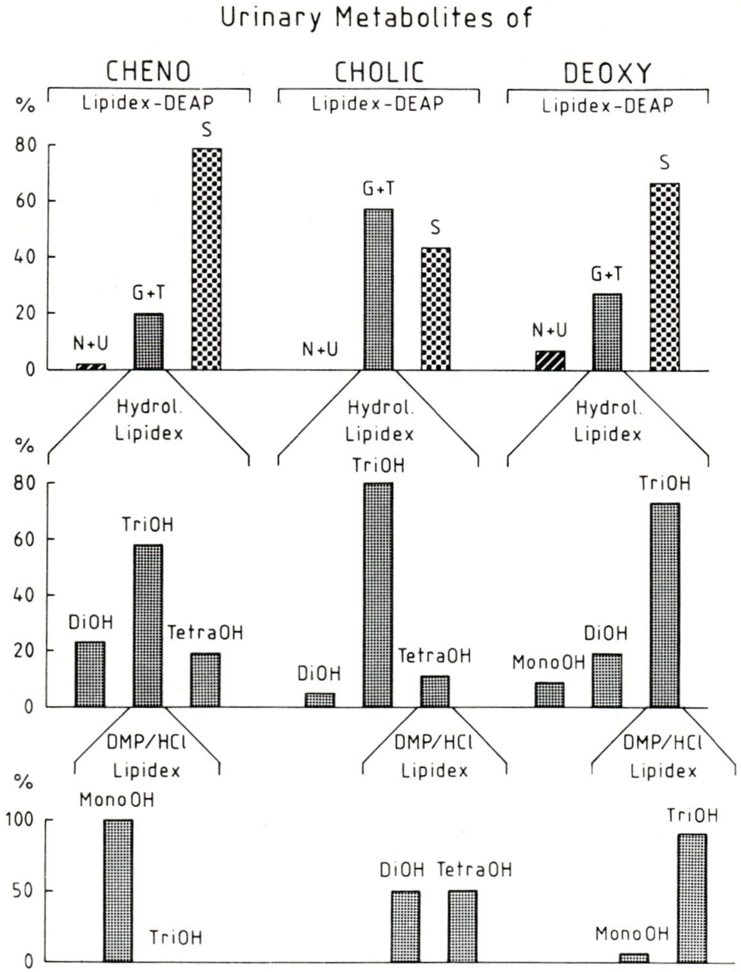

Figure 2 *Upper bars:* percentage distribution of radioactivity between neutral (N), unconjugated (U), glycine (G) and taurine (T) conjugated, and sulphated (S) bile acids in urine following administration of ^{14}C-labelled CDCA, CA and DCA. *Middle bars:* percentage distribution of radioactivity from the hydrolysed G+T fractions between mono-, di-, tri- and tetrahydroxycholanoates separated on Lipidex 5000. *Lower bars:* percentage distribution of radioactivity between mono-, di-, tri-and tetrahydroxycholanoates following reaction of the hydroxylated metabolites with dimethoxypropane

had retention times (t_R (HiEff 8 BP): 0.80; t_R (SE–30): 1.25) and mass spectrum identical with those of the TMS ether of 1,3,7,12-tetrahydroxycholanoate, tentatively identified in a previous study[2]. The specific radioactivity was closely similar to that of CA. The other three tetrahydroxycholanoates were not definitely identified. However, GC/MS data for one of them is compatible with a 6β-hydroxycholic acid structure.

About 20% of the metabolites of DCA appeared in the glycine- and taurine-conjugated fractions, where most of the radioactivity was associated with trihydroxycholanoates. The predominant labelled compound had the GC/MS characteristics of 1,3,12-trihydroxycholanoate tentatively identified in a previous study[2]. Comparison with authentic material, prepared by microbial hydroxylation of DCA[7], showed that the structure was 1β,3α,12α-trihydroxy-5β-cholanoic acid. The specific radioactivity was similar to that of DCA. A minor metabolite had the GC/MS characteristics (as methyl ester TMS ether) of 3α,6α,12α-trihydroxy-5β-cholanoic acid[8].

DISCUSSION

This study has shown that the 'unusual' bile acids excreted in urine of humans can be formed by 1- and 6-hydroxylation of the common biliary bile acids. Judging from the specific radioactivities, the common bile acids appear to be the sole precursors of the 1- and 6-hydroxylated bile acids.

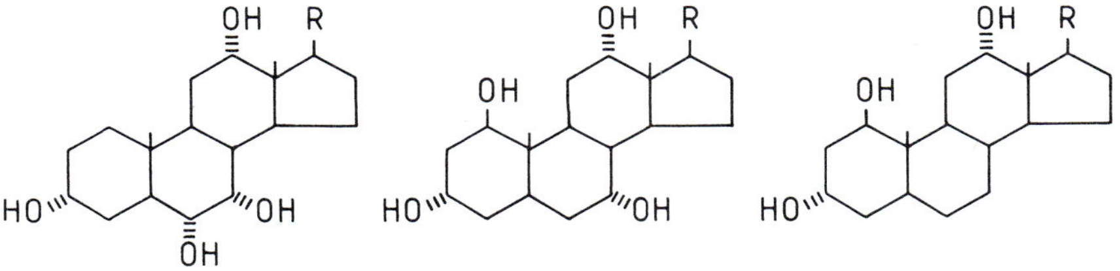

Figure 3 Major hydroxylated metabolites of CA (left and middle) and of DCA (right). The stereochemistry of the l-hydroxylated CA metabolite is tentative and is supported by retention times and the analogous hydroxylation of DCA

CDCA was hydroxylated in the 6α-position, whereas DCA was predominantly hydroxylated in the 1β-position (Figure 3). Cholic acid was hydroxylated both in 1ξ- and 6α-positions (Figure 3). This indicates that the presence of a 7α- or 12α-hydroxy group in the substrate is of importance for the interaction with the hydroxylase(s) involved. Although the stereochemistry of the hydroxyl groups in the 1-hydroxylated metabolite of CA has not been determined, the analogous 1β-hydroxylations of DCA and 3α,17α,20β,21-tetrahydroxy-5β-pregnan-11-one[9] makes it reasonable to assume that the CA metabolite is 1β,3α,7α,12α-tetrahydroxy-5β-cholanoic acid.

It is likely that hydroxylations other than those demonstrated in the three patients of this study take place. DCA was probably hydroxylated in the 6α-position. The importance of this reaction could be greater than apparent, since 3α,6α,12α-trihydroxy-5β-cholanoic acid was recently found to be excreted as a glucuronide in urine[8], and glucuronides were not included in this study. The isomeric 3α,6β,12α-trihydroxy-5β-cholanoic acid frequently occurs in urine[2,5,6] indicating possible 6β-hydroxylation. One of the CA metabolites observed in this study had GC/MS properties compatible with a 6β-hydroxycholic acid structure. CDCA may become 1-hydroxylated since some patients with liver disease excrete a bile acid tentatively identified as 1,3,7-trihydroxycholanoic acid[5].

Hyocholic and 1β,3α,12α-trihydroxy-5β-cholanoic acids are found in urine from most healthy subjects[2]. This is in contrast to the hydroxylated metabolites of CA which are below the detection limit when a routine analysis is performed[2]. Small amounts are found in pregnant women[6], and the excretion increases in cholestasis[5,6]. Several factors may be responsible for this increase, e.g. lowered biliary excretion compared to other bile acids, changes in mode of conjugation resulting in increased renal clearance rates, enhanced hydroxylase activities, increased concentrations of substrates for the hydroxylase(s). The simplest explanation may be that cholestasis increases the concentration of primary bile acids in the liver so that more substrate is available for the hydroxylase(s). This would also explain the finding that when the primary bile acids and their hydroxylated metabolites increase in urine, there is no increase of 1β-hydroxydeoxycholic acid when DCA excretion remains unchanged[5,6].

The hydroxylations described have not previously been reported to occur in man. This is probably explained by the fact that previous studies have not included metabolites excreted in urine. A comparison of bile acid patterns in bile and urine reveals striking differences. Besides the well-known predominance of sulphates in urine[10] there is a marked enrichment of hydroxylated bile acids in urine[1-6]. Since bile acids are most likely hydroxylated in the liver, the high relative excretion in urine is probably due to a high renal clearance of these metabolites.

Acknowledgments

This work was supported by grants from the Danish Medical Research Council (Nos. 512–6675 and 15474) and the Swedish Medical Research Council (No. 03X–219).

References

1. Almé, B., Bremmelgaard, A., Sjövall, J. and Thomassen, P. (1974). Complexity of the bile acid mixture in human urine. In Matern, S., Hackenschmidt, J., Back, P. and Gerok, W. (eds.). *Advances in Bile Acid Research*, pp. 145–147. (Stuttgart: F. K. Schattauer Verlag)
2. Almé, B., Bremmelgaard, A., Sjövall, J. and Thomassen, P. (1977). Analysis of metabolic profiles of bile acids in urine using a lipophilic anion exchanger and computerized gas–liquid chromatography–mass spectrometry. *J. Lipid Res.*, **18,** 339
3. Summerfield, J. A., Billing, B. H. and Shackleton, C. H. L. (1976). Identification of bile acids in the serum and urine in cholestasis. *Biochem. J.*, **154,** 507
4. van Berge Henegouwen, G. P., Brandt, K.-H., Eyssen, H. and Parmentier, G. (1976). Sulphated and unsulphated bile acids in serum, bile and urine of patients with cholestasis. *Gut*, **17,** 861
5. Bremmelgaard, A. and Sjövall, J. (1979). Bile acid profiles in urine of patients with liver diseases. *Eur. J. Clin. Invest.*, **9,** 341
6. Thomassen, P. A. (1979). Urinary bile acids in late pregnancy and in recurrent cholestasis of pregnancy. *Eur. J. Clin. Invest.*, **9,** 425
7. Carlström, K., Kirk, D. N. and Sjövall, J. (1981). Microbial synthesis of 1- and 15-hydroxylated bile acids. (Submitted for *J. Lipid Res.*)

8. Almé, B. and Sjövall, J. (1980). Analysis of bile acid glucuronides in urine. Identification of 3α,6α,12α-trihydroxy-5β-cholanoic acid. *J. Steroid Biochem.*, **13,** 907
9. Schneider, J. J and Bhacca, N. S. B. (1966). 1β-Hydroxylation of 3α,17α,20β,21-tetrahydroxy-5β-pregnan-11-one and of other 5β-steroids in man and by surviving liver slices of the guinea pig. *J. Biol. Chem.*, **241,** 5313
10. Makino, I., Hashimoto, H., Shinozaki, K., Yoshino, K. and Nakagawa, S. (1975). Sulfated and unsulfated bile acids in urine, serum and bile of patients with hepatobiliary diseases. *Gastroenterology*, **68,** 545

15
Characterization of bile acid UDP-glucuronyltransferase from human liver

H. MATERN, S. MATERN AND W. GEROK

INTRODUCTION

Bile acid glucuronides were detected in man about 6 years ago[1,2]. However the enzyme catalysing the glucuronidation of bile acids in man, the bile acid UDP-glucuronyltransferase, has only recently been characterized from human liver[3], since hitherto no sensitive assay for determination of this enzyme from small specimens of human liver was available. In this chapter the bile acid UDP-glucuronyltransferase from human liver is characterized in regard to catalytic properties and the affinity to different bile acids. Furthermore the influence of exogenous and endogenous substrates of UDP-glucuronyltransferase(s) on the activity of bile acid UDP-glucuronyltransferase in human liver is described.

MATERIALS AND METHODS

Specimens of human liver were obtained for histological examination from surgical patients who had undergone laparotomy for cholecystectomy because of cholelithiasis. Only laparotomy specimens with normal hepatic histology were used. A 10% liver homogenate (wet weight/volume) was prepared with 0.25 M sucrose in 5 mM Tris-HCl (pH 7.4) using a glass homogenizer with a Teflon pestle.

For the determination of bile acid UDP-glucuronyltransferase activity, human liver homogenate corresponding to about 2 mg liver (wet weight) was incubated for 30 min at 37 °C in a reaction mixture containing 0.5 mM [^{14}C]chenodeoxycholic acid (0.8 μCi/μmol), 9 mM UDP-glucuronic acid, 5 mM $MgCl_2$, 5 mM saccharolactone and 0.1 M imidazol-HCl (pH 6.8), and the formation of chenodeoxycholic acid (CDCA) glucuronide was measured[3]. As shown for microsomal UDP-glucuronyltransferase(s)[4], the bile acid UDP-glucuronyltransferase was activated by the addition of detergents[3]. The enzyme was found to be in the fully activated state at saturating substrate concentration (0.5 mmol/l CDCA) due to the surface-active effect of the bile acid[3]. Therefore, the bile acid UDP-glucuronyltransferase has only been assayed in the fully activated state which was achieved either by 0.5 mmol/l CDCA as substrate or by the presence of 0.01 % (v/v) Triton X-100 at <0.5 mmol/l CDCA[3].

Bilirubin UDP-glucuronyltransferase was determined as described by Black *et al.*[5] with the following modifications: the final concentrations of bilirubin and of UDP-glucuronic acid were 0.17 mmol/l and 9 mmol/l, respectively; the reaction mixture contained 0.1 mol/l imidazole-HCl (pH 6.7) as buffer.

Materials were the same as previously described[3].

RESULTS AND DISCUSSION

The effect of pH on bile acid UDP-glucuronyltransferase activity from human liver is shown in Figure 1. The enzyme exhibited a sharp optimum of activity at pH 6.7.

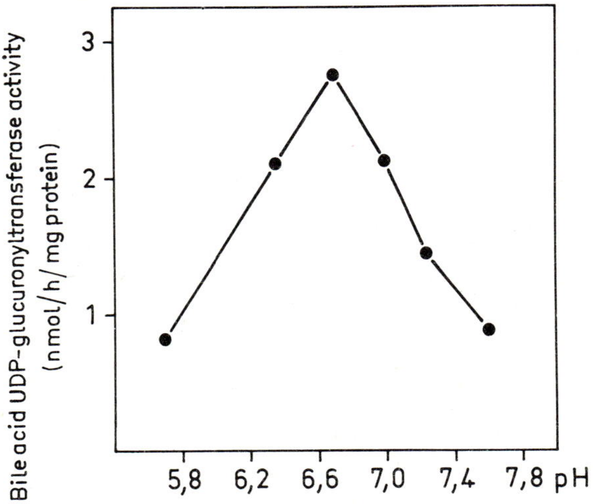

Figure 1 Effect of pH on bile acid UDP-glucuronyltransferase activity from human liver. Enzyme activity was determined as described in Materials and Methods except that 0.1 M potassium phosphate buffers were used. Duplicate incubation mixtures (UDP-glucuronic acid omitted) served for determination of pH

The Lineweaver–Burk plot of the initial rates of enzyme activity as a function of varying concentrations of chenodeoxycholic acid in the presence of 0.01 % Triton X-100 yielded a straight line from which the apparent K_m was calculated to be 0.083 mmol/l CDCA (Figure 2). The V_{max} was 2.4 nmol h^{-1} mg protein^{-1}. When UDP-glucuronic acid was used as the variable substrate and chenodeoxycholic acid was kept constant at 0.5 mmol/l, the apparent K_m for UDP-glucuronic acid was determined to be 0.96 mmol/l (not shown).

The affinity of the enzyme to different bile acids has been investigated by studying the influence of various bile acids on the glucuronidation of CDCA (Table 1). The affinity of the unconjugated bile acids to the enzyme decreased

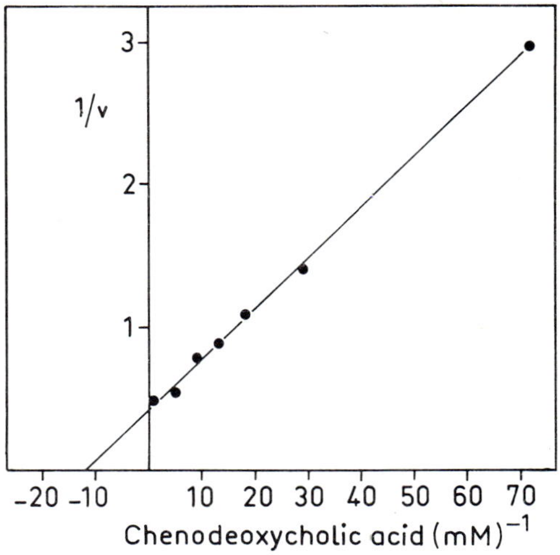

Figure 2 Lineweaver–Burk plot of the dependence of bile acid UDP-glucuronyltransferase activity (initial rates) on chenodeoxycholic acid concentration. For experimental details see Materials and Methods. (v = nmol h^{-1} mg protein^{-1})

with increasing number of hydroxyl groups in the bile acid skeleton. The glucuronidation of CDCA was inhibited in the presence of 0.1 mM lithocholic acid by 62%, whereas only 16% inhibition of CDCA glucuronidation was observed by 0.1 mM cholic acid (CA). The degree of inhibition of CDCA glucuronidation observed in the presence of dihydroxylated bile acids shows that the affinity of the bile acids to the enzyme seems to depend not only on

Table 1 Effect of bile acids on the glucuronidation of chenodeoxycholic acid

Bile acid	*Bile acid concentration* (mmol/l)	*Percentage inhibition of chenodeoxycholic acid glucuronidation in the presence of*		
		Unconjugated bile acid	*Glycine-conjugated bile acid*	*Taurine-conjugated bile acid*
Lithocholic acid (3α-ol)	0.1	62	51	58
	0.5	—	91	98
Chenodeoxycholic acid (3α,7α-ol)	0.1	—	28	33
	0.5	—	76	90
Ursodeoxycholic acid (3α,7β-ol)	0.1	27	17	—
	0.5	69	25	—
Deoxycholic acid (3α,12α-ol)	0.1	42	45	51
	0.5	99	91	99
Cholic acid (3α,7α,12α-ol)	0.1	16	15	19
	0.5	21	24	44

Enzyme activity was assayed in the presence of 0.5 mM chenodeoxycholic acid as described in Materials and Methods. Lithocholic acid (unconjugated or conjugated with glycine or taurine) was dissolved in ethylene glycol containing 1% (v/v) ethanolamine (final concentration solvent 19.2% (v/v)). The position and configuration of the hydroxyl groups in the acid bile skeleton are given in parentheses the number, but also on the position and configuration, of hydroxyl groups in the bile acid skeleton. Compared to the corresponding unconjugated bile acids, the affinity of the glycine-conjugated bile acids to the enzyme was similar or lower, whereas the taurine-conjugated bile acids showed a similar or higher affinity to the enzyme (Table 1).

A variety of foreign and endogenous compounds are known to be substrates of UDP-glucuronyltransferase(s)[6,7]. In human liver evidence exists that there is more than one UDP-glucuronyltransferase, e.g. morphine and bilirubin may be glucuronidated by separate forms of enzymes[8]. Since in animal experiments monohydroxylated bile acids have been shown to be hepatotoxic[9], it is clinically important to know whether drugs or endogenous compounds compete with bile acids for the same active site on UDP-glucuronyltransferase. Therefore the effect of morphine, bilirubin, oestradiol and testosterone on the glucuronidation of CDCA in human liver was investigated. As shown in Table 2, 15 mM morphine had no effect on the activity of bile acid UDP-glucuronyltransferase, whereas the glucuronidation of CDCA was inhibited by testosterone, bilirubin and oestradiol. Inhibition

Table 2 Effect of exogenous and endogenous substrates of UDP-glucuronyltransferase(s) on the glucuronidation of chenodeoxycholic acid

Additions to assay	*Concentrations* (mmol/l)	*Bile acid UDP-glucuronyltransferase activity* (*percentage of control without addition*)
None	—	100
Morphine	15	103
Bilirubin	0.25	66
Oestradiol-17β	0.25	55
Testosterone	4	43

For the determination of enzyme activity, see Materials and Methods. Bilirubin, oestradiol-17β and testosterone were dissolved as described for lithocholic acid in the legend to Table 1

kinetics were performed with these substrates according to Dixon (Figure 3) and to Lineweaver–Burk (not shown). Bilirubin (Figure 3A) and oestradiol (Figure 3B) competitively inhibited the glucuronidation of CDCA with apparent K_i values of 0.28 mM for bilirubin and 0.26 mM for oestradiol. Testosterone exhibited a non-competitive inhibition pattern with an apparent K_i value of 2.2 mM testosterone (Figure 3C). Furthermore, it could be shown that the glucuronidation of CDCA was not only inhibited by bilirubin, but that conversely, the glucuronidation of bilirubin was inhibited by 40% in the presence of 1 mM CDCA at pH 6.7. These studies suggest that in human liver bile acids, bilirubin and oestradiol may be glucuronidated by the same enzyme, whereas morphine and testosterone may be substrates for a separate or different form(s) of UDP-glucuronyltransferase(s). However, definite proof can only be obtained from specificity studies with the purified UDP-glucuronyltransferase, which are now in progress.

The inhibition of bile acid UDP-glucuronyltransferase activity by bilirubin and oestradiol, and conversely the inhibition of bilirubin UDP-glucuronyltransferase activity by CDCA, might be of pathogenic significance. During

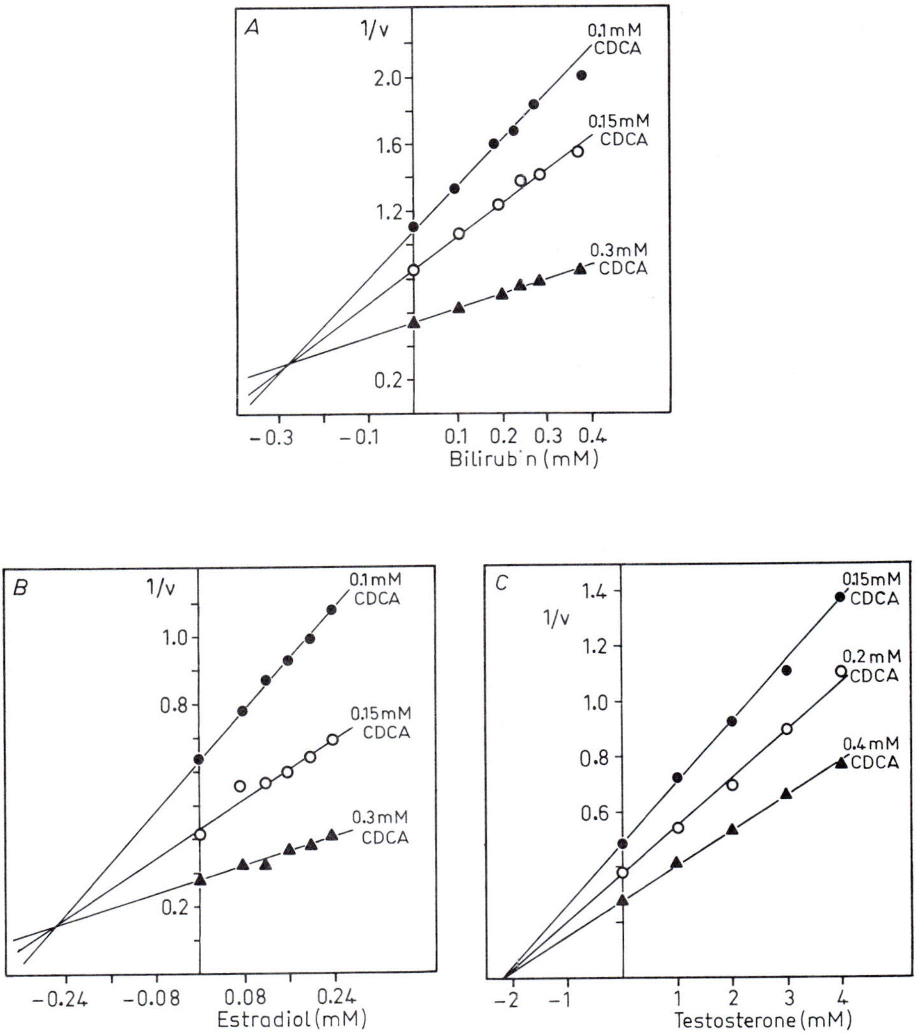

Figure 3 Inhibition of bile acid UDP-glucuronyltransferase by bilirubin (A), oestradiol-17β (B) and testosterone (C) (Dixon plots). The concentrations of CDCA used are shown in the figure. Bilirubin, oestradiol and testosterone were dissolved as described in the legend to Table 2. For the determination of enzyme activity, see Material and Methods. Triton X-100 was added to the reaction mixtures in a final concentration of 0.01% (v/v) (v = nmol h^{-1} mg $protein^{-1}$)

treatment of patients with CDCA for gallstone dissolution unconjugated bilirubin was found to be elevated in serum[10,11]. One explanation for this finding could be that CDCA competes with bilirubin for the active site of UDP-glucuronyltransferase resulting in decreased bilirubin glucuronidation. Whether or not the inhibition of the glucuronidation of bile acids by bilirubin and oestradiol plays a pathogenic role in the development or maintenance of cholestasis seen during pregnancy or oral contraceptive therapy has to be clarified.

Acknowledgments

This work was supported by the Deutsche Forschungsgemeinschaft (Grant no. De 113/26-3). The excellent technical assistance of Mrs Ch. Schelzig is gratefully acknowledged.

References

1. Back, P., Spaczinski, K. and Gerok, W. (1974). Bile-salt glucuronides in urine. *Hoppe-Seyler's Z. Physiol. Chem.*, **355**, 749
2. Fröhling, W. and Stiehl, A. (1975). Bile salt glucuronides in man: identification and quantitative analysis. In Matern, S., Hackenschmidt, J., Back, P. and Gerok, W. (eds.). *Advances in Bile Acid Research*, pp. 153–156. (Stuttgart: Schattauer)
3. Matern, H., Matern, S., Schelzig, Ch. and Gerok, W. (1980). Bile acid UDP-glucuronyltransferase from human liver. Properties and studies on aglycone substrate specificity. *FEBS Lett.*, **118**, 251
4. Winsnes, A. (1969). Studies on the activation in vitro of glucuronyltransferase. *Biochim. Biophys. Acta*, **191**, 279
5. Black, M., Billing, B. H. and Heirwegh, K. P. M. (1970). Determination of bilirubin UDP-glucuronyltransferase activity in needle-biopsy specimens of human liver. *Clin. Chim. Acta*, **29**, 27
6. Dutton, G. J. (1966). The biosynthesis of glucuronides. In Dutton, G. J. (ed.). *Glucuronic Acid*, pp. 185–299. (New York: Academic Press)
7. Dutton, G. J. and Burchell, B. (1977). Newer aspects of glucuronidation. In Bridges, J. W. and Chasseaud, L. F. (eds.). *Progress in Drug Metabolism*. Vol. 2, p. 1. (London: John Wiley)
8. Bock, K. W., Brunner, G., Hoensch, H. and Josting, D. (1978). Determination of microsomal UDP-glucuronyltransferase in needle-biopsy specimens of human liver. *Eur. J. Clin. Pharmacol.*, **14**, 367
9. Matern, S. and Gerok, W. (1979). Pathophysiology of the enterohepatic circulation of bile acids. *Rev. Physiol. Biochem. Pharmacol.*, **85**, 125
10. Thistle, J. L. and Hofmann, A. F. (1973). Efficacy and specificity of chenodeoxycholic acid therapy for dissolving gallstones. *N. Engl. J. Med.*, **289**, 655
11. Capron, J. P., Dupas, J. L., Capron-Chivrac, D., Aubin, J. B. and Delamarre, J. (1979). Unconjugated hyperbilirubinaemia during treatment with chenodeoxycholic acid. *Gastroenterology*, **77**, 121

16
Bile acid kinetics in pregnancy and in women receiving contraceptive steroids (CS)

F. KERN, Jr., G. EVERSON, B. DEMARK,
P. A. SZCZEPANIK AND P. KLEIN

For several years we have studied the mechanisms by which pregnancy and contraceptive steroids (CS) increase the risk of cholesterol gallstones. As part of a larger study, bile acid kinetic studies have been completed in 16 non-pregnant young women, 18 pregnant women, and 9 taking CS (1 mg norethindrone and 0.05 mg mestranol). All subjects were young (20–30), Caucasian, and non-obese. We gave [^{13}C]cholic acid (CA) and [^{13}C]chenodeoxycholic acid (CDCA) orally and measured isotope ratios by GC/MS of duodenal bile acids daily for 4–5 days. Bile acid kinetics were calculated according to Lindstedt.

RESULTS

In both groups of experimental subjects the total bile acid pool was significantly larger than in non-pregnant controls (controls 72.4 ± 4.9 μmole/kg, CS 103.8 ± 8.1, $p<0.005$; pregnant 110.1 ± 10.6, $p<0.004$). In non-pregnant women the CA pool was 28.2 ± 2.9 compared with 42.9 ± 4.9 ($p<0.01$) in those taking CS and 50.9 ± 5.2 ($p< <0.001$) in pregnant subjects. There was no serial change during pregnancy. CDCA pool size, on the other hand, responded differently. It was 28.8 ± 1.9 mole/kg in non-pregnant women, 37.1 ± 4.1 (p = n.s.) in those taking CS and in pregnant subjects it was larger than in control subjects only in the first trimester (46.6 ± 6.7, $p<0.02$). In the second and third trimesters it was 33.0 ± 2.9 and 30.0 ± 5.3, respectively (p = n.s.). The fractional turnover rate (FTR) of both bile acids was slower in both groups than in non-pregnant subjects. Throughout pregnancy CA FTR was significantly lower than in controls, but CDCA FTR was significantly slower only in the second trimester. CA synthesis rate was 28% higher in the CS and 35% higher during pregnancy than in control subjects. The synthesis rate of CDCA was not affected by CS. It was the same during pregnancy as in control subjects except that it was lower in the second trimester (control 8.8 ± 0.9 mole kg^{-1} day^{-1}; second trimester 4.9 ± 0.5, $p<0.005$).

The change in ratio of CA to CDCA in the bile acid pool may affect the coupling of biliary lipids during secretion, causing an increase in biliary cholesterol secretion.

17
Lithocholate sulphation as a predictor of chenodeoxycholate-induced serum transaminase elevations

L. J. SCHOENFIELD, S. O. SUE, B. J. PEARLMAN,
J. W. MARKS, G. G. BONORRIS, P. VARADY AND
J. M. LACHIN

Chenodeoxycholic acid (CDCA), through its metabolite, lithocholic acid (LCA), is hepatotoxic in certain species. The significance of serum transaminase elevations in 25% of humans ingesting CDCA is unknown, but efficient hepatic sulphation of LCA may protect against hepatic injury.

AIM

To determine if a low capacity to sulphate LCA predisposes to CDC-induced transaminase elevations.

DESIGN

Pre-treatment sulphation capacity (SC) was estimated in 63 randomly selected gallstone patients in a double-blind randomized trial of CDCA, 750 or 375 mg/day or placebo; in 22 of these, SC was repeated at 1 year; in four, SC was done at 2 years only. SGOT and SGPT were determined every 3 months; elevation was defined as $>150\%$ of normal upper limit in asymptomatic patients.

METHODS

Ten μCi of [^{3}H]glyco-LCA (specific activity 40 mCi/mg) was ingested 10–12 h before fasting duodenal biliary drainage. Bile acids in bile were separated by thin-layer chromatography. SC was estimated as percentage of total radioactivity (scintillation counting) in sulphated glyco-LC. Standard deviation for duplicate SC determinations ($n = 89$) was 1.4%.

RESULTS

Pre-treatment SC (60.7 $\pm$ 1.7 SEM) exhibited a break in the population

SECTION 2
Absorption

18
Physical – chemical basis for dissimilar intraluminal solubilities and intestinal absorption efficiencies of chenodeoxycholic and ursodeoxycholic acids

M. C. CAREY AND H. IGIMI

INTRODUCTION

Organic chemists have customarily employed the term 'bile acid' as a generic term for the cholanoic class of biological compounds. It is our belief that the physiologist and clinician should confine the use of this term for the undissociated or protonated (HA) form of these compounds, whether conjugated or unconjugated, and to employ the term 'bile salt' to distinguish the dissociated or ionized bile acid anion (A^-), whether conjugated or unconjugated. This terminology may appear at first confusing, but a solid rationale for this distinction is seen when the general physical–chemical and pathophysiological properties of the bile acids (HA) are compared with these

Table 1 General properties of bile acids (HA) and bile salts (A^-)

	Bile acids (COOH)	*Bile salts* (COO^-/SO_3^-)
Class	polar lipid, class I – insoluble non-swelling amphiphile	polar lipid, class III – soluble amphiphile
Aqueous solubility	10^{-6}–0.5×10^{-3} mol/l	1–2 M (CMC; 0.6–5 mmol/l)
Organic solvent solubility	high in non-polar solvents; low in polar solvents	high in polar solvents; low in non-polar solvents
Membrane solubility	High; diffuses through, no solubilization	High; saturates and solubilizes
Micelles	Do not form (high solubility *in* micelles)	micelles form (high solubility *as* micelles)
Occurrence	colon $^{++++}$ portal vein $^{+}$ systemic blood $^{+}$ hepatocyte $^{+}$ bile $^{-}$	small bowel $^{++++}$ portal vein $^{+++}$ systemic blood $^{+}$ hepatocyte $^{+}$ bile $^{++++}$
Membrane toxicity	'Yes'	'No'

properties of bile salts (A^-) (Table 1). Protonated bile acids are very insoluble in water and hence neither form micelles nor act as detergent-like molecules. In contrast, the K^+ and Na^+ salts of the common bile acid anions are detergents which are very water-soluble by virtue of forming micelles. At the maximum monomeric solubility of the anions (the CMC) the solubilities of bile salts are 10–500-fold greater than the monomeric solubility of the corresponding protonated bile acids. At concentrations above the CMC, bile acids can be solubilized by bile salt micelles to form mixed micelles composed of the anions (A^-) and their acids (HA) and thus aqueous HA solubilities can be dramatically increased. For this reason, considerable quantities of bile acids can be solubilized in the biliary tree and in the gastrointestinal tract even though they would otherwise precipitate from solution. On account of the relatively high pK'_a values of all unconjugated and glycine conjugated bile salts (Table 2), the pH ranges over which the corresponding bile acids

Table 2 Dissociation constants of bile acids

$$pK'_a = \text{pH at which } \frac{50\%\ A^-(\text{salt})}{50\%\ \text{HA(acid)}}$$

pK'_a values

free bile acids	=	5–6.5
glycine conjugates	=	3.8–5.2
taurine conjugates	=	?(1.0–2.0)

pK'_a values of free bile acids
CDCA > DCA > UDCA > CA

pK'_a values of glycine conjugates
GDCA > GUDCA > GCDCA > GCA

precipitate (pHppt) from solution, fall within the pH range commonly experienced throughout the gastrointestinal tract (Table 3). Thus in the acid environment of the stomach, both unconjugated (free) and glycine-conjugated bile salts become protonated, exceed their aqueous solubilities and precipitate from solution. This occurs during oral bile acid therapy and during gastro-duodenal reflux of secreted bile. In the duodenum, free bile acids precipitate even at normal pH (5.0–6.5), e.g. in bacterial overgrowth syndromes and

Table 3 Equilibrium precipitation pH (pHppt) of bile acids

pHppt = pH at which system is saturated with [HA]aq + [HA]micellar

pHppt values (> CMC)

free bile acids	=	6.4–8.1
glycine conjugates	=	4.3–7.4
taurine conjugates	=	sol. at pH 1.0

pHppt of free bile acids
UDCA > CDCA > DCA > CA

pHppt of glycine conjugates
GUDCA > GCDCA = GDCA > GCA

during ingestion of unconjugated bile acids. A proportion of the glycine conjugates can also precipitate in certain disease states when the duodenum is more acid, such as in the Zollinger–Ellison syndrome and in chronic pancreatic insufficiency states of any aetiology. In the caecum and colon bacterial enzymatic action results in the formation of a considerable amount of deconjugated or free bile salts. The free bile acids will precipitate from solution when the colonic pH falls below their pHppt values (Table 3).

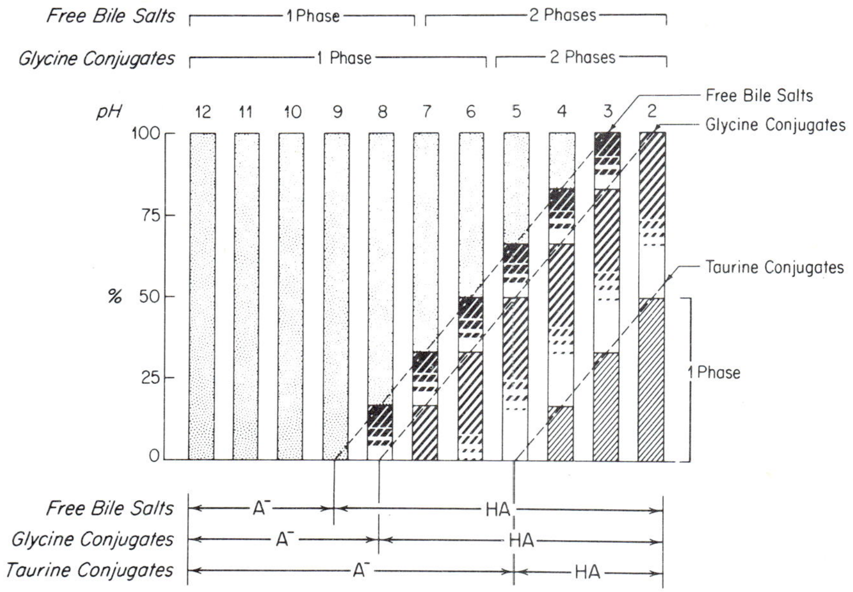

Figure 1 Equilibrium physical states and percentage of bile salts in ionized (A^-) and protonated (HA) form as a function of pH

Figure 1, which summarizes these concepts, is based upon *in vitro* titration studies of the common bile salts carried out by Ekwall and colleagues[1,2], Small[3] and Igimi and Carey[4]. From the graph plotted here, the percentage of free, glycine-, and taurine-conjugated bile salts which exist in ionized (A^-) and un-ionized (HA) form and the physical state of the systems can be readily estimated at all physiological pH values. It is apparent that when titrated with a mineral acid like HCl, protonation of free bile salts begins at pH 9.0, glycine conjugates at pH 8.0 and taurine conjugates at $\approx$pH 4.0–5.0. On account of the high solubility of bile acids in bile salt micelles, precipitation of the HA form (indicated by the two-phase bracket) does not commence until pH 7.25 $\pm$ 0.85 in the case of free bile salts, pH 5.85 $\pm$ 1.5 in the case of the glycine conjugates. However, even when partially protonated, taurine conjugates remain in micellar solution down to pH values as low as 1. Further, the pK'_a values of taurine conjugates are not known with certainty since they cannot be titrated to completion with HCl[3,4].

APPLICATION OF THESE PRINCIPLES TO THE SOLUBILITIES OF CHENODEOXYCHOLIC ACID (CDCA) AND URSODEOXYCHOLIC ACID (UDCA)

Because both cholelitholytic bile acids are administered orally in the unconjugated form and since the sodium salts of UDCA and its conjugates display a poorer capacity than the sodium salts of the CDCA species to solubilize cholesterol, it became important to study the ionization properties and physical state of these systems as a function of pH in order to determine if differences existed in the micellar solubilization of their bile acids. We studied the free (unconjugated) species as well as their glycine conjugates by potentiometric titration with HCl. The methods and results have been detailed in an earlier publication[4] and only the pertinent findings will be summarized here.

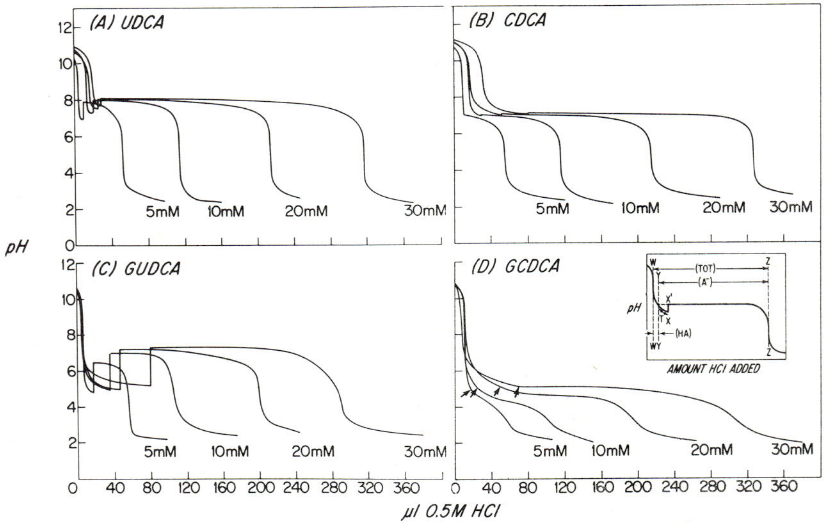

Figure 2 Potentiometric titration curves of free and glycine (G)-conjugated chenodeoxycholic (CDCA) and ursodeoxycholic (UDCA) acids. Inset in (D): typical titration curve for free and glycine-conjugated bile acids with notation as explained in the text. The arrows on the GCDCA curves (D) indicate the point of HA precipitation

Figure 2 shows potentiometric titration curves for all four bile salts in H_2O at 37 °C. The inset in panel (D) represents a hypothetical titration curve for the titration with HCl of an unconjugated or glycine-conjugated bile salt in concentrations above its CMC. The amount of HCl added between points W and Z represents the total amount of HCl (TOT) required to titrate an equivalent amount of bile salt. This chemical reaction is shown by the equation

$$NA^+A^- + HCl \rightarrow HA + Na^+Cl^- \quad (1)$$

If such an experiment is carried out under equilibrium conditions the total moles of HCl consumed between points W and Z, divided by the total moles of bile salt added (from the gravimetric and molecular weights) should be unity. As the titration is continued past the point Y, the titration curve becomes concave. In the region marked T, the solution displays a bluish opalescence (Tyndall effect) and at point X without, further addition of HCl, the pH rises sharply to an equilibrium value of X′. At this pH the solution becomes a two-phase system composed of precipitated HA crystals and A^- micelles containing solubilized HA molecules. More and more HA crystals are precipitated with further additions of HCl. Since these added protons precipitate as part of the insoluble (HA) phase, the pH demonstrates a plateau, i.e. the two-phase system behaves as a buffer. Between points Y and X, the one-phase solution is supersaturated with HA and not in thermodynamic equilibrium. Therefore, extrapolation of the plateau section of the curve to the initial concave part, i.e. from point X′ to point Y, gives the pH at which HA precipitation would have occurred in the theoretical absence of supersaturation. Provided the total bile salt concentration is above the CMC, this gives a good estimate of the solubility of HA (W–Y) in the system, i.e. in micelles of A^- (Y–Z) plus the intermicellar solution. If the bile salt concentration is below the CMC, the amount of HCl consumed from W–Y provides an estimate of the true aqueous solubility of HA. The theoretical curve is reproduced faithfully in the titration curves of CDCA, UDCA and GUDCA (G prefix indicates glycine conjugate) (A, B and C respectively) but not in the case of GCDCA (D) where no supersaturation is observed. The arrows point to the region on these curves where a strong Tyndall effect was first observed and which was taken as the point of HA precipitation. Finally, each curve can be employed to estimate the pK'_a of the particular bile salt from the formula proposed by Back and Steenberg:

$$pK'_a = pHy + \log \frac{HA}{TOT\text{-}HA} + \frac{0.5\sqrt{\mu}}{1 + \sqrt{\mu}} \quad (2)$$

where pHy is the pH at point Y (Figure 2D), HA is the amount of HCl added from point W to Y, TOT is the total amount of HCl required to carry the reaction in equation 1 to completion, i.e. from W to Z, and μ is the total solute ionic strength at point Y.

The equilibrium pHppt values and apparent pK (pK'_a) values for all four bile salts as functions of bile salt concentration (H_2O, 37 °C) are plotted in Figure 3. For comparable bile salt concentrations, the HA species of UDCA and GUDCA precipitate at higher pH values than the HA species of CDCA and GCDCA despite similar pK'_a values. The physical–chemical reason why the pHppt of the UDCA and GUDCA species should be greater by ≈ 2 pH units than the corresponding pK'_a values in contrast <1 pH unit difference in the case of CDCA and GCDCA can be appreciated from the plot in Figure 4. Here, equilibrium bile acid (HA) solubilities are shown as functions of the total bile salt concentration. The curves show break points at the apparent CMCs of each bile salt; thereafter, linear increases in HA solubilities occur. Above the CMC, HA solubility increases dramatically in the case of GCDCA and CDCA, but with UDCA and GUDCA, HA solubility increases only slightly. Below the apparent CMC values the horizontal slopes give an estimate of the HA solubilities in water. These values are close to those

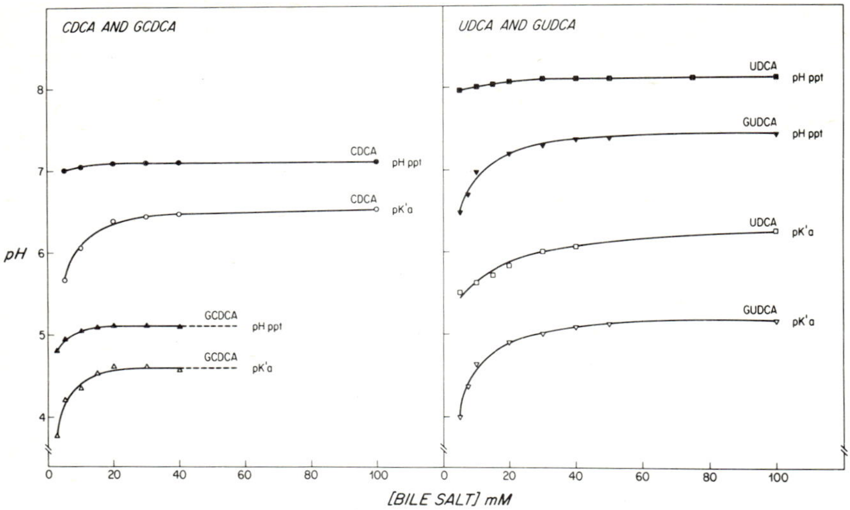

Figure 3 Equilibrium precipitation pH (pHppt) and apparent p*K* (pK'_a) values as functions of bile salt concentration (H_2O, 37 °C)

derived directly (37 °C, pH 2.4) employing radiolabelled compounds (CDCA: 256 μmol/l, UDCA, 53 μmol/l). Above the apparent CMC values the slopes of the curves provide an estimate of the mean bile salt : bile acid saturation ratios in the micelles, i.e. the number of bile salt molecules required to carry one HA molecule in micellar solution. These calculations show that five or six molecules of GCDCA and CDCA, but 235 and 90 GUDCA and UDCA molecules, respectively, are required to carry one HA molecule in aqueous solution. Therefore, since UDCA and GUDCA micelles are saturated with their respective HA species much more readily than micelles or CDCA and GCDCA, the pHppt of the former are appreciably higher than the latter since protonation of both species begins at the same pH (Figure 2).

It is our belief that these electrochemical differences are quite important pathophysiologically. For example when titrated in a bile salt mixture composed of UDCA and CDCA conjugates or a normal conjugated bile salt mixture with and without lecithin or mono-olein, UDCA is much less soluble than CDCA and in addition induces the systems to gel at ≈ pH 6.6–6.8. In contrast, CDCA when titrated in artificial bile does not induce gel formation and HA precipitation occurs at a lower pH. These studies alone would preclude the use of the sodium salt of UDCA as a direct intraductal gallstone solvent. Such considerations also suggest that absorption of orally administered UDCA from the duodeno-jejunum may not be as efficient as CDCA since dissolution in a conjugated bile salt mixture at duodenal pH would be slow or impossible. Further, as is well known, CDCA is a powerful colonic secretagogue whereas UDCA is not. Based on our *in vitro* results, we can hypothesize that at a bulk aqueous colonic pH of ≈7, UDCA will be precipitated completely from solution as insoluble HA crystals with only ≈53 μmol/l of the HA species remaining in the aqueous phase (Figure 5).

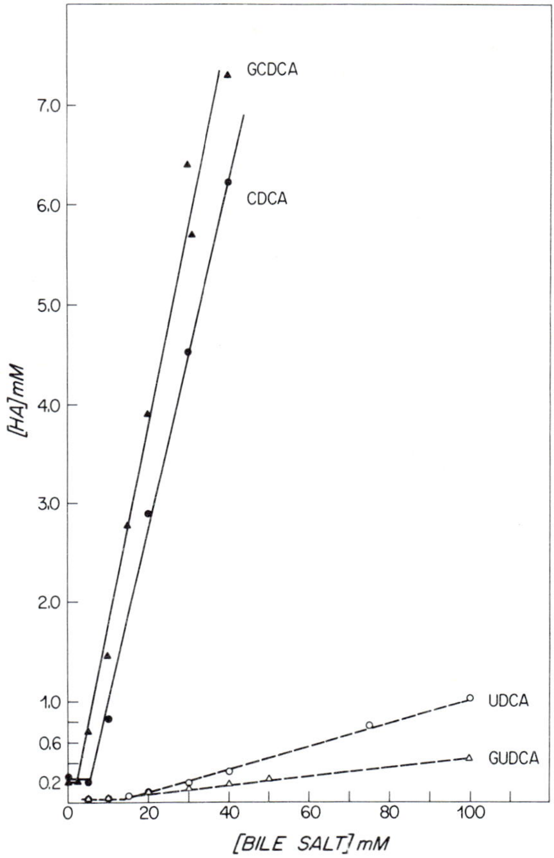

Figure 4 Equilibrium bile acid (HA) solubilities as functions of bile salt concentration (H_2O, 37 °C)

Under the same conditions CDCA remains quite soluble, both as A^- micelles saturated with HA and as monomeric A^- (the CMC, 1–2 mmol/l) and HA (256 μmol/l) in the intermicellar solution. Since bile salt solubility is necessary for the exhibition of secretogenic properties, these considerations provide a physical–chemical hypothesis for the infrequent occurrence of diarrhoea in patients on UDCA therapy for gallstone dissolution.

THE IMPORTANT EFFECTS OF CALCIUM IONS ON GUDCA AND GCDCA SOLUBILITIES

Because the glycine to taurine ratio of conjugated bile salts in bile increases markedly with prolonged bile acid therapy, it is theoretically possible that the free bile acids or the calcium salts of GUDCA or GCDCA might precipitate from bile onto the surface of gallstones and retard if not terminate dissolution.

This idea is further supported by the clinical observation that partial dissolution of radiolucent gallstones is far more common than complete dissolution, and the anecdotal reports that calcified shells may appear on the surface of gallstones in a small percentage of patients during both CDCA and UDCA dissolution therapy. We therefore carried out potentiometric studies of 100 mmol/l GUDCA and GCDCA solutions in the presence of 5 mmol/l $CaCl_2$ in 0.15 mol/l NaCl at 37 °C. We found that this concentration of calcium actually 'salted in' GUDCA by lowering the pHppt from 7.4 to 7.2, doubling the solubility of the HA species in GUDCA micelles and inducing a depression of the pK'_a (7.2 *vs.* 7.4). In contrast, 5 mmol/l $CaCl_2$ induced a 100 mmol/l GCDCA solution (0.15 mol/l NaCl, 37 °C) to gel and precipitate at pH 5.1. Further when the solutions were held at pH 8, precipitation of solid crystals occurred in 100 mmol/l GCDCA solutions (0.15 mol/l NaCl, 37 °C) with the addition of 10 mmol/l $CaCl_2$ and these crystalline precipitates were shown to be the calcium salts of GCDCA. In contrast equimolar concentrations of GUDCA under the same conditions could not be precipitated with 20 mmol/l $CaCl_2$. Furthermore, when precipitation of GUDCA was induced by lowering the pH, the crystals were shown to be that of the protonated acid form of GUDCA and not the calcium salt. We predict that if glycine-conjugated bile salts precipitate from bile or gut luminal contents, it is likely that the calcium salts of GCDCA and the protonated acid form of GUDCA will precipitate. This is consonant with the well-known observation that the more polar an ionic amphiphile the less well it binds Ca^{2+} ions. In this regard, GUDCA has been shown by a number of chromato-

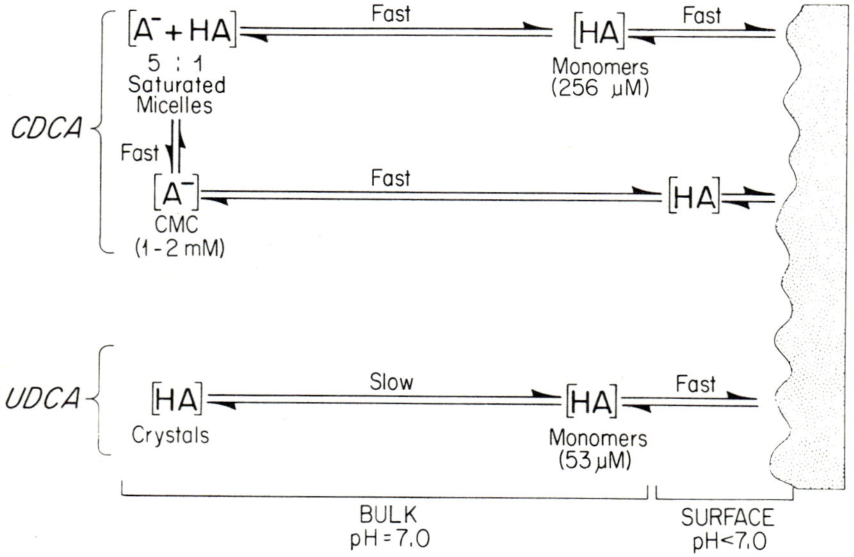

Figure 5 Hypothetical physical states of UDCA and CDCA in the colonic lumen at a bulk pH of 7.0 (see text for explanation)

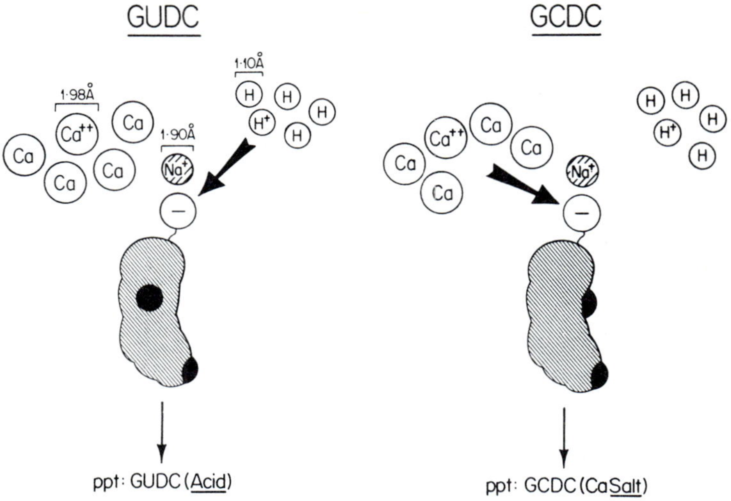

Figure 6 Competition of Ca^{2+} and H^{+} ions for the carboxylate groups of GCDCA and GUDCA. As the pH of the systems is lowered below ≈pH 7.1–7.2 in the presence of added Ca^{2+}, our experiments suggest that the calcium salt of GCDCA and the HA form of GUDCA precipitate

graphic methods to be much more polar than GCDCA[6]. The relevance of these *in vitro* observations to the deployment of UDCA and CDCA in gallstone dissolution must await future studies. However, it is likely that the electrochemical and molecular logic of the molecules will be expressed clinically.

Acknowledgments

Figures 2–5 are reproduced from Ref. 4 with permission of the copyright owner, Lipid Research, Inc. Supported in part by NIH Research Grant AM 18559 and Research Career Development Award AM 00195 (M. C. Carey). Dr I. Igimi's permanent address is Department of Surgery, Fukuoka University School of Medicine, Fukuoka, Japan.

References

1. Ekwall, P., Rosendahl, T. and Löfmann, N. (1957). Studies on bile acid salt solutions. I. The dissociation constant of the cholic and desoxycholic acids. *Acta Chem. Scand.*, **11,** 590
2. Ekwall, P., Rosendahl, T. and Sten, A. (1958). Studies on bile acid salt solutions. II. The solubility of cholic acid in sodium cholate solutions and that of desoxycholic acid in sodium desoxycholate solutions. *Acta Chem. Scand.*, **12,** 1622
3. Small, D. M. (1971). The physical chemistry of cholanic acids. In Nair, P. P. and Kritchevsky, D. (eds.). *The Bile Acids*, vol. 1, pp. 249–356. (New York: Plenum Press)
4. Igimi, H. and Carey, M. C. (1980). pH-solubility relations of chenodeoxycholic and ursodeoxycholic acids: physical–chemical basis for dissimilar solution and membrane phenomena. *J. Lipid Res.*, **21,** 72

5. Back, E. and Steenberg, B. (1950). Simultaneous determination of ionization constant, solubility product and solubility for slightly soluble acids and bases. Electrolytic constants for abietic acid. *Acta Chem. Scand.*, **4,** 810
6. Carey, M. C., Montet, J.-C., Phillips, M. C., Armstrong, M. J. and Mazer, N. A. (1981). Thermodynamic and molecular basis for dissimilar cholesterol solubilizing capacities by micellar solutions of bile salts: the cases of sodium chenodeoxycholate, sodium ursodeoxycholate and their glycine and taurine conjugates. *Biochemistry* (in press)

19
The influence of bile acid pool composition on the regulation of cholesterol absorption

M. PONZ DE LEON AND N. CARULLI

INTRODUCTION

It has been well documented, in the last few years, that the administration of either chenodeoxycholic acid (CDCA) or ursodeoxycholic acid (UDCA) causes a reduction of biliary cholesterol secretion, a decrease of bile saturation and may induce the dissolution of gallstones[1–5]. It has been suggested that all these effects could be due to the inhibition of hepatic cholesterogenesis, since the activity of hydroxymethyl-glutaryl coenzyme A (HMG-CoA) reductase, the rate-limiting enzyme in cholesterol synthesis[6], has been found constantly reduced during CDCA treatment[7,8] (both in animals and man) and, according to some authors at least, also during long-term UDCA therapy[9,10].

However, several recent observations cast some doubt on this interpretation of the data. Thus it has been shown by two independent groups that only a small fraction of biliary cholesterol (20–30%) is newly synthesized in the liver, the major portion coming from other sources, i.e. serum lipoproteins[11,12]. Similarly, no relation has been found, in the rat, between the rate of hepatic cholesterogenesis and the secretion of biliary cholesterol[13]. Furthermore, during treatment with CDCA no relation has been found between biliary cholesterol secretion and HMG-CoA reductase activity[14]. Finally, in the past few years evidence has been provided, by Dietschy and co-workers, that bile acids *per se* do not seem to affect the rate of hepatic cholesterogenesis[15]. Taken together these observations strongly suggest that CDCA and UDCA might have other mechanisms of action in desaturating bile and dissolving gallstones.

On the other hand, recent studies have shown that feeding large amounts of cholesterol may induce a supersaturation of bile both in animals and man[16]; consequently, it is not surprising that a decrease of bile saturation has been reported during the administration of β-sitosterol, which competitively inhibits cholesterol absorption[17]. These and other observations stimulated us to investigate the effect of CDCA and UDCA feeding on the absorption of dietary cholesterol. The study has been subsequently extended to deoxycholic acid (DCA) and cholic acid (CA) in order to provide a complete picture of the effect of individual bile acid pool expansion on the absorption of dietary cholesterol.

METHODS AND RESULTS

The design of the first part of our study is shown in Table 1. Twenty-two volunteers, most of whom were patients with gallstones, were hospitalized

Table 1 Protocol I. Twenty-two volunteers were put on a standard diet containing a constant amount of calories and cholesterol per day

Days	*Procedures*
1	Given a standard breakfast with 500 mg cholesterol 5 μCi [^{14}C]cholesterol 10 μCi [^{3}H]sitosterol faecal samples collected for 4–6 days and cholesterol absorption estimated from the recovered radioactivity
6–7	CDCA (11 patients) or UDCA (11) administration started (15 mg kg^{-1} day^{-1})
25–27	Cholesterol absorption restudied
Serum lipids, biliary lipid and bile acid composition also studied before and after treatment	

and put on a standard diet providing a constant amount of cholesterol and calories per day. After approximately 1 week, on the first day of the study, the patients were given a standard breakfast containing 500 mg of cholesterol, 5 μCi of [^{14}C]cholesterol and 10 μCi of [^{3}H]sitosterol, the latter as a non-absorbable marker to correct losses of cholesterol not due to absorption. On this day no other food containing cholesterol was given to the patients. All faecal samples were then collected and dietary cholesterol absorption was estimated from the recovered radioactivity[18]. After faecal samples collection, on the 7th day of the study 11 patients were put on CDCA and 11 on UDCA, both at the dose of 15 mg kg^{-1} day^{-1}. After approximately 3 weeks of treatment cholesterol absorption was restudied in each patient. Serum lipids, biliary lipids and bile acid composition were also studied before and after treatment.

As expected the fed bile acid became the most abundant in the pool, whereas the fraction of the other bile acids was markedly reduced. Bile cholesterol saturation, calculated according to Carey[19], was significantly reduced after both treatments. Serum cholesterol and triglyceride levels were virtually unaffected by both bile acids feeding. Figure 1 summarizes the effect of bile acid feeding on dietary cholesterol absorption expressed as a percentage of the administered dose. Treatment of either CDCA or UDCA was associated with a reduction of dietary cholesterol absorption in almost all patients, from a mean pre-treatment value of approximately 35–40% to a mean post-treatment value of 15–20% of the given dose, the difference being statistical significant at 1% levels[20,21].

This first part of the study can be summarized as follows: when given in doses effective to desaturate bile and dissolve gallstones, both CDCA and UDCA cause a marked reduction of dietary cholesterol absorption, in the order of 50% of the administered dose. We speculated that this effect could probably contribute to the desaturating properties of these two bile acids.

In the second part of the study we tried to define the possible mechanisms whereby CDCA and UDCA depress dietary cholesterol absorption. A second

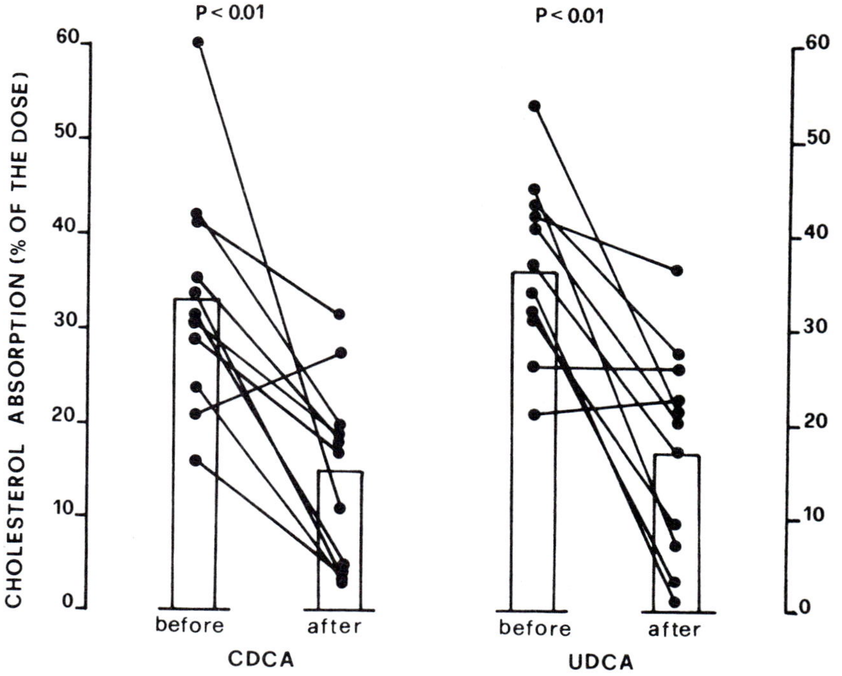

Figure 1 Effect of CDCA and UDCA feeding on dietary cholesterol absorption.

purpose was also to discover whether this effect on cholesterol absorption could be related to bile desaturation.

In theory, treatment with CDCA or UDCA could decrease cholesterol absorption by several mechanisms. First, these two bile acids could directly damage the intestinal mucosa, leading to a decreased absorption. This interpretation seemed to us improbable since, to our knowledge, gastro-intestinal lesions have not been reported in patients treated with bile acids and, in addition, malabsorption of other nutrients has never been documented. Second, CDCA and UDCA could reduce cholesterol absorption by decreasing the intestinal transit time, which animal studies have suggested to be one of the factors regulating cholesterol absorption[22]. Indeed, the pattern of faecal sterol excretion in patients treated with CDCA suggested that the administration of this bile acid could have decreased the intestinal transit time; however, sterol excretion was entirely normal with UDCA[21], so that this interpretation seems hardly tenable, though the problem deserves further study. Third, the presence of large amounts of free bile acids in the upper intestine (as is the case in patients treated with bile acids) could theoretically lead to an impaired micellar solubilization of cholesterol and, ultimately, to cholesterol malabsorption[20]. This possibility seems even more pertinent for UDCA, whose capacity to solubilize lipids into mixed micelles is less than the other bile acids[19]. However, preliminary studies in our laboratory, in which cholesterol absorption has been studied after single doses of CDCA without any pretreatment with bile acids, showed no changes of the absorption values (unpublished observations), making this interpretation unlikely. Finally, CDCA and UDCA might decrease cholesterol absorption by reducing the size of the CA pool, an event which has been constantly observed during the administration of dihydroxy bile acids. In this respect, animal studies have shown that feeding CA leads to an increase of cholesterol absorption, an effect which has not been usually observed with dihydroxylated bile acids.

We focused our attention on this last hypothetical mechanism and, consequently, we studied the effect of either DCA (another dihydroxy bile acid) or CA pool expansion on dietary cholesterol absorption in man.

Table 2 Protocol II. Twenty-one volunteers (11 male, 20 female; age range 23–65) were put on a standard diet containing a constant amount of cholesterol and calories per day

Days	*Procedures*
1	cholesterol absorption studied
5–7	administration of 5–10 μCi of [^{14}C]CA or DCA duodenal intubation bile lipid composition bile acid composition bile acid pool size
8–9	started treatment with bile acids
30–35	cholesterol absorption, bile lipid composition, bile acid composition and pool size restudied in each subject

The protocol of the study is shown in Table 2. Twenty-one volunteers, most of whom were patients with gallstones, were put on a standard diet as in the previous study. On the first day of the investigation labelled sterols were given and cholesterol absorption was studied as already described. After complete recovery of the labelled sterols, patients were given 5 μCi of [^{14}C]CA or DCA at 8 pm. On the following morning a bile sample was taken, bile composition was studied with standard techniques[23], bile acid composition by GLC, total and individual bile acid pool size following the isotope dilution principle (as recently described by Duane *et al.*[24]). Thereafter eight patients started to ingest DCA (15 mg kg^{-1} day^{-1}); nine patients were given oral ampicillin (2–4 g daily) for 4 days, then CA was added (15 mg kg^{-1} day^{-1}). We reasoned that the contemporary administration of CA plus broad-spectrum antibiotics could suffice to expand CA pool size by inhibiting many strains of intestinal bacteria responsible for the degradation of CA to DCA. Indeed, in previous studies in which CA was given alone the fraction of DCA in the pool was often greater than that of CA, so that bile did not enrich consistently with trihydroxylated bile acids. Finally, four patients were given ampicillin alone.

The effect of bile acid feeding on biliary bile acid composition, expressed as percentages of total, are shown in Table 3. As expected, after DCA feeding this became the most abundant bile acid, whereas the fraction of the others was significantly reduced. Similarly, after CA plus ampicillin the fraction of

Table 3 Effect of DCA and CA pool expansion on total bile acid pool size, bile acid composition, cholesterol absorption and bile saturation

Treatments	*Total bile acid pool* (mg)		*DCA* (% of total)		*CA* (% of total)		*CDCA* (% of total)		*Cholesterol absorption* (%)		*Saturation index* (Carey)	
	B	*A*	*B*	*A*	*B*	*A*	*B*	*A*	*B*	*A*	*B*	*A*
DCA Mean ± SD	2921 ± 882	3145 ± 1720	21 ± 10	78 ± 12	31 ± 10	8.0 ± 7	48 ± 12	11 ± 6	38 ± 12	19 ± 6	1.53 ± 0.40	2.38 ± 0.7
CA + Ampicillin	2492 ± 1475	4589 ± 1589	15 ± 8	22 ± 12	34 ± 15	60 ± 18	41 ± 9	13 ± 7	29 ± 7	46 ± 11	1.21 ± 0.21	0.92 ± 0.20

B = before treatment; *A* = after treatment

CA in the pool increased, reaching nearly 60% of the total; again the fraction of the other bile acids was more or less reduced.

DCA feeding did not affect total bile acid pool size (Table 3) but, as expected, DCA pool size increased 5-fold, reaching 80% of total. In contrast, total bile acid pool was significantly increased after CA + ampicillin (Table 3), and this was mainly due to a 3-fold increase of CA pool.

Dietary cholesterol absorption was significantly reduced ($p < 0.01$) after DCA feeding, from a mean of 38 ± 12% to a mean of 19.0 ± 6.0 of the administered dose, thus, DCA feeding caused a reduction of cholesterol absorption of the same order of magnitude as that seen after CDCA or UDCA. In contrast, CA pool expansion was associated with a significant rise of cholesterol absorption in all treated patients, from 29 ± 7.0% to a mean post-treatment value of 46 ± 11% of the given dose (Table 3, $p < 0.02$).

In the four investigated patients, ampicillin feeding did not induce any consistent change of dietary cholesterol absorption.

Table 3 also shows the effect of DCA and CA pool expansion on bile lipid composition, expressed as 'saturation index' and calculated according to Carey[19]. DCA pool expansion was associated with a significant increase of bile saturation (1.53 ± 0.40 before and 2.38 ± 0.7 after treatment); in contrast, a significant reduction of bile saturation was observed after CA pool expansion (1.21 ± 0.21 before and 0.92 ± 0.20 after treatment) ($p < 0.02$ for both bile acids feeding).

SUMMARY AND CONCLUSIONS

CDCA, UDCA and DCA pool expansion is associated with a significant reduction of dietary cholesterol absorption but with different effects on bile saturation, since CDCA and UDCA desaturate bile, whereas DCA tends to supersaturate bile or, according to other authors[25], does not induce any change. The expansion of CA pool size increases dietary cholesterol absorption and bile saturation tends to decrease (though with a large inter-individual variation).

In conclusion: dietary cholesterol absorption, in man, is closely dependent on bile acid pool composition. When bile enriches with dihydroxy bile acids and the fraction of trihydroxylated bile acids decreases, cholesterol absorption tends to decrease. In contrast, when CA pool size is selectively expanded dietary cholesterol absorption tends to rise. It follows that the size of CA pool probably plays a key role in promoting cholesterol absorption, presumably owing to its specific effect on the intestinal cholesterol esterase, as many animal studies have indicated[26]. The action of individual bile acid feeding on cholesterol absorption cannot explain the effect of CDCA and UDCA on bile saturation and gallstone dissolution.

REFERENCES

1. Danzinger, R. G., Hofmann, A. F., Thistle, J. L. *et al.* (1973). Effect of oral chenodeoxycholic acid on bile acid kinetics and biliary lipid composition in women with cholelithiasis. *J. Clin. Invest.*, **52,** 2809

2. Mok, H. Y. I., Bell, G. C. and Dowling, R. H. (1974). Effect of different doses of chenodeoxycholic acid on bile lipid composition and on the frequency of side effects in patients with gallstones. *Lancet*, **2,** 253
3. Northfield, T. C., LaRusso, N. F., Hofmann, A. F. *et al.* (1975). Effect of chenodeoxycholic acid treatment in gallstone patients. *Gut*, **16,** 12.
4. Makino, I. and Nakagawa, S. (1978). Changes of biliary lipids and biliary bile acid composition in patients after administration of ursodeoxycholic acid. *J. Lipid Res.*, **19,** 723
5. Stiehl, A., Czygan, P. and Kommerel, B. *et al.* (1978). Ursodeoxycholic acid versus chenodeoxycholic acid. Comparison of their effects on bile lipid composition in patients with gallstones. *Gastroenterology*, **75,** 1016
6. Wilson, J. D. (1972). The role of bile acid in the overall regulation of steroid metabolism. *Arch. Intern. Med.*, **130,** 493
7. Coyne, M. J., Bonorris, G. G., Goldstein, L. J. *et al.* (1976). Effect of chenodeoxycholic acid and phenobarbital on the rate-limiting enzymes of hepatic cholesterol and bile acid synthesis in patients with gallstones. *J. Lab. Clin. Med.*, **87,** 281
8. Carulli, N., Zironi, F., Ponz de Leon, M. *et al.* (1978). Comparative effects of short term feeding of chenodeoxycholic acid and ursodeoxycholic acid on hepatic sterol metabolism in man (Abstr.). *Gut*, **19,** A994
9. Maton, P. N., Murphy, G. M. and Dowling, R. H. (1977). Ursodeoxycholic acid treatment of gallstones. Dose–response study and possible mechanism of action. *Lancet*, **2,** 1297
10. Fedorowski, T., Salen, G., Zaki, F. G. *et al.* (1978). Comparative effects of ursodeoxycholic acid and chenodeoxycholic acid in the rhesus monkey. *Gastroenterology*, **74,** 75
11. Schwartz, C. C., Halloran, L. G., Vlahcevic, Z. R. *et al.* (1978). Multicompartimental analysis of cholesterol metabolism in man. Characterization of the hepatic bile acid and biliary cholesterol precursor sites. *J. Clin. Invest.*, **61,** 408
12. Long, T. T., Jacoi, L., Stevens, R. *et al.* (1978). The sources of rat biliary cholesterol and bile acid. *J. Lipid Res.*, **19,** 872
13. Key, P. H., Bonorris, G. G., Marks, J. W. *et al.* (1978). Mechanisms of cholesterol desaturation of bile by chenodeoxycholic acid in gallstone patients (Abstr.). *Gastroenterology*, **74,** 1161
14. Turley, S. D. and Dietschy, J. M. (1978). Regulation of biliary cholesterol output in the rat: dissociation from the rate of cholesterol synthesis and the size of the cholesterol esters pool in the liver (abstr.). *Gastroenterology*, **74,** 1106
15. Nervi, F. O. and Dietschy, J. M. (1978). The mechanisms of the inter-relationship between bile acid and chylomicron mediated regulation of hepatic cholesterol synthesis in the liver of the rat. *J. Clin. Invest.*, **61,** 895
16. DenBesten, L., Connor, W. E. and Shieleybell, B. S. (1973). The effect of dietary cholesterol on the composition of human bile. *Surgery*, **73,** 266
17. Begemann, F., Bandomer, G. and Herget, H. J. (1978). The influence of beta-sitosterol on biliary cholesterol saturation and bile acid kinetics in man. *Scand. J. Gastroenterol.*, **13,** 57
18. Borgstrom, B. (1969). Quantification of cholesterol absorption in man by faecal analysis after the feeding of a single isotope-labelled meal. *J. Lipid Res.*, **10,** 331
19. Carey, M. C. (1978). Critical tables for calculating the cholesterol saturation of native bile. *J. Lipid Res.*, **19,** 945
20. Ponz de Leon, M., Carulli, N., Loria, P. *et al.* (1979). The effect of chenodeoxycholic acid (CDCA) on cholesterol absorption. *Gastroenterology*, **77,** 223
21. Ponz de Leon, M., Carulli, N., Loria, P. *et al.* (1980). Cholesterol absorption during bile acid feeding: effect of ursodeoxycholic acid (UDCA) administration. *Gastroenterology*, **78,** 214
22. Traber, M. G. and Ostwald, R. (1978). Cholesterol absorption and steroid excretion in cholesterol fed guinea pig. *J. Lipid Res.*, **19,** 448
23. Ponz de Leon, M., Ferenderes, R. and Carulli, N. (1978). Bile lipid composition and bile acid pool size in diabetes. *Am. J. Dig. Dis.*, **23,** 710
24. Duane, W. C., Adler, R. D., Bennion, L. J. *et al.* (1975). Determination of bile acid pool

size in man: a simplified method with advantages of increased precision, shortened analysis time and decreased isotope exposure. *J. Lipid Res.*, **16,** 155

25. LaRusso, N. F., Szczepanic, P. and Hofmann, A. F. (1977). Effect of deoxycholic acid ingestion on bile acid metabolism and biliary lipid secretion in normal subjects. *Gastroenterology*, **72,** 132
26. Vahouny, G. V., Weersing, S. and Treadwell, C. R. (1965). Function of specific bile acids in cholesterol esterase activity *in vitro*. *Biochim. Biophys. Acta*, **98,** 607

20
Effect of ursodeoxycholic and chenodeoxycholic acid on cholesterol absorption in patients with cholelithiasis

N. F. LARUSSO AND J. L. THISTLE

INTRODUCTION

Ingestion of 10–15 mg/kg daily of chenodeoxycholic acid (CDCA) or ursodeoxycholic acid (UDCA) by gallstone patients reduces biliary cholesterol secretion by the liver and results in bile unsaturated in cholesterol and gallstone dissolution[1–4]. The mechanism by which hepatic cholesterol secretion is suppressed has not been established, but a reduction in intestinal cholesterol absorption has been proposed[5,6]. We therefore investigated the hypothesis that intestinal absorption of cholesterol is suppressed by chronic administration of litholytic bile acids using an isotope ratio method for measuring cholesterol absorption which had been previously validated in humans[7].

METHODS

Five non-obese Caucasian patients (three men, two women) with radiolucent gallstones and well-visualized gallbladders were studied before and after 6–8 weeks of CDCA and UDCA (13 mg kg^{-1} day^{-1}) administered in random order. Three microcuries of [4-^{14}C]cholesterol were ingested in milk simultaneously with the intravenous administration of 3 μCi of [1,2-^{3}H]-cholesterol; cholesterol absorption was calculated from the difference in the plasma ^{14}C and ^{3}H during days 3–8 following administration. [^{3}H]cholesterol required extensive purification by thin-layer chromatography; its biological stability was documented both in rats and humans by a constant plasma ^{3}H/^{14}C ratio after co-administration of the isotopes intravenously. To document compliance and demonstrate bile acid-induced changes in biliary lipid and bile acid composition, fasting gallbladder bile samples were obtained by duodenal intubation following stimulation of gallbladder contraction by intravenous cholecystokinin–pancreozymin after each study.

RESULTS

The ^{14}C and ^{3}H plasma decay curves became parallel after 3 days in all patients; therefore the calculated cholesterol absorption was similar on days 3–8 in each study.

After administration of CDCA and UDCA, the administered bile acid became the predominant bile acid in bile. Before treatment, all patients had bile which was supersaturated in cholesterol (138 ± 9%, mean ± SEM) according to the solubility limits proposed by Dam and Hegardt. Cholesterol saturation decreased significantly in all patients after administration of either CDCA (102 ± 10%) or UDCA (87 ± 9%). Finally, cholesterol absorption was not different before (45.5 ± 4.3%, mean ± SEM) or after CDCA (42.7 ± 5.1) or UDCA (46.8 ± 3.7%) administration.

CONCLUSIONS

These results suggest that in non-obese patients with cholesterol cholelithiasis, chronic administration of 13 mg kg^{-1} day^{-1} of UDCA or CDCA unsaturates bile without affecting intestinal absorption of cholesterol. The major mechanism whereby these litholytic bile acids inhibit biliary secretion of cholesterol therefore does not appear to require suppression of intestinal cholesterol absorption.

References

1. Thistle, J. L., Hofmann, A. F., Ott, B. J. *et al.* (1978). Chenotherapy for gallstones. I. Efficacy and safety. *J. Am. Med. Assoc.*, **239,** 1138
2. Makino, I., Shinozaki, K., Yoshino, K. *et al.* (1975). Dissolution of cholesterol gallstones by long-term administration of ursodeoxycholic acid. *Jpn. J. Gastroenterol.*, **72,** 690
3. LaRusso, N. F., Hoffman, N. E., Hofmann, A. F. *et al.* (1975). Effect of primary bile acid metabolism and biliary lipid secretion in gallstone patients. *Gastroenterology*, **69,** 1301
4. Von Bergmann, K., Gustsfeld, M., Schulze-Hagen, K., *et al.* (1978). Comparison of urso- versus chenodeoxycholic acid on biliary lipid secretion in man. *Gastroenterology*, **75,** 955
5. Ponz de Leon, M., Carulli, N., Loria, P. *et al.* (1979). The effect of chenodeoxycholic acid (CDCA) on cholesterol absorption. *Gastroenterology*, **77,** 223
6. Ponz de Leon, M., Carulli, N., Loria, P. *et al.* (1980). Cholesterol absorption during bile acid feeding. Effect of ursodeoxycholic acid (UDCA) administration. *Gastroenterology*, **78,** 214
7. Samuel, P., Crouse, J. R. and Ahrens, E. H. (1978). Evaluation of an isotope ratio method for measurement of cholesterol absorption in man. *J. Lipid Res.*, **19,** 82

21
Effect of primary and secondary bile acid administration on intestinal absorption of cholesterol in man

C. SAMA AND N. F. LARUSSO

It is well known that chronic administration of chenodeoxycholic acid (CDCA), but not cholic acid (CA)[1] and deoxycholic acid (DCA)[2], reduces hepatic cholesterol secretion[3,4], decreases biliary cholesterol saturation[5,6] and dissolves cholesterol gallstones[6,7].

The postulated mechanisms by which CDCA might unsaturate bile include: (a) inhibition of hepatic cholesterol synthesis; (b) alteration in biliary bile acid/cholesterol coupling; and (c) reduction in intestinal cholesterol absorption.

As far as this last hypothesis is concerned, the effects of bile acids on intestinal cholesterol absorption have been recently studied by many authors[8–11], with conflicting results.

We report the results of studies in humans on the effect of CDCA, CA and DCA on the intestinal absorption of [^{3}H]cholesterol in a 20 cm duodenal segment during a 24 h perfusion study.

MATERIALS AND METHODS

Six non-obese Caucasians with radiolucent gallstones were studied before and after three months of CDCA and CA administration (15 mg kg^{-1} day^{-1}), and seven healthy volunteers were studied before and after 6 weeks of DCA administration (10 mg kg^{-1} day^{-1}). The dose of CDCA given was sufficient to unsaturate bile in cholesterol in all gallstone patients. The hourly absorption of [^{3}H]cholesterol was measured during a 24 h period in a 20 cm duodenal segment by use of an intestinal perfusion technique, previously described in detail[1]. The perfusate contained [^{3}H]cholesterol as an absorption marker and PEG as a recovery marker. (Results for biliary bile acid and lipid composition before and after primary and secondary bile acid administration, and for serum lipid levels before and after DCA administration, have been previously published[1,2]. Calculations of cholesterol absorption were made using data from these same patients.) Values of cholesterol absorption were calculated by the following equation:

Hourly cholesterol absorption (%) = 1 − (dpm[^{3}H]cholesterol in the aspirate/PEG in the aspirate) × (PEG in the perfusate/dpm[^{3}H]cholesterol in the perfusate) × 100.

Fasting serum cholesterol and triglyceride levels were also measured before and after bile acid administration.

RESULTS

In gallstone patients, absorption of cholesterol in the duodenum, expressed as the mean (±SEM) percentage of [^{3}H]cholesterol absorbed hourly for 24 h, was not significantly different before (18.2 ± 3.1%) and after CDCA (19.4 ± 4.9%) or CA (25.6 ± 5.9%) administration. Moreover, CDCA and CA administration did not affect serum lipid levels. In contrast DCA administration to healthy volunteers suppressed [^{3}H]cholesterol absorption (13.2 ± 3.2%) compared with that of pretreatment period (26.5 ± 3.8%) and decreased serum cholesterol levels by 15%; serum triglyceride levels remained unchanged.

CONCLUSIONS

Our results suggest that CDCA unsaturates bile in cholesterol by a mechanism other than inhibition of cholesterol absorption.

The data also indicate that the hypocholesterolaemic effect of DCA is due to the inhibition of intestinal absorption of cholesterol.

References

1. LaRusso, N. F., Hoffman, N. E., Hofmann, A. F. *et al.* (1975). Effect of primary bile acid ingestion on bile acid metabolism and biliary lipid secretion in gallstone patients. *Gastroenterology*, **69,** 1301
2. LaRusso, N. F., Szczepanik, P. A. and Hofmann, A. F. (1977). Effect of deoxycholic acid ingestion on bile acid metabolism and biliary lipid secretion in normal subjects. *Gastroenterology*, **72,** 132
3. Northfield, T. C., LaRusso, N. F. and Hofmann, A. F. (1975). Biliary lipid output during three meals and an overnight fast. II. Effect of chenodeoxycholic acid treatment in gallstone subjects. *Gut*, **16,** 12
4. Adler, R. D., Bennion, L. J., Douane, W. C. *et al.* (1975). Effects of low doses of chenodeoxycholic acid feeding on biliary lipid metabolism. *Gastroenterology*, **68,** 326
5. Thistle, J. L. and Schoenfield, J. L. (1971). Induced alterations in composition of bile of person having cholelithiasis. *Gastroenterology*, **61,** 488
6. Danzinger, R. G., Hofmann, A. F., Schoenfield, L. J. *et al.* (1972). Dissolution of cholesterol gallstones by chenodeoxycholic acid. *N. Engl. J. Med.*, **286,** 1
7. Bell, G. D., Whitney, B. and Dowling, R. H. (1972). Gallstone dissolution in man using chenodeoxycholic acid. *Lancet*, **2,** 1213
8. Tangedhal, T. N., Thistle, J. L., Hofmann, A. F. *et al.* (1979). Effect of β-sitosterol alone or in combination with chenic acid on cholesterol saturation of bile and cholesterol absorption in gallstone patients. *Gastroenterology*, **76,** 1341
9. Ponz de Leon, M., Carulli, N., Loria, P., *et al.* (1979). The effect of chenodeoxycholic acid (CDCA) on cholesterol absorption. *Gastroenterology*, **77,** 223
10. Einarsson, K. and Grundy, S. M. (1980). Effects of feeding cholic acid and chenodeoxycholic acid on cholesterol absorption and hepatic secretion of biliary lipids in man. *J. Lipid Res.*, **21,** 23
11. Mok, H. Y. I. and Grundy, S. M. (1980). Cholesterol and bile acid absorption during bile acid therapy in obese subjects undergoing weight reduction. *Gastroenterology*, **78,** 62

SECTION 3
Biliary Secretion

22
The cytoskeleton and secretion of biliary lipids

S. ERLINGER, M. DUBIN AND M. DUMONT

INTRODUCTION

There is increasing evidence that cytoskeletal and contractile elements in hepatocytes may have a role in secretion. Cytochalasin B and phalloidin, two agents interfering with the structure and function of microfilaments, induced cholestasis in the isolated rat liver preparation and in the rat *in vivo*[1,2], suggesting that microfilament dysfunction may cause cholestasis. Colchicine, an anti-microtubular agent, which was reported to have no effect on bile flow in the rat *in vivo*[3] has been shown to decrease bile flow in the isolated perfused rat liver[4] and to depress taurocholate-induced bile flow *in vivo*[5]. These studies were undertaken to examine the influence of phalloidin and colchicine on biliary lipid secretion in rats.

MATERIAL AND METHODS

Experimental protocols

Experiments were performed in male albino rats (Charles River, St-Aubin-les-Elbeuf, France) weighing from 175 to 250 g. *Phalloidin* (Boehringer, Mannheim, West Germany) was dissolved in a dimethylformamide/NaCl (0.15 mol/l) solution (1 : 50, v/v) at a concentration of 0.2 mg/ml, and a daily dose of 50 μg/100 g body weight was injected intraperitoneally for 1, 3 or 7 days. The experiments were performed on the next day. Control rats received the solvent alone and it was verified that bile flow and biliary lipids in these controls were not different from those of animals having received NaCl alone. *Colchicine* (Sigma, St Louis, Mo., USA) was dissolved in NaCl 0.15 mol/l and injected intravenously, at the dose of 0.2 mg/100 g body weight. The experiments were performed 3 h after the injection. Control animals studied under the same conditions received NaCl alone.

For the study of bile secretion, the rats were anaesthetized with pentobarbital (Nembutal, Abbott, St-Rémy-sur-Avre, France), 5 mg/100 g body weight, intraperitoneally. The rectal temperature was monitored throughout the experiments and maintained at 38 $\pm$ 0.5 °C on a heating table. The jugular vein was cannulated with a polyethylene catheter and used for injections. The common bile duct was cannulated with a polyethylene PE 1 catheter (Biotrol, Paris, France).

For measurements of basal bile secretion, bile was collected in pre-weighed tubes for three 10 min periods immediately after cannulation. The values taken for each animal are the means of these three measurements. For measurement of bile acid-stimulated bile secretion, after the 30 min basal bile flow period, an intravenous injection of sodium taurocholate (Maybridge, Tintagel, UK) at the dose of 10 μmol/100 g body weight was administered and bile was collected in pre-weighed tubes for 1 min (or 2 min) periods for a period of 10 min after injection. Because of the small amount of bile in some samples, bile collected from four animals was pooled and three series of four animals were studied.

Analytical methods

Bile acid concentration in bile was measured by a standard enzymatic technique using 3α-hydroxysteroid dehydrogenase. Phospholipid concentration was measured by the colorimetric technique of Bartlett, and cholesterol concentration was measured by gas–liquid chromatography. Cholesterol saturation index of bile was calculated from the tables of Carey[6].

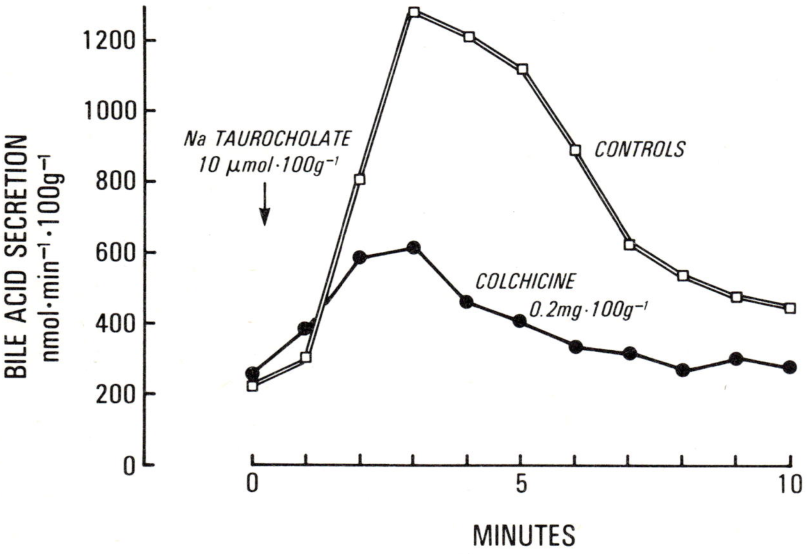

Figure 1 Influence of colchicine on bile acid secretion after a bile acid load. Colchicine was administered 3 h before the experiment. After the 30 min basal period, an injection of Na-taurocholate was administered (arrow). Bile was collected during 1 min periods. Each point represents the mean of six animals

RESULTS

Influence of colchicine on bile acid and biliary lipid secretion

The influence of colchicine on bile acid secretion is shown in Figure 1: colchicine had no detectable effect on basal bile acid secretion; however taurocholate-induced bile acid secretion was markedly lower in colchicine-treated animals than in controls. While in the controls bile acid secretion

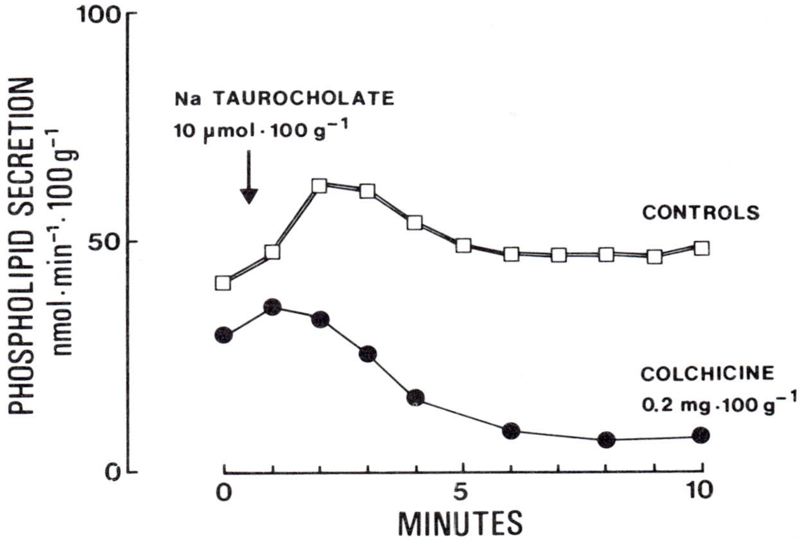

Figure 2 Influence of colchicine on phospholipid secretion after a bile acid load. Same experimental conditions as on Figure 1. In colchicine-treated animals, bile was collected during 1 min periods for the first 4 min, and every 2 min thereafter. Each point represents the mean of three series of four animals

increased 4-fold after the injection of sodium taurocholate, it increased by only 50% in the animals treated with colchicine. The influence of colchicine on biliary phospholipid secretion is shown in Figure 2: both basal and taurocholate-induced phospholipid secretion were lower in colchicine-treated animals than in controls. The influence of colchicine on cholesterol secretion is shown in Figure 3: again, both basal and taurocholate-induced cholesterol secretion were lower in colchicine-treated animals than in controls; almost no increase in cholesterol secretion after the injection of sodium taurocholate was observed in the colchicine-treated animals.

In the controls bile acid, phospholipid and cholesterol secretion returned to control values 10 min after the injection of sodium taurocholate; in contrast, in the colchicine-treated animals it was apparent that phospholipid and cholesterol secretion rates were lower 10 min after the injection of sodium taurocholate than during the basal period.

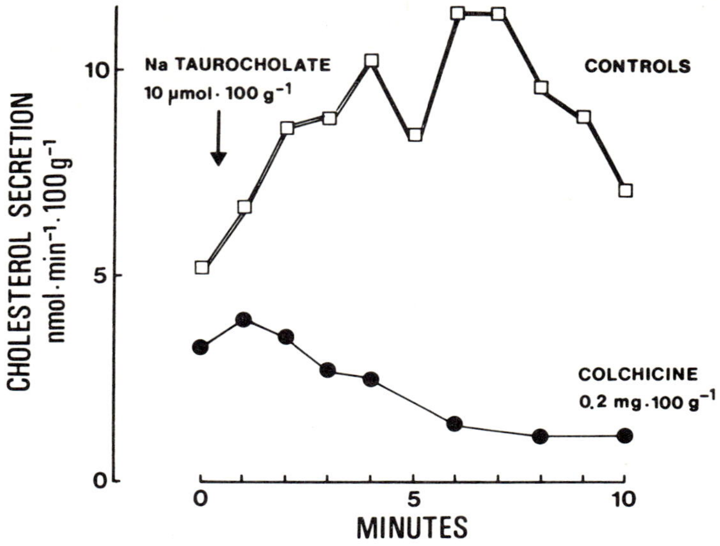

Figure 3 Influence of colchicine on cholesterol secretion after a bile acid load. Same experimental conditions and same number of animals as on Figure 2

Influence of phalloidin on biliary bile acids, phospholipids and cholesterol

In the rats treated with phalloidin for 1, 3 or 7 days, bile acid and phospholipid concentrations were not significantly modified (data not shown). In contrast, cholesterol concentration in bile was lower in phalloidin-treated animals than in controls; the difference was statistically significant at 3 and 7 days. As a result, the molar percentage of cholesterol (data not shown) and the cholesterol saturation index (Figure 4) decreased progressively: the mean decrease was 8.8% after 1 day, 51.7% after 3 days and 58.7% after 7 days. As shown previously[2], bile flow was significantly decreased, so that secretion rates of phospholipid and cholesterol were significantly lower in phalloidin-treated animals than in controls.

DISCUSSION

These experiments have shown colchicine administration in rat decreases markedly the choleretic response to a bile acid load, as shown previously[5]. In addition it decreases the enhancement of bile acid, phospholipid and cholesterol secretion observed normally after a bile acid injection. In these experiments basal phospholipid and cholesterol secretion rates were also slightly decreased. These observations strongly suggest that microtubule dysfunction is associated with a decreased biliary secretion of water, bile acids and lipids after a bile acid load. This is consistent with recent findings on lipoprotein secretion in the rat *in vivo*, suggesting that a minimum number of microtubules is required for lipoprotein secretion to proceed normally[7].

We also observed that phalloidin, also shown previously to decrease bile flow and bile acid secretion[2], decreased selectively cholesterol concentration in bile, while bile acid and phospholipid concentration remained unchanged. (Because of the decrease in bile flow, the biliary outputs of phospholipids and cholesterol were decreased with a predominant decrease in cholesterol output.) The reason for the selective decrease in cholesterol concentration in bile is not known. Among the theoretical possibilities are an effect on synthesis, an interference with mixed micelle formation, or an interference with secretion itself. It has been proposed that the micellar solubilization of cholesterol occurs within the canalicular membrane[8] and dramatic changes in the ultrastructural appearance of the plasma membrane have been observed after phalloidin administration[2,9,10], especially of its canalicular portion. It is therefore conceivable that microfilament dysfunction, either directly or through changes in the plasma membrane, could alter cholesterol secretion. These results provide circumstantial evidence for the view that microtubules on the one hand, and microfilaments on the other hand, may play a role in the secretion of biliary lipids.

Since, however, both colchicine and phalloidin – in addition to their effects on microtubules and microfilaments (respectively) – may alter the plasma membrane, it is difficult to decide whether the alterations in biliary

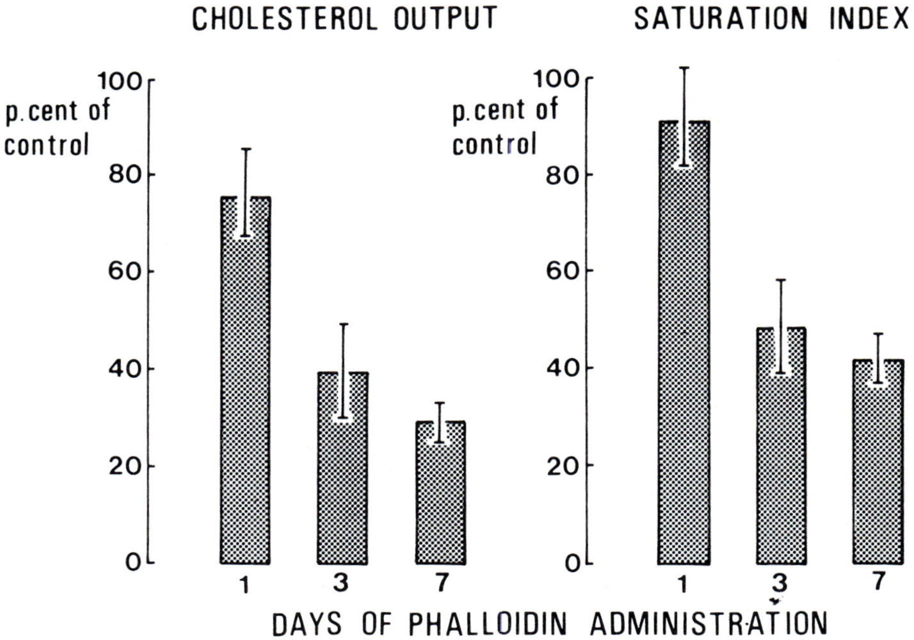

Figure 4 Influence of phalloidin on cholesterol secretion and cholesterol saturation index of bile. Animals were treated with phalloidin (50 μg/100 g) for 1, 3 or 7 days and studied 1 day after the last injection. Controls were studied simultaneously. Bars represent the means ± 1 SEM of seven animals at 1 day, six animals at 3 days and 10 animals at 7 days. The decrease in saturation index is significant at 3 days ($p < 0.05$) and 7 days ($p < 0.001$)

lipid secretion reported here are due to microtubule and microfilament dysfunction (or, alternatively, to changes in the plasma membrane).

A preliminary report of the results regarding phalloidin has appeared[11].

Acknowledgment

This work was supported in part by grant INSERM CRL 77.5.122.7.

References

1. Phillips, M. J., Oda, M., Mak, E.,, Fisher, M. M. and Jeejeebhoy, K. N. (1975). Microfilament dysfunction as a possible cause of intrahepatic cholestasis. *Gastroenterology*, **69,** 48
2. Dubin, M., Maurice, M., Feldmann, G. and Erlinger, S. (1978). Phalloidin-induced cholestasis in the rat: relation to changes in microfilaments. *Gastroenterology*, **75,** 450
3. Stein, O., Sanger, L. and Stein, Y. (1974). Colchicine-induced inhibition of lipoprotein and protein secretion into the serum and lack of interference with secretion of biliary phospholipids and cholesterol by rat liver *in vivo. J. Cell Biol.*, **62,** 90
4. Gregory, D. H., Vlahcevic, Z. R., Prugh, M. F. and Swell, L. (1978). Mechanism of secretion of biliary lipids: role of a microtubular system in hepatocellular transport of biliary lipids in the rat. *Gastroenterology*, **74,** 93
5. Dubin, M., Maurice, M., Feldmann, G. and Erlinger, S. (1980). Influence of colchicine and phalloidin on bile secretion and hepatic ultrastructure in the rat. Possible interaction between microtubules and microfilaments. *Gastroenterology*, **79,** 646
6. Carey, M. C. (1978). Critical tables for calculating the cholesterol saturation of native bile. *J. Lipid Res.*, **19,** 945
7. Reaven, E. P. and Reaven, G. M. (1980). Evidence that microtubules play a permissive role in hepatocyte very low density lipoprotein secretion. *J. Cell Biol.*, **84,** 28
8. Carey, M. C. and Small, D. M. (1972). Micelle formation by bile salts. Physical–chemical and thermodynamic considerations. *Arch. Intern. Med.*, **130,** 506
9. Gabbiani, G., Montesano, R., Tuchweber, B., Salas, M. and Orci, L. (1975). Phalloidin-induced hyperplasia of actin filaments in rat hepatocytes. *Lab. Invest.*, **33,** 562
10. Agostini, B., Govindan, V. M. and Hofmann, W. (1975). Morphological changes induced by phalloidin in the rat liver. In Keppler, D. (ed.), *Pathogenesis and Mechanisms of Liver Cell Necrosis*, pp. 175–192. (Lancaster: MTP Press)
11. Dubin, M. and Erlinger, S. (1980). Influence of phalloidin on biliary lipid secretion in rats. *Clin. Sci.*, **58,** 545

23
Studies on the relationship between mixed lipid biliary micelles, pigment and protein in bile
Physicochemical interactions in bile

A. REUBEN, K. E. HOWELL AND J. L. BOYER

INTRODUCTION

Bile consists of an aqueous solution of inorganic salts, organic anions, bile salts, lipids and proteins[1]. Theoretically, many different interactions could occur between these constituents. To date most experiments have been designed to study the nature and properties of the micellar aggregates of bile salts, phospholipids and cholesterol in bile[2-4]. Although the presence of lipid–protein–pigment complexes in bile was proposed over 25 years ago[5], it was not until recently that there was evidence for the associations between mixed lipid micelles and organic anions in bile[6] as well as the existence of specific[7,8] and non-specific lipid–protein complexes[9,10]. To test these possibilities further, we examined the interactions between lipids, pigment and proteins in bile using gel filtration chromatography, pre-equilibrating the columns with a wide range of bile salt concentrations. We took advantage of the fact that the size of mixed lipid micelles varies with the intermicellar bile salt concentrations[11], and therefore the elution profiles of the lipid micelles could be varied.

METHODS

Bile was collected at room temperature by biliary cannulation from fed, male Sprague-Dawley rats, anaesthetized with sodium pentobarbital (50 mg/kg). Samples of 0.4–2.0 ml (1–5% bed volume) were applied to Sephadex G100 chromatography columns. The latter were pre-equilibrated with an electrolyte–bile salt solution of the same composition that was subsequently used for elution. The electrolyte concentrations of this solution (Na^+ 125 mmol/l, Cl^- 105 mmol/l, K^+ 5 mmol/l, HCO_3^- 25 mmol/l) were physiological for rat bile[6]. Different concentrations of sodium taurocholate (NaTC 5–60 mmol/l) were used for elution in order to vary the bile salt lipid micelle size sufficiently to alter its elution profile for comparison with the profiles of bile pigment and proteins.

Table 1 Elution coefficients (K_{av}) of biliary mixed lipid micelles and bile pigment, according to the bile salt concentration (mmol/l NaTC) used for column pre-equilibration and elution

Bile salt concentration (mmol/l NaTC)	*Elution coefficient* (K_{av}) *Mixed lipid micelles*	*Bile pigment*
5	0.07 ± 0.03 (4)	0.87 – (2)
10	0.14 – (2)	0.84 – (2)
15	0.21 ± 0.01 (4)	0.74 ± 0.66 (4)
20	0.33 – (2)	0.76 – (2)
30	0.37 ± 0.04 (6)	0.68 – (2)
40	0.50 – (2)	0.62 – (2)
60	0.46 ± 0.03 (5)	0.65 ± 0.09 (5)

Mean values are shown with ± standard deviation, where appropriate. Figures in parentheses indicate number of studies.

In the elution fractions phospholipid was analysed chemically[12], cholesterol was detected by gas–liquid chromatography[13], bile salts were determined using an enzyme assay[14], bile pigment was quantified by absorption spectrophotometry at 400 nm and total proteins were measured by a Coomassie Blue binding reaction[15] as well as SDS-polyacrylamide gel electrophoresis (SDS-PAGE) for separation of individual components[16]. In each chromatography experiment, the void volume of the column (V_o) was determined with blue dextran (MW 2×10^6) and the total bed volume (V_t) was measured with [^{14}C]sucrose. An elution coefficient, which can vary from zero to unity (the approximate distribution coefficient K_{av}[17]), was calculated for both mixed lipid micelles and bile pigments, from the formula $K_{av} = (V_e - V_o)/(V_t - V_o)$, where V_e is the peak elution volume of the bile lipid micelles or pigment, respectively[17]. Low K_{av} values characterize high molecular weight compounds which are rapidly eluted from the column, whilst high K_{av} values reflect low molecular weight substances which elute slowly.

RESULTS

In each gel filtration experiment peak separation was obtained for proteins, lipids and bile pigments throughout the whole range of bile salt concentrations used. Phospholipid and cholesterol co-eluted in a single peak within the included volume of the column, under all conditions tested, confirming that the biliary mixed lipid micelles were isolated intact. The elution profile of these micelles varied with the eluant bile salt concentration, as shown by the corresponding elution coefficients in Table 1. Mixed lipid micelles were largest with the low bile salt concentrations (low K_{av}) and decreased progressively in size, as the bile salt concentration was increased, reaching a limit in 30–40 mmol/l NaTC. The bile pigment always eluted after the mixed lipid micelles but within the total volume of the column, indicating the presence of aggregates. Monomeric bilirubin has a molecular weight of 585, and therefore would be expected to elute in the total volume of the column. However, in direct contrast to the lipid micelles, there was a progressive increase in size (reducing K_{av}) of these pigment aggregates as the eluant bile salt concentration was increased. The only similarity in size between the lipid micelles and bile pigment aggregates was seen when high bile salt concentrations were used (40–60 mmol/l NaTC).

Over 80% of the biliary proteins separated from the lipid and pigments in the void volume of the columns, irrespective of the eluant bile salt concentration. This indicates that the majority of the proteins are present in a molecular weight form of 70 000–100 000 daltons or greater. Analysis by SDS-PAGE detected over 15 separate bands in these fractions, ranging from a molecular weight of ~10 000 to ~200 000 daltons. Very few intermediate and small molecular weight proteins (approximately 15 000 daltons) were detected in later elution fractions, i.e. eluted as would be predicted according to their molecular weight. In contrast to the marked changes in the micelle and pigment elution profiles, no change in the protein pattern was seen with different bile salt concentrations.

DISCUSSION

Using gel filtration chromatography of rat bile, no association could be demonstrated between the lipid micelles, pigments and proteins when physiological concentrations of bile salt were used to pre-equilibrate and elute the columns. This finding conflicts with the results of many published studies in which macromolecular complexes of these constituents were isolated from bile[5,7–9,18–20]. However, it is possible that in previous studies such complexes were artifactually produced by the experimental methods employed. Strong electrostatic forces[5,7,9], adsorbent media[5,9] and isolation in bile salt-free conditions[5,7,9,10] all tend to dissociate bile salts from the lipids, resulting in liposome formation[4] which, in the adsence of bile salts, non-specifically binds protein and/or pigment. In the present study, anionic binding to the Sephadex gel is minimized by equilibrating the column with bile salts prior to use[21,22], so that the components of bile are separated according to molecular size. The isolation of pigment aggregates which were smaller than lipid micelles was also achieved, confirming previous findings[6]. Although the sizes of these bile pigment aggregates and lipid micelles clearly differ at physiological bile salt concentrations between 5 and 30 mmol/l, they co-elute when higher bile salt concentrations are used (40–60 mmol/l). The similarity in the elution profile of the lipid micelle and pigment aggregates at these higher bile salt concentrations could be misinterpreted as the binding of organic anions to lipid micelles, as has recently been reported[6].

Although complexes of proteins and lipids have not been found in this study, the existence of lipid-free protein aggregates in bile is suggested by the SDS-PAGE analysis of biliary proteins following gel filtration. The current study, however, offers no explanation for these bile protein aggregates but suggests that they have no significant association with the bile lipid micelle.

Acknowledgment

This work was supported by USPHS Grant AM 25636. Dr Reuben is supported, in part, by a British Medical Research Council Eli Lilly award and an American Liver Foundation Fellow Supplement Award.

References

1. Forker, E. (1977). Mechanism of hepatic bile formation. *Ann. Rev. Physiol.*, **39,** 323
2. Admirand, W. M. and Small, D. M. (1968). The physicochemical basis of cholesterol gallstone formation in man. *J. Clin. Invest.*, **47,** 1043
3. Holzbach, R. T., Marsh, M., Olszewski, M. and Holan, K. (1973). Cholesterol solubility in bile. Evidence that supersaturated bile is frequent in healthy man. *J. Clin. Invest.*, **52,** 1467
4. Mazer, N. A., Benedek, G. B. and Carey, M. C. (1980). Quasi elastic light-scattering studies of aqueous biliary lipid systems. Mixed micelle formation in bile salt-lecithin solutions. *Biochemistry*, **19,** 601
5. Verschure, J. C. M. (1956). Electro-chromograms of human bile. *Clin. Chem. Acta*, **1,** 38
6. Scharschmidt, B. F. and Schmid, R. (1978). The micellar sink. A quantitative assessment of the association of organic anions with mixed micelles and other macromolecular aggregates in rat bile. *J. Clin. Invest.*, **62,** 1122
7. Lafont, H., Lairon, D., Domingo, N., Nalbone, G. and Hauton, J. C. (1974). Does a lecithin–polypeptide association in bile originate from membrane structural sub-units? *Biochimie*, **56,** 465
8. Nalbone, G., Lafont, H., Vigne, J. L., Domingo, N., Lairon, D., Chabert, C., Lechene, P. and Hauton, J. C. (1979). The apoprotein fraction of the bile lipoprotein complex: isolation, partial characterization and phospholipid binding properties. *Biochimie*, **61,** 1029
9. Manzato, E., Fellin, R., Baggio, G., Walch, S., Neubeck, W. and Seidel, D. (1976). Formation of lipoprotein-X. Its relationship to bile compounds. *J. Clin. Invest.*, **57,** 1248
10. Holzbach, R. T., Claffey, W. J., Freedman, M. R., Corbusier, C. S., Pickrel, S. G., Wieland, H. and Seidel, D. (1980). Protein–lipid complexes in human bile. *Gastroenterology*, **78,** 1308 (abstr.)
11. Small, D. M. (1977). Bile salts of the blood. High density lipoprotein systems and cholesterol removal. In Bianchi, L., Gerok, W. and Sickinger, K. (eds.) *Liver and Bile*, pp. 89–100. (Lancaster: MTP Press)
12. Bartlett, G. R. (1959). Phosphorus assay in column chromatography. *J. Biol. Chem.*, **234,** 466
13. Hardison, W. G. M. and Apter, J. T. (1972). Micellar theory of biliary cholesterol excretion. *Am. J. Physiol.*, **222,** 61
14. Boyer, J. L., Scheig, R. L. and Klatskin, G. (1970). The effect of sodium taurocholate on the hepatic metabolism of sulfobromophthalein sodium (BSP). The role of bile flow. *J. Clin. Invest.*, **49,** 206
15. Bradford, M. (1976). A rapid and sensitive method for the quantitation of microgram quantities of protein utilizing the principle of protein-dye binding. *Anal. Biochem.*, **72,** 248
16. Maizel, J. V., Jr. (1971). Polyacrylamide gel electrophoresis of viral proteins. In Maramorosh, K. and Kiprowski, H. (eds.). *Methods in Virology*. Vol. 5, pp. 179–246. (New York: Academic Press)
17. Laurent, T. C. and Killander, J. (1964). A theory of gel filtration and its experimental verification. *J. Chromatog.*, **14,** 317
18. Bouchier, I. A. D. and Cooperband, S. R. (1967). Isolation and characterization of a macromolecular aggregate associated with bilirubin. *Clin. Chem. Acta.*, **15,** 291
19. Juniper, K. (1965). Physicochemical characteristics of bile and their relation to gallstone formation. *Am. J. Med.*, **39,** 98
20. Nakayama, F. (1966). Nature of cholesterol complexing macromolecular fractions in bile. *Clin. Chem. Acta*, **13,** 212
21. Borgstrom, B. (1965). The dimensions of the bile salt micelle. Measurement by gel filtration. *Biochem. Biophys. Acta*, **106,** 171
22. Carbis, R. A., Rodda, S. J. and Hampson, A. W. (1979). Adsorption of deoxycholate on Sephadex G-25. *J. Chromatog.*, **173,** 182

24
Measurement of the contribution of newly synthesized cholesterol to biliary cholesterol using [^{3}H]water

S. D. TURLEY AND J. M. DIETSCHY

INTRODUCTION

The origin of biliary cholesterol and the factors which ultimately dictate the rate of biliary cholesterol secretion are poorly understood. The cholesterol secreted in bile must be derived from either dietary or newly synthesized cholesterol, or both. There are however, very few definitive data in any species on the proportion of biliary cholesterol derived from each source.

The direct secretion of newly synthesized cholesterol into bile has been demonstrated both in man and the rat by administering precursors such as labelled mevalonate or acetate[1–3]. However, the contribution of newly synthesized cholesterol to biliary cholesterol cannot be accurately quantitated using such data because of the unknown degree of intracellular dilution which such labelled precursors undergo.

Such problems can, however, be avoided by using [^{3}H]water as the precursor. Since [^{3}H]water readily penetrates most cell membranes the specific activity (SA) of total body water rapidly becomes constant and remains so for many hours providing the animal is not given any fluids. The ^{3}H of [^{3}H]water is incorporated into the sterol molecule either directly or after equilibration with the reductive H of NADH[4,5]. At least in the liver, approximately 22 μg atoms of ^{3}H are inserted into each μmol of cholesterol[5]. Thus, using this relationship the [^{3}H]sterol content of bile can be converted into an absolute content of newly synthesized cholesterol.

The objectives of the present studies were: to establish whether biliary cholesterol is derived from a pool of sterol that is separate from the general pool of cholesterol in the hepatocyte, to quantitate the proportion of biliary cholesterol that is derived directly from newly synthesized cholesterol, and to determine whether this proportion is influenced by the rate of hepatic cholesterol synthesis.

MATERIALS AND METHODS

Animal preparations

Female Sprague-Dawley-derived rats (Charles River Breeding Laboratories, Inc., Wilmington, MA), originally purchased in the weight range of

125–150 g, were housed in a room with alternating 12 h periods of light (1500–0300 hours) and darkness (0300–1500 hours) and were allowed free access to water and rat chow (Wayne Laboratory Animal Diets, Allied Mills, Inc., Chicago, IL) for at least 2 weeks before being used in specific experiments. All rats were fed plain chow except in one experiment in which groups of rats were fed plain chow containing either 3% (w/w) cholestyramine (Mead Johnson Research Center, Evansville, IN) or 0.25% (w/w) cholesterol (Byron Chemical Company, Inc., Long Island City 1, NY) for 14 days. In another experiment rats which had been fed plain chow were fasted for 48 h before use.

In the basic protocol used to measure the proportion of biliary cholesterol that was newly synthesized, rats were fitted with a femoral vein catheter and administered 100 mCi of [^{3}H]water as a bolus. After 6 h the rats were anaesthetized again, a catheter placed in the common bile duct and bile was collected for the following 4 h, either at hourly intervals or as a single sample.

This protocol was modified slightly in two studies involving the measurement of the SA of sterols in the bile, plasma and tissues. In one of these studies bile was collected from separate groups of rats during either the 1st, 2nd, 3rd or 4th hours of biliary diversion. Each group was then killed at the end of its respective collection period and the SA of free and esterified cholesterol in the liver, plasma and bile was measured. In the other study, biliary diversion was again commenced 6 h after administration of the [^{3}H]water but the collection of bile was not started until 90 min later. The bile was collected for 1 h, the rats were then killed and samples of plasma, liver and various extrahepatic tissues obtained for measurement of the SA of sterols.

In another series of experiments the contribution of newly synthesized cholesterol to biliary cholesterol was measured in rats in which biliary bile acid output was varied over a wide range. In these experiments the rats were administered 100 mCi of [^{3}H]water immediately following the commencement of biliary diversion. Over the following 8 h one group of rats received a continuous intravenous infusion of sodium taurocholate (Calbiochem, San Diego, CA) at a rate of 20 μmol/h. To minimize any change in plasma water SA during this time the volume infused was only 0.24 ml/h. Bile was collected at hourly intervals.

Determination of the rate of hepatic sterol synthesis *in vivo*

As described in detail elsewhere, rats which had been subjected to the various dietary manipulations were administered intravenously 25 mCi of [^{3}H]water as a bolus and were killed 60 min later[6]. The blood and liver were removed and the SA of plasma water and the [^{3}H]digitonin precipitable sterol ([^{3}H]DPS) content of the liver were determined[6] ([^{3}H]DPS refers to sterols in which the ^{3}H from [^{3}H]water has been incorporated).

Isolation and purification of [^{3}H]DPS

In addition to the samples of liver, aliquots of bile to which carrier cholesterol had been added were also saponified. The sterols were then quantitatively extracted using petroleum ether and precipitated as the digitonides as previously described in detail[6]. The digitonide precipitates were washed, dried under vacuum at 80 °C and then dissolved in pyridine. The free sterols were quantitatively extracted with diethyl ether, taken to dryness under air and then placed in a vacuum oven at 80 °C for an additional hour following which scintillation solution was added and the samples assayed for their ^3H content[6].

Assay of SA of cholesterol in bile, plasma and tissues

Aliquots of bile, plasma, liver and various extrahepatic tissues were added to chloroform : methanol (2 : 1 v/v) and heated on a steambath. The free and esterified sterols were then separated on silicic acid : celite columns[7]. After saponification the sterols were precipitated as the digitonides and aliquots taken for determination of ^3H content and mass.

Assay of biliary lipid levels

Aliquots of bile were taken for the determination of [^3H]DPS as described above, and for the quantitation of total cholesterol content. In this procedure the cholesterol was extracted and isolated as the digitonide and then assayed using the $FeCl_3$–H_2SO_4 method[8]. The same colorimetric procedure was used to measure the mass of sterol in the free and esterified cholesterol fractions of the bile, plasma and various tissues. The concentration of total bile acids in bile was determined using the hydroxysteroid dehydrogenase assay as described in detail elsewhere[9]. Biliary phospholipid concentration was assayed by colorimetric determination of inorganic phosphate[10].

Calculations

The equations used to calculate the SA of plasma water and to convert the [^3H]DPS content of liver to a corresponding rate of incorporation of [^3H]water have been described in detail previously[6].

The amount of newly synthesized cholesterol in bile was calculated using the following equation:

$$\frac{(\text{ct/min [}^3\text{H]DPS/ml bile}) \ (1.45)}{(\text{SA plasma water}) \ (18) \ (1000)}$$

The [^3H]DPS content of the bile was first converted to an equivalent rate of incorporation of [^3H]water by dividing by the SA of plasma water. The nmol of [^3H]water incorporated was then converted to the equivalent number of C_2 units by multiplying by 1.45 (1.45 nmol of acetyl CoA units are incorporated into DPS for each nmol [^3H]water[5]). Since 18 μmol of acetyl CoA are needed for the synthesis of 1 μmol of cholesterol the number of C_2 units incorporated was converted to nmol of cholesterol synthesized by dividing the value by 18. The units were then changed to μmol by dividing by 1000. This value, when divided by the total cholesterol content of bile, also expressed as μmol/ml, and multiplied by 100, gave the percentage of biliary cholesterol that was newly synthesized.

Where appropriate, mean values ± 1 SEM for groups of data are given. Differences in mean values were tested for significance using the unpaired Student's *t* test. For correlating two variables a linear regression line was fitted by the method of least squares to the data obtained from individual animals and has the usual form $y = a \pm bx$.

RESULTS

In preliminary experiments not reported here, but described in detail elsewhere, it was established that following the intravenous administration of a bolus of [^{3}H]water to rats, the SA of plasma water rapidly attained a constant value which remained unchanged[11] for at least the following 8 h. In the same experiment it was also shown that the SA of liver water rapidly reached the same value as found in the plasma, indicating complete equilibration of the liver water with that in the plasma. In a separate group of studies it was also established that when rats were restrained and subjected to total biliary

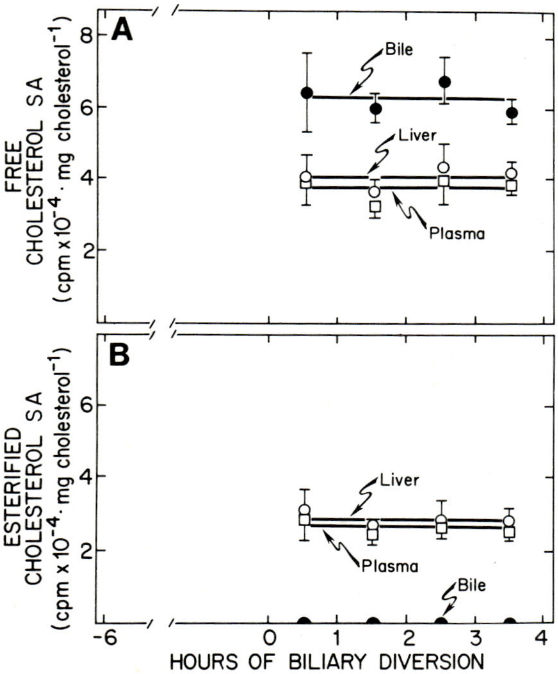

Figure 1 Specific activity of free and esterified cholesterol in the bile, liver and plasma over a 4 h period in rats administered [^{3}H]water 6 h before the commencement of biliary diversion. In this experiment rats were administered 100 mCi of [^{3}H]water and 6 h later were subjected to total biliary diversion. Bile was collected from separate groups of rats during either the 1st, 2nd, 3rd or 4th hours of diversion. Each group was killed at the end of its respective collection period and the SA of free and esterified cholesterol in the bile, liver and plasma was measured. The values represent the mean ± 1 SEM of data obtained in four animals. The SA of free cholesterol in bile was significantly different from that of the liver at each time point at the $p < 0.05$ level

diversion over an 8 h period, the rate of cholesterol synthesis in the liver, as measured by both *in vitro* and *in vivo* procedures, did not change significantly[11].

The first series of experiments was carried out to examine whether the cholesterol secreted in bile could be traced to a pool of sterol functionally distinct from the general pool of cholesterol in the hepatocyte. Rats were given [^{3}H]water and 6 h later were subjected to total biliary diversion for 4 h. The SA of both free and esterified cholesterol in the bile, liver and plasma was measured at hourly intervals in separate groups of rats. As shown in panel A of Figure 1 the SA of free cholesterol in bile was, on average, 55% higher ($p < 0.05$) than that in the liver over the 4 h period. Although the SA of plasma free cholesterol was consistently lower than that of the liver, the difference was not statistically significant. The average SA of esterified cholesterol in the liver and plasma also did not differ significantly (panel B).

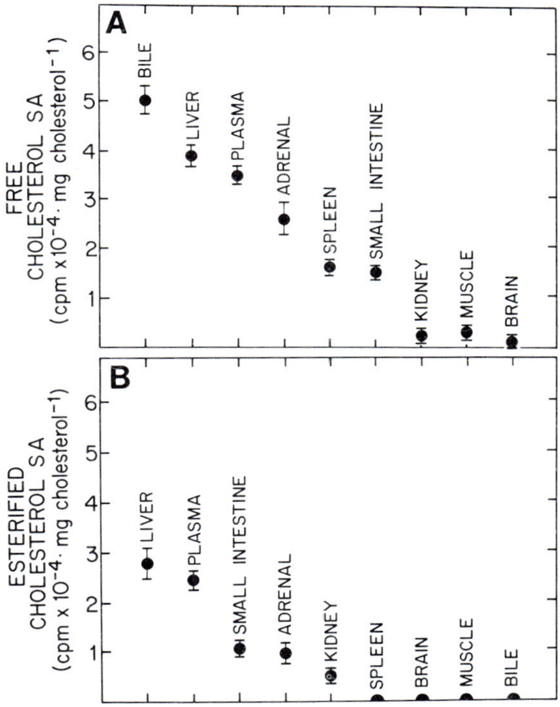

Figure 2 Specific activity of free and esterified cholesterol in the bile, plasma and various tissues at a single time point in rats administered [^{3}H]water 6 h before the commencement of biliary diversion. In this experiment biliary diversion was again commenced 6 h after administration of the [^{3}H]water but the collection of bile was not started until 90 min later. The bile was collected for 1 h, the rats were then killed and samples of plasma, liver and various extrahepatic tissues were obtained for measurement of the SA of sterols. The values represent the mean ± 1 SEM of data obtained in six animals. The SA of the free cholesterol in bile is significantly different from that in the liver, plasma and other tissues at the $p < 0.05$ level

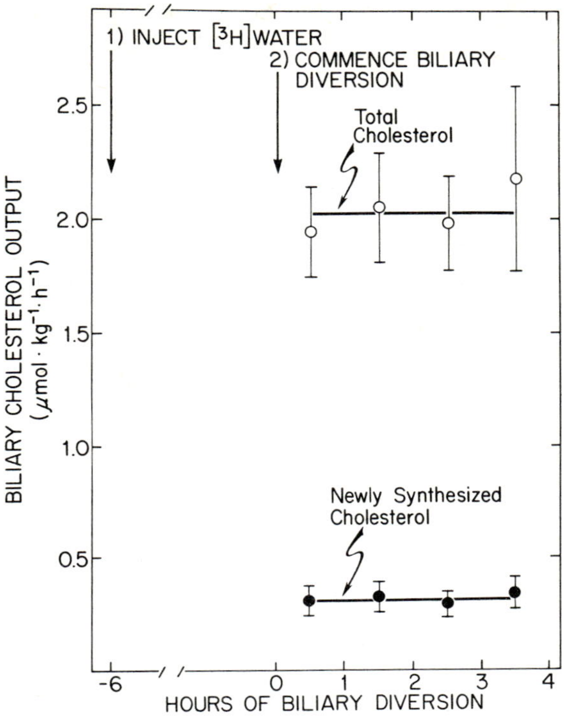

Figure 3 Biliary secretion rates of total and newly synthesized cholesterol over 4 h in rats administered [^{3}H]water 6 h before the commencement of total biliary diversion. The values represent the mean ± 1 SEM of data obtained in four animals

However, the SA of the esterified fraction in both the liver and plasma was only about 70% of that in free cholesterol. In a similar experiment the SA of free and esterified cholesterol in the bile, liver, plasma and several extrahepatic tissues was measured at a single time-point. Rats that had been administered [^{3}H]water 6 h earlier were subjected to total biliary diversion and bile was collected for only 1 h starting 90 min after the commencement of diversion. The rats were then killed and samples of plasma, liver and various extrahepatic tissues were obtained. As shown in panel A of Figure 2 the SA of biliary free cholesterol exceeded not only that of the liver and plasma, but also that of all the other tissues examined. Thus, it was about 3-fold greater than the SA of free cholesterol in the spleen and small intestine and 17- to 55-fold higher than that in the kidney, thigh muscle and brain. The data in panel B show that the SA of esterified cholesterol was highest in the liver and plasma although, again, these values were less than those found in the free cholesterol fraction of these samples. The SA of esterified cholesterol in the small intestine, adrenal gland and kidney was much less than that in the liver and plasma. Radiolabelled esterified cholesterol was not detected in the bile, spleen, muscle or brain.

The results of the first experiment in which the contribution of newly synthesized cholesterol to total biliary cholesterol output was measured over a 4 h period of biliary diversion is shown in Figure 3. The output of both total and labelled cholesterol remained constant during this time with the proportion of the total that was newly synthesized averaging 16%. In this experiment the rats had been fed plain chow and thus had normal rates of hepatic cholesterol synthesis.

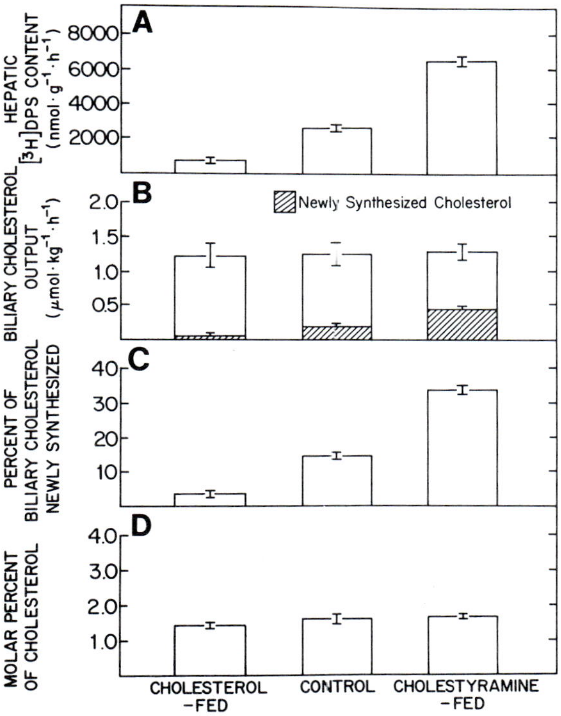

Figure 4 Effect of feeding cholesterol and cholestyramine on hepatic [^{3}H]DPS content, biliary secretion rates of total and newly synthesized cholesterol and the molar percentage of cholesterol in bile. In the experiment shown in panel A the rats were administered 25 mCi of [^{3}H]water, killed 1 h later and the [^{3}H]DPS content of the liver was measured. The data represent the mean ± 1 SEM of determinations in five animals. In the experiment shown in the other panels, rats which had been fed the various diets were given [^{3}H]water and 6 h later were subjected to total biliary diversion for 4 h. The values represent the mean ± 1 SEM of data obtained in six animals. The values for hepatic [^{3}H]DPS content, biliary secretion rates of newly synthesized cholesterol and the percentage of biliary cholesterol newly synthesized in the cholesterol-fed and cholestyramine-fed groups are significantly different from the corresponding control values at the $p < 0.05$ level

The next series of experiments examined the effect of varying the rate of hepatic cholesterol synthesis on the amount of newly synthesized cholesterol secreted in bile. Thus, rats which had either been fed diets containing added cholesterol or cholestyramine, or which had been fasted for 48 h, as well as respective control animals, were subjected to the protocol described in Figure 3. The results of the experiment with the cholesterol and cholestyramine-fed rats are shown in Figure 4. The data in panel A represent the hepatic [^{3}H]DPS contents of rats fed these diets as well as of control animals. As discussed previously the [^{3}H]DPS content can be taken as a measure of the rate of hepatic cholesterol synthesis[12]. Cholesterol feeding suppressed the rate of hepatic sterol synthesis 73%, whereas cholestyramine feeding enhanced the rate 2.5-fold. The data in panel B show the rates of biliary secretion of both total and newly synthesized cholesterol. These values represent the average rates over a 4 h period of bile collection. The amount of newly synthesized sterol in the bile of the cholesterol-fed group was decreased by 76%, whereas in the cholestyramine-fed animals it was increased 2.3-fold compared to the control value. However, the total cholesterol secretion rate was not different in the three groups of animals. The percentage of biliary cholesterol that was newly synthesized in each group is given in panel C. In the control animals this value was 14.9%, whereas in the rats fed cholesterol and cholestyramine the values were 3.5% and 34.1%, respectively. Although the data are not shown, the rates of output of bile acid and phospholipid in the bile of the cholesterol- and cholestyramine-fed rats were not significantly different from

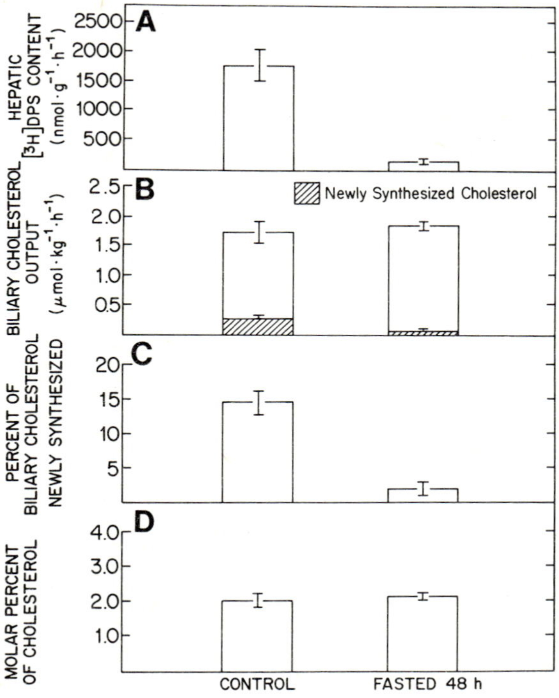

Figure 5 Effect of fasting on hepatic [^{3}H]DPS content, biliary secretion rates of total and newly synthesized cholesterol and the molar percentage of cholesterol in bile. The experimental procedures were the same as those described in the legend to Figure 4. All values represent the mean ± 1 SEM of data obtained in five animals. The values for hepatic [^{3}H]DPS content, biliary secretion rates of newly synthesized cholesterol and the percentage of biliary cholesterol newly synthesized in the fasted group are significantly different from the corresponding control values at the $p < 0.05$ level

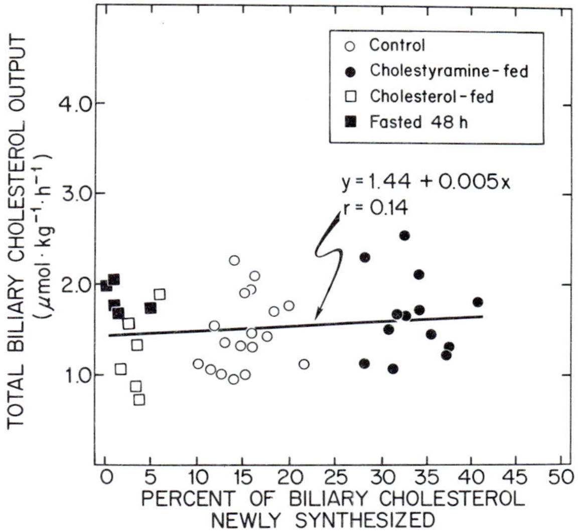

Figure 6 Total biliary cholesterol output as a function of the proportion of biliary cholesterol that is newly synthesized. These data represent the rates of biliary cholesterol output and the percentage of biliary cholesterol derived from newly synthesized sterol in individual animals that had either been fed the cholestyramine or cholesterol diets, or which had been fasted for 48 h as well as controls. There are points for a total of 42 animals. The slope of the regression line is not significantly different from the *x*-axis

those in the control animals. Thus, since total cholesterol output was also unchanged the molar percentage of cholesterol in the bile, as indicated in panel D, was similar in all three groups.

The data for the fasted animals and their respective control group are given in Figure 5. As indicated in panel A the rate of hepatic cholesterol synthesis was suppressed 94% in the fasted group. In these animals the amount of newly synthesized sterol in the bile was decreased by 88% compared to the value for the controls but there was no change in total cholesterol secretion (panel B). Thus, as shown in panel C, only 1.7% of biliary cholesterol was newly synthesized in the fasted animals compared to 14.5% in the control group. Although the data are not shown, biliary phospholipid output was slightly elevated in the fasted group but bile acid output was unchanged. Thus, while there was a rise in the relative phospholipid content of the bile this was offset mainly by a decrease in the relative content of bile acid so that, as shown in panel D, the molar percentage of cholesterol in the fasted group did not differ significantly from that in the controls. Plasma cholesterol levels in the fasted animals (45.5 ± 5.0 mg/dl) were significantly lower than those in the control group (76.5 ± 4.3 mg/dl).

In Figure 6 the rate of total biliary cholesterol output has been plotted as a function of the percentage of biliary cholesterol that was newly synthesized in the same animal. These data include those shown in panels B and C of both Figures 4 and 5, as well as some additional values for control and cholestyramine-fed rats. It is clearly evident that varying the proportion of biliary cholesterol derived from newly synthesized sterol from 0.2 to 42% had no effect on total biliary cholesterol output.

In the final series of experiments rats that had been fed plain chow were administered [^{3}H]water immediately following the commencement of total biliary diversion. Over the following 8 h one group was given a continuous infusion of bile acid at a rate that was sufficient not only to maintain biliary cholesterol output at a more stable level but also to drive the overall rate of cholesterol secretion to values higher than normal. The other group was not given any bile acid, thus allowing almost complete depletion of the bile acid pool over the 8 h period. In all animals the biliary secretion rates of total and newly synthesized cholesterol as well as bile acid were measured in the 7th and 8th hours of diversion. In the group in which the bile acid pool was almost depleted, the average rate of bile acid output in the 7th and 8th hours of diversion was 30 ± 5 μmol kg^{-1} h^{-1}. The corresponding rate of total cholesterol output was 0.65 ± 0.10 μmol kg^{-1} h^{-1}, of which 17.7% was newly synthesized. In the rats given bile acid the average bile acid output during this period was 147 ± 12 μmol kg^{-1} h^{-1}, and the corresponding total cholesterol output was 3.46 μmol kg^{-1} h^{-1}, which was more than 5-fold greater than the output of cholesterol in the bile acid-depleted animals. The output of labelled cholesterol was also increased about 5-fold by bile acid infusion and so the contribution of newly synthesized cholesterol to biliary cholesterol was again 17.4%. In a separate group of experiments it was shown that the rate of hepatic cholesterol synthesis in bile acid-infused animals was not significantly different from that in the bile acid-depleted group.

DISCUSSION

The present lack of definitive data on the quantity of cholesterol that the liver synthesizes and then secretes directly across the canalicular membrane into bile is due partly to the limited number of methods that can be used to make such quantitative measurements. Although labelled sterol rapidly appears in bile following the administration of ^{14}C-labelled precursors such as acetate of mevalonate, such data cannot be used to determine the proportion of biliary cholesterol that is newly synthesized because these substrates undergo a variable and unknown degree of intracellular dilution. Thus, calculations based upon such measurements will invariably grossly underestimate the true amount of newly synthesized cholesterol transported into bile.

Such problems can be circumvented by using [^{3}H]water as the precursor because it rapidly equilibrates with total body water resulting in a uniform and measurable SA. The amount of newly synthesized sterol secreted into bile can thus be quantitated directly using [^{3}H]water providing that several conditions are fulfilled. First, the SA of water in the plasma must be the same as that of intracellular water. Second, the SA of plasma water must remain constant throughout the period in which the rate of incorporation of [^{3}H]water into sterols is being measured. Third, the rate of cholesterol synthesis in the liver must remain constant over the same period. Fourth, the relative rates of incorporation of ^{3}H and C into the cholesterol molecule must be known. Each of these conditions has been met in the present studies. The specific experiments relating to the first three of these conditions have been discussed in detail elsewhere[11]. The conversion of the [^{3}H]DPS content of bile into an absolute quantity of newly synthesized cholesterol was made using a value of 1.45 for the C/^{3}H incorporation ratio. This value was derived from previously published studies[5].

Utilizing this technique the present studies have provided experimental information on four major aspects of the regulation of biliary cholesterol secretion. The first conclusion to be drawn from these studies is that biliary cholesterol in the rat is derived from a subcompartment of the liver cell that is not in equilibrium with the hepatic cholesterol pool as a whole. This conclusion derives from the finding that the SA of biliary cholesterol was consistently and significantly higher than that of the liver, plasma and various extrahepatic tissues.

The second conclusion concerns the source of newly synthesized cholesterol that enters into the pool of free cholesterol from which biliary cholesterol is derived. Such [^{3}H]DPS could have been synthesized locally within the liver cell. Alternatively, it may have been delivered to the liver either from the intestine or some other extrahepatic tissue. However, in previous studies it was shown that the amount of [^{3}H]DPS in the blood is a linear function of the rate of sterol synthesis in the liver[6,12]. When hepatic [^{3}H]DPS synthesis is eliminated by the infusion of chylomicrons or by surgically removing the liver, essentially no [^{3}H]DPS appears in the blood[6,12]. This occurs even though sterol synthesis in the extrahepatic tissues is unchanged under these experimental conditions. Apparently the [^{3}H]DPS is mixed with a large pool of unlabelled cholesterol in these tissues so that relatively little appears in the blood. In the present study, even 6–10 h after the administration of [^{3}H]water, the SA of cholesterol in the extrahepatic tissues was very low (Figure 2). Thus it is unlikely that [^{3}H]DPS synthesized in the extrahepatic tissues contributes significantly to the labelled sterol in the pool of cholesterol from which biliary cholesterol is derived. Instead, most of the newly synthesized sterol that enters this pool and subsequently appears in bile must be derived from *de novo* cholesterol synthesis in the liver.

The third conclusion concerns the importance of the contribution of newly synthesized sterol to this pool in determining the actual rate of biliary cholesterol secretion. In the control animal with an intermediate rate of hepatic cholesterol synthesis approximately 16–18% of biliary cholesterol is newly synthesized, the remaining 82–84% consists of preformed, unlabelled cholesterol. A similar percentage for the contribution of newly synthesized sterol to biliary cholesterol has been reported in rats treated with triparanol, where it was found that desmosterol made up approximately 28% of biliary sterols[13]. The present studies further established that the proportion of biliary cholesterol that was newly synthesized could be varied from 0.2 to 42% and that the amount of newly synthesized cholesterol in bile correlated directly with the rate of hepatic cholesterol synthesis. However, despite the marked variation in the contribution of newly synthesized cholesterol to bile, total biliary cholesterol output and the molar percentage of cholesterol in bile remained constant. From this finding, and from other related data published elsewhere, it can be concluded that the rate of biliary cholesterol secretion is independent of the rate of cholesterol synthesis in the whole animal or in the liver[14] and, further, is unaffected by the amount of newly synthesized cholesterol entering the precursor pool for biliary cholesterol.

The final conclusion to be drawn from these studies is that while biliary cholesterol output is independent of the rate of cholesterol synthesis in any compartment of the body, it is tightly coupled to the absolute rate of bile acid output. Thus in the final series of experiments the absolute output of biliary cholesterol in control animals was varied over more than a 5-fold range by varying the output of bile acid. Despite this the contribution of newly synthesized cholesterol to biliary cholesterol remained constant at about 17%. Furthermore, when the contribution of newly synthesized cholesterol to biliary cholesterol was suppressed by feeding cholesterol or fasting (Figures 4 and 5) or enhanced by cholestyramine feeding (Figure 4), the absolute output of biliary cholesterol remained tightly coupled to bile acid output. Thus it can be concluded that while the rate of hepatic cholesterol synthesis determines the relative contribution of newly synthesized cholesterol to biliary cholesterol, it is the rate of bile acid output that determines the absolute rate of biliary cholesterol secretion.

Acknowledgments

The authors wish to acknowledge the excellent technical assistance of John Dermody, Larry Diana, and Kathy Johnson, and the help of Dorothy Dunham in the preparation of the manuscript. We also wish to thank Dr K. W. Wheeler at the Mead Johnson Research Center for a generous gift of cholestyramine. These studies were supported by US Public Health Service Research Grants AM 19329 and HL 09610.

References

1. Gregory, D. H., Vlahcevic, Z. R., Schatzki, P. and Swell, L. (1975). Mechanism of secretion of biliary lipids. I. Role of bile canalicular and microsomal membranes in the synthesis and transport of biliary lecithin and cholesterol. *J. Clin. Invest.*, **55**, 105
2. Schwartz, C. C., Vlahcevic, Z. R., Halloran, L. G., Gregory, D. H., Meek, J. B. and Swell, L. (1975). Evidence for the existence of definitive hepatic cholesterol precursor compartments for bile acids and biliary cholesterol in man. *Gastroenterology*, **69**, 1379
3. Normann, P. T. and Norum, K. R. (1976). Newly synthesized hepatic cholesterol as precursor for cholesterol and bile acids in rat bile. *Scand. J. Gastroenterol.*, **11**, 427
4. Lakshmanan, M. R. and Veech, R. L. (1977). Measurement of rate of rat liver sterol synthesis in vivo using tritiated water. *J. Biol. Chem.*, **252**, 4667
5. Andersen, J. M. and Dietschy, J. M. (1979). Absolute rates of cholesterol synthesis in extrahepatic tissues measured with ^{3}H-labelled water and ^{14}C-labelled substrates. *J. Lipid Res.*, **20**, 740
6. Jeske, D. J. and Dietschy, J. M. (1980). Regulation of rates of cholesterol synthesis *in vivo* in the liver and carcass of the rat measured using [^{3}H]water. *J. Lipid Res.*, **21**, 364
7. Andersen, J. M. and Dietschy, J. M. (1978). Relative importance of high and low density lipoproteins in the regulation of cholesterol synthesis in the adrenal gland, ovary, and testis of the rat. *J. Biol. Chem.*, **253**, 9024
8. Tonks, D. B. (1967). The estimation of cholesterol in serum: a classification and critical review of methods. *Clin. Biochem.*, **1**, 12

9. Turley, S. D. and Dietschy, J. M. (1978). Re-evaluation of the 3α-hydroxysteroid dehydrogenase assay for total bile acids in bile. *J. Lipid Res.*, **19,** 924
10. Chalvardjian, A. and Rudnicki, E. (1970). Determination of lipid phosphorus in the nanomolar range. *Anal. Biochem.*, **36,** 225
11. Turley, S. D. and Dietschy, J. M. (1981). The contribution of newly synthesized cholesterol to biliary cholesterol in the rat. *J. Biol. Chem.*, **256,** 2438
12. Turley, S. D., Andersen, J. M. and Dietschy, J. M. (1981). Rates of sterol synthesis and uptake in the major organs of the rat *in vivo*. *J. Lipid Res.* (In press)
13. Long, T. T., Jakoi, L., Stevens, R. and Quarfordt, S. (1978). The sources of rat biliary cholesterol and bile acid. *J. Lipid Res.*, **19,** 872
14. Turley, S. D. and Dietschy, J. M. (1979). Regulation of biliary cholesterol output in the rat: dissociation from the rate of hepatic cholesterol synthesis, the size of the hepatic cholesteryl ester pool, and the hepatic uptake of chylomicron cholesterol. *J. Lipid Res.*, **20,** 923

25
Bile salt–lipid interactions: the effect of sodium taurocholate (NaTC) on the permeability of lipid bilayers to water and urea

R. A. SMALLWOOD, C. J. RESTALL AND D. CHAPMAN

INTRODUCTION

The formation of bile is an important function of the liver in all classes of vertebrates. A major stimulus to bile water production is the active secretion of bile salts from the liver cell into the lumen of the biliary canaliculus. Water then enters the canaliculus passively, consequent upon the active transport of solute, so that bile becomes isosmotic with plasma[1,2]. In most species studied, there is a substantial bile salt-independent fraction (so called) of bile water, which does not depend on the osmotic effect of the secreted bile salt. Both bile salt-'dependent' and 'independent' fractions may in fact be modified by prior infusions of bile salt, suggesting that bile salt may modify liver cell membranes, either functionally or structurally[3]. In addition to influencing water movement, bile salts stimulate the secretion of phospholipid and cholesterol into bile[4]. The exact origin of these two biliary lipids is uncertain, but both the canalicular membrane[4] and membranes within the liver cell[5] are possible sources. There is evidence that other constituents in bile are removed from the canalicular membrane by bile salts, e.g. various glycoprotein enzymes present on the outer surface of the membrane[6]. Thus, the movement of water and other bile constituents from the liver cell into bile appears to be intimately associated with the interaction of bile salt with liver cell membranes.

The present study was designed to examine the influence of the bile salt sodium taurocholate on the movement of water and urea through lipid bilayers, using multilamellar liposomes of purified egg yolk lecithin.

MATERIALS AND METHODS

Materials

Egg yolk lecithin (EYL) (grade IX Sigma) was purified essentially as described by Singleton[7]. The resulting material was found to be homogeneous by thin-layer chromatography using the solvent system chloroform : methanol : water (65 : 25 : 4 v/v/v) on silica gel G plates.

Dipalmitoylphosphatidylcholine (DPPC), cholesterol, dicetylphosphate and 1,6-diphenyl-1,3,5-hexatriene (DPH) were all obtained from Sigma. Gramicidin A was obtained from Koch-Light Laboratories and sodium taurocholate from Calbiochem. All other reagents used were of analytical grade.

Liposome preparation

Multilamellar liposomes were prepared by methods similar to those used by Bangham *et al.*[8]. Solutions of EYL, dicetylphosphate, cholesterol and sodium taurocholate were prepared in chloroform : methanol (2 : 1 v/v). Appropriate amounts of each solution were added to 100 ml round-bottomed flasks and coprecipitated by removing the solvent under a stream of nitrogen. The resulting thin film of lipid coating the walls of the flask was resuspended in distilled water by gentle shaking. The following liposome suspensions were prepared: (1) EYL alone, (2) EYL : cholesterol 2 : 1, and (3) mixtures of (1) or (2) with sodium taurocholate using lipid : bile salt ratios of 40 : 1, 20 : 1, 10 : 1 and 5 : 1. The liposome suspensions contained 10 μmol EYL/ml water, so that taurocholate concentrations ranged from 0.25 to 2.0 mmol/l. The use of these concentrations and lipid : bile salt ratios ensured that the composition of the mixtures lay outside the mixed micellar phase boundary, in the region of the taurocholate–lecithin phase diagram where only liposomes and bilayers are formed[9]. Dicetylphosphate (5 mol% of total lipid) was incorporated into all EYL liposomes in order to give the bilayers a net negative charge. Without dicetylphosphate, neutral lipids such as EYL produce liposomes with small interlamellar spaces, and as a consequence the osmotic swelling effects are small and not readily detected. Gramicidin A was incorporated into the bilayers (at molar ratios of 40 : 1, 20 : 1, 10 : 1) using the same procedure as described for the incorporation of bile salt.

Permeability studies

Changes in 'apparent absorption' of liposome suspensions were measured in all cases at 25 °C using a Pye-Unicam spectrophotometer[10] operating at 450 nm. 0.2 ml of each liposome suspension was rapidly dispersed in 2.0 ml of 0.1 M urea using a simple injection system. Using this system it was possible to produce intimate mixing of the lipid with the urea within a second. Consequently we were able to monitor the rapid absorption changes due to liposome shrinkage as well as the slower changes due to the subsequent swelling as urea entered the liposome. To obtain the baseline absorption, i.e. the absorption due to the liposomes prior to any changes induced by shrinkage or swelling, 0.2 ml of lipid suspension was injected into 2 ml of distilled water. The baseline absorption (OD_{base}) was taken as the mean of three separate injections.

Physical studies

Fluorescence polarization studies were performed at 25 °C using an Elscint MV1-a Microviscosimeter. Lipid samples were prepared as for the permeability studies, with the exception that the final suspension contained approximately 0.1 mg lipid/ml water. Diphenyl hexatriene (DPH) was added to the dispersion at a lipid : probe ratio of 500 : 1 by adding an aliquot of DPH solution in tetrahydrofuran. To ensure that light-scattering was not causing any depolarization, samples were measured at two dilutions. Identical readings were obtained in each case.

Calorimetric studies were performed using a Perkin-Elmer DSC2 differential scanning calorimeter. Samples of DPPC and DPPC–taurocholate mixtures were dispersed in excess water and transferred to Perkin-Elmer 'volatile' sample pans. Two ratios of lipid : bile salt were investigated – 20 : 1 and 10 : 1. The instrument was calibrated using standards of naphthalene and indium. The areas of the transition endotherm peaks were determined by weighing paper cut-outs of the peaks. The phospholipid content of each pan was determined after calorimetry by solubilizing the pan contents in 1% w/v SDS at 70 °C. The fatty acids present were analysed by quantitative gas–liquid chromatography using an internal standard of heptadecanoic acid. The chromatograph employed was a Pye-Unicam Model 204 equipped with a column of 15% polyethyleneglycol adipate on Gas–Chrom Z.

RESULTS

Permeability studies

EYL and EYL : cholesterol (2 : 1) *liposomes*

The changes in apparent absorption in EYL and EYL : cholesterol (1 : 1) liposomes (with entrapped water) after sudden dispersion in 0.1 M urea are shown in Figure 1. There is a rapid increase in optical density (OD) due to the shrinkage of liposomes as water moves out into the surrounding medium. Subsequently the liposomes begin to swell as the slower movement of urea into the interlamellar spaces occurs. From the semi-logarithmic plot this second process is well described by a single exponential. The effects of cholesterol are:

(1) to slow the rate of attainment of the maximum OD (ΔA_{max}) (i.e. the time to ΔA_{max} (t_{max}) is longer); and

(2) to increase the half-life time ($t_{\frac{1}{2}}$) of the terminal exponential (Figure 1).

If the assumption is made that the system is going from state I to state II with a rate constant k_1 and then from state II to state III with rate constant k_2, the experimental curve would be expected to describe a function of the form:

$$A_{(t)} = \Delta A \cdot \frac{k_1}{k_1 - k_2}\left(\exp^{-k_2 t} - \exp^{-k_1 t}\right) \tag{1}$$

where $A(_t)$ is the time-dependent absorption and ΔA is the maximum absorption that would be obtained if state II were not decaying to state III. However, as the two processes are occurring simultaneously, the true value

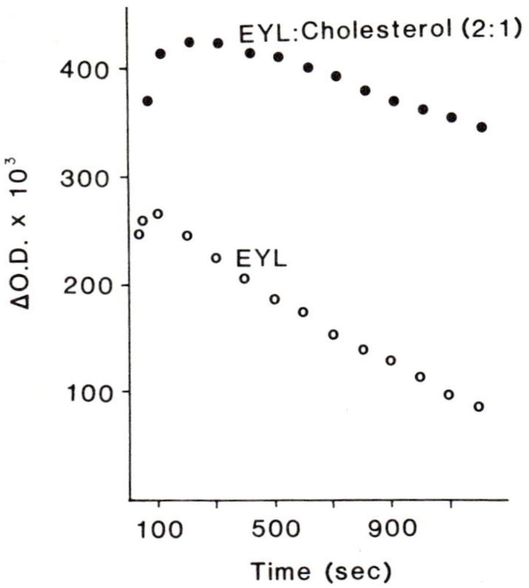

Figure 1 Time-dependent absorption changes in EYL liposomes (○) and EYL : cholesterol (2 : 1) liposomes (●) following rapid dispersion in 0.1 M urea. The larger OD values of the cholesterol-containing samples are due to the greater light-scattering caused by the presence of cholesterol

of ΔA is never attained. It is possible to calculate it, though, from the observed value using the relation:

$$\Delta A = A_{max} \cdot \frac{k_2 - k_1}{k_1} \left(\exp^{-k_1 t_{max}} - \exp^{-k_2 t_{max}} \right) \tag{2}$$

where A_{max} is the observed maximum absorption and t_{max} is the time to

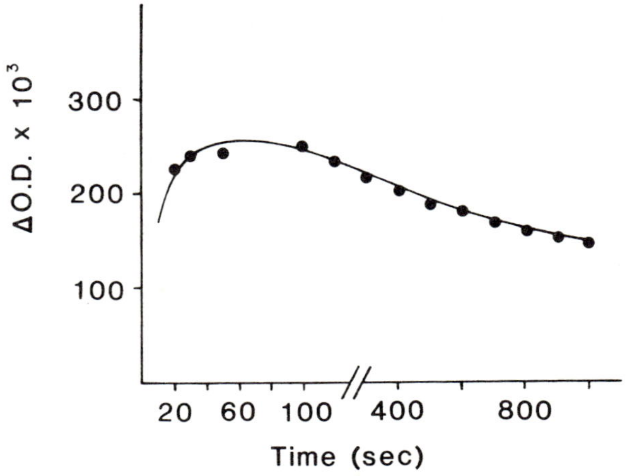

Figure 2 Comparison of the theoretical absorption changes predicted by the two-exponential function (shown as the solid line) with the experimental obtained values. The sample comprised EYL liposomes formed in distilled water and then rapidly dispersed in 0.1 M urea

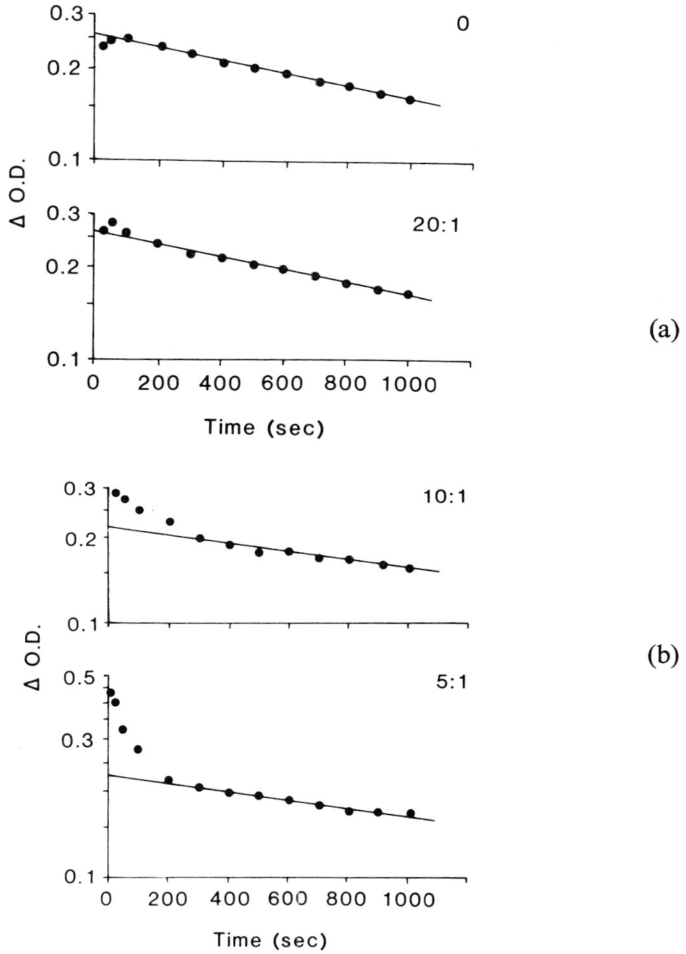

Figure 3 Time-dependent absorption changes in EYL liposomes containing differing amounts of sodium taurocholate after dispersion in 0.1 M urea. The phospholipid : bile salt ratios are as indicated

A_{max}. The value of k_2 can be obtained from the value of $t_{\frac{1}{2}}$ for the process state II to state III at long times where the contribution of k_1 is small, since for a first-order reaction[2] $k_2 = \ln 2/t_{\frac{1}{2}}$. The value of t_{max} can also be obtained experimentally. Knowing these two values an estimate of k_1 can be made by solving the relation:

$$t_{max} = \frac{\ln k_1/k_2}{k_1 - k_2} \quad (3)$$

for k_1 by iteration. Substituting the estimated k_1 in equation (2) enables the value of ΔA to be obtained and hence equation (1) to be solved. A comparison of the theoretical curve obtained by the above procedure is shown in Figure 2 together with the experimental data. It can be seen that excellent agreement is obtained between the theoretical curve (solid line) and the experimental data points, indicating that the system is well described by a two-exponential process.

Liposomes incorporating taurocholate

The presence of taurocholate in the EYL liposome suspension alters the kinetic pattern of water and urea movement (Figure 3a,b). The system can no longer be described by a two-exponential process. The presence of taurocholate superimposes a relatively short-lived initial effect, which increases with increasing amounts of bile salt. This effect is evident, although less pronounced, in liposomes containing cholesterol (Figure 4a,b). As the mole fraction of taurocholate increases, t_{max} decreases. A measure of the

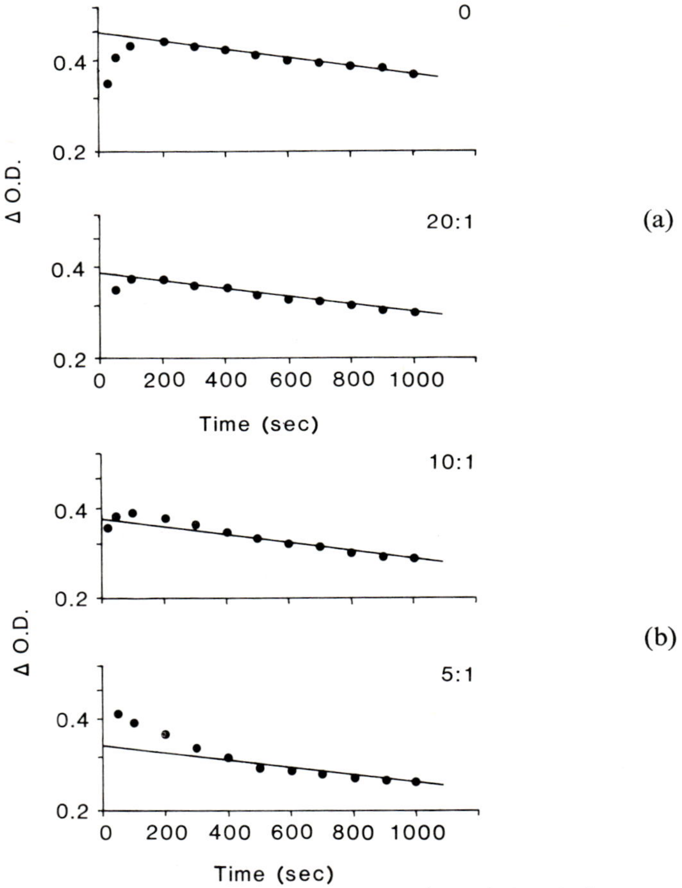

Figure 4 Time-dependent absorption changes in EYL : cholesterol (2 : 1) liposomes containing differing amounts of sodium taurocholate after dispersion in 0.1 M urea. The phospholipid : bile salt ratios are as indicated

amplitude of the bile salt effect can be calculated as follows; At time intervals t_{1-n}, a series of values of f can be calculated from the observed absorption changes when no bile salt is present.

$$f = \frac{A^{\text{meas}}}{A^{\text{ex}}} \quad (4)$$

where A^{meas} is the measured absorption and A^{ex} is the expected absorption if the process were following the same kinetics as seen in the absence of bile salt, i.e. the two-exponential processes shown in Figure 1.

A^{meas} and A^{ex} values are measured at several points for each sample containing taurocholate, and the expression $(A^{\text{meas}} - A^{\text{ex}}) \cdot f$ is calculated for each point. The y-intercept of the line joining these points, plotted logarithmically, can be used as a measure of the amplitude of the bile salt effect. Figure 5 shows that the effect (E) is approximately linear over the range of phospholipid : bile salt ratios used.

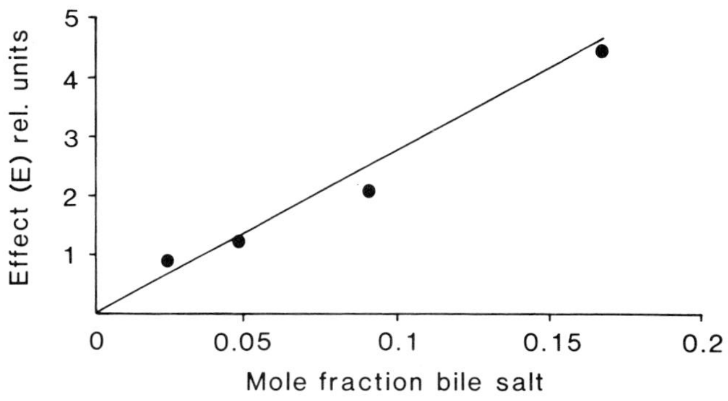

Figure 5 The relationship between the magnitude of the bile salt effect (E) and the mole fraction of bile salt present

Gramicidin A studies

The incorporation of gramicidin A into the lipid bilayers produces changes in the apparent absorption curve similar to those seen with taurocholate. The predominant effect is produced early in the experiment. The efflux of water is more rapid with gramicidin present, as is the influx of urea. Compared with the bile salt the gramicidin effect is more pronounced, and results in the system returning almost to the initial absorption within the period of study. Even with the highest bile salt concentrations used, relaxation of the system was only 60% achieved within 1000 s.

It should be noted that the effects of both taurocholate and gramicidin A are most pronounced in the first 200–300 s, and that thereafter the swelling process continues as though neither taurocholate nor polypeptide were present. This most probably reflects the kinetics of the processes concerned. The rapid movement of urea and water through, for example, the gramicidin A channel, will be perceived early in the course of the experiment. However, one would expect that at a given time during the experiment the process of shrinkage and swelling will be nearer completion when gramicidin A or taurocholate is present. This has proved to be the case. For example, at 1000 s, EYL liposomes have only swollen to 40–50% of their original state. In contrast, EYL : gramicidin A 10 : 1 liposomes are 80–85% swollen.

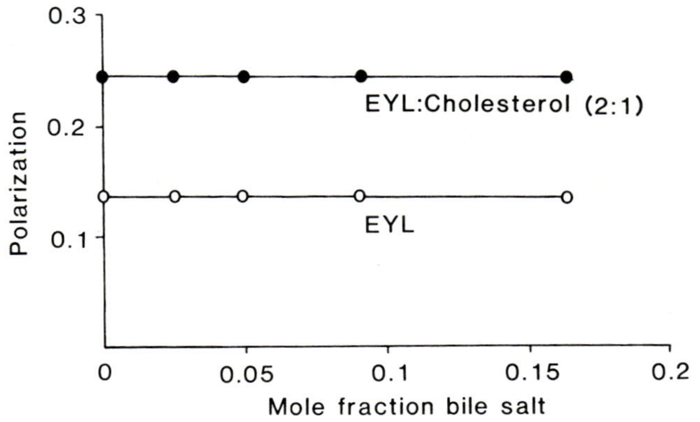

Figure 6 The dependence of the fluorescence polarization (*P*), measured at 25 °C, on the mole fraction of bile salt (sodium taurocholate) for (○) EYL liposomes and (□) EYL : cholesterol (2 : 1) liposomes

Physical studies

Figure 6 shows the dependence of DPH fluorescence polarization (*P*) where $P = (I_{II} - I_I)/(I_{II} + I_I)$ on the bile salt concentration in both EYL and EYL–cholesterol liposomes. The well-known ordering effect of cholesterol on fluid lipid bilayers is evident in the higher *P* values seen in the EYL–cholesterol liposomes. Increasing the molar proportion of bile salt to a lipid : bile salt ratio of 5 : 1 has no effect on the DPH polarization, whether or not cholesterol is present in the bilayer.

The calorometric heating curves for the DPPC–taurocholate mixtures showed no evidence of having changed in shape relative to the pure lipid, nor was there any change in the gel to liquid crystal (T_C) transition temperature. Calculation of the transition enthalpy gave values of 8.7, 7.9 and 8.5 kcal/mol for the pure lipid, DPPC : taurocholate 20 : 1 and DPPC : taurocholate 10 : 1 respectively. Thus taurocholate did not cause any appreciable reduction in the transition enthalpy such as is normally obtained when intrinsic molecules are present in the bilayer.

DISCUSSION

We have shown that it is possible to characterize the shrinkage and swelling of a simple liposome system in response to osmotic stimuli by an exponential function. Using this model as a basis for further investigations we have shown that the introduction of the bile salt, sodium taurocholate, affects the permeability of the liposomes both to water and urea. As the proportion of bile salt increases, the amplitude of the effect increases in a manner which is directly proportional to the mole fraction of bile salt. A similar change is observed when cholesterol is present in the bilayer, but the taurocholate effect is less pronounced. This might be expected from the known membrane stabilizing effect of cholesterol[11,12]. Thus, the time taken to reach maximum absorption (t_{max}) decreases in EYL–cholesterol liposomes with increasing amounts of taurocholate, but is appreciably longer than with the corresponding liposomes containing EYL alone.

In order to understand the molecular details of the effect of taurocholate on these membranes we have compared the behaviour with that shown by gramicidin A. Gramicidin A is known to increase the permeability of lecithin liposomes to small hydrophilic solutes[13,14]. It is thought that gramicidin A exists as a dimer within the bilayer, and that a transmembrane channel is thereby formed for the passage of hydrophilic molecules. The similarity of the taurocholate and gramicidin A effects in our test system suggested the possibility that taurocholate might also insert into the bilayer and form similar channels. Indeed, the studies of Mazer *et al.*[9,15] and of Small[16] on ternary systems of bile salt, lecithin and water have led them to suggest that in both lamellar and micellar phases, bile salt may exist as dimers within lipid bilayers. They envisage that the molecules would be hydrogen bonded through their hydroxyl groups, with their hydrophobic backs facing the lipid chains in the bilayer. Coincidence of dimers in the inner and outer halves of the bilayer would thus form a transmembrane hydrophilic pathway which would facilitate the passage of hydrophilic molecules.

However, the calorimetry and fluorescent probe studies do not support this model. Calorimetric heating curves for DPPC bilayers containing gramicidin A (10 : 1 molar ratio) show a marked effect on the transition endotherm of DPPC, with a marked increase in transition width and a loss of enthalpy[17]. In contrast, no such effect was observed with taurocholate on the transition endotherm. The fluorescence data also failed to show any change in the observed polarization when taurocholate was present.

It seems clear that in our system taurocholate does not increase the permeability of the lipid bilayer by staying in the bilayer and forming a channel, in the manner of gramicidin A. The change in the kinetics of water and urea movement suggests a second process superimposed on the slower diffusion which is seen in the absence of taurocholate. This suggests a transient disturbance of the lipid bilayer which is localized and which does not alter the overall characteristics of the membrane.

These findings may have interesting implications for understanding water transport which occurs where a membrane is exposed to bile salts *in vivo*. The brush border of small intestinal absorptive cells is such a membrane. Liver cell membranes, in particular the canalicular portion of the plasma membrane, are also confronted with large amounts of bile salts.

There is evidence to suggest that, *in vivo*, sodium taurocholate may alter liver cell secretory membranes, thereby modifying both bile salt-'dependent' and bile salt-'independent' fractions of canalicular bile[3]. Liver and intestinal plasma membranes are involved in the translocation of water and other hydrophilic molecules in substantial amounts. For example, 1–1.5 l of bile are formed on average each day, while 7–8 l of water cross the epithelium of the small bowel[18]. The presence of bile salt may well play an important role in modulating the movement of water at these sites.

Acknowledgment

The help and advice of Dr Winfreid Hoffman are gratefully acknowledged. This study was in part supported by the National Health and Medical Research Council of Australia.

References

1. Sperber, I. (1965). Biliary excretion of organic anions and its influence on bile flow. In Taylor, W. (ed.). *The Biliary System*, pp. 456–467. (Oxford: Blackwell)
2. Wheeler, H. O. (1972). Secretion of bile acids by the liver and their role in the formation of hepatic bile. *Arch. Intern. Med.*, **130,** 533
3. Baker, A. L., Wood, R. A. B., Moossa, A. R. and Boyer, J. L. (1979). Sodium taurocholate modifies the bile acid-independent fraction of canalicular bile flow in the rhesus monkey. *J. Clin. Invest.*, **64,** 312
4. Wheeler, H. O. and King, K. K. (1972). Biliary excretion of lecithin and cholesterol in the dog. *J. Clin. Invest.*, **51,** 1337
5. Gregory, D. H., Vlahcevic, Z. R., Schatzki, P. and Swell, L. (1975). Mechanisms of secretion of biliary lipids. I. Role of bile canalicular and microsomal membranes in the synthesis and transport of biliary lecithin and cholesterol. *J. Clin. Invest.*, **55,** 105
6. Evans, W. H., Kremmer, T. and Culvenor, J. G. (1976). Role of membranes in bile formation. Comparison of the composition of bile and a liver bile-canalicular subfraction. *Biochem. J.*, **154,** 589
7. Singleton, W. S., Gray, M. S., Brown, M. L. and White, J. L. (1965). Chromatographically homogeneous lecithin from egg phospholipids. *J. Am. Oil. Chem. Soc.*, **42,** 53
8. Bangham, A. D., Standish, M. M. and Watkins, J. C. (1965). Diffusion of univalent ions across the lamellae of swollen phospholipids. *J. Mol. Biol.*, **13,** 238
10. Bangham, A. D., deGier, J. and Grenville, G. D. (1967). Osmotic properties and water permeability of phospholipid liquid crystals. *Chem. Phys. Lipids*, **1,** 225
11. Ladbrooke, B. D., Williams, R. M. and Chapman, D. (1968). Studies on lecithin–cholesterol–water interactions by differential scanning calorimetry and X-ray diffraction. *Biochim. Biophys. Acta*, **150,** 333
12. Singer, M. A. (1973). Transfer of anions across phospholipid membranes. *Can. J. Physiol. Pharmacol.*, **51,** 523
13. Cohen, B. E. (1975). The permeability of liposomes to nonelectrolytes. I. Activation energies for permeation. *J. Membrane Biol.*, **20,** 205
14. Cohen, B. E. (1975). The permeability of liposomes to nonelectrolytes. II. The effect of nystatin and gramicidin A. *J. Membrane Biol.*, **20,** 235
15. Mazer, N. A., Benedek, G. B. and Carey, M. C. (1976). The size and shape of bile salt (BS), BS-lecithin (L) and BS-L cholesterol (Ch) micelles using quasielastic light scattering spectroscopy. *Gastroenterology*, **70,** 998
17. Chapman, D., Cornell, B. A., Eliasz, A. W. and Perry, A. (1977). Interactions of helical polypeptide segments which span the hydrocarbon region of lipid bilayers. Studies of the gramicidin A lipid–water system. *J. Mol. Biol.*, **113,** 517
18. Phillips, S. F. (1972). Diarrhea: A current view of the pathophysiology. *Gastroenterology*, **63,** 495

26
Effects of lactulose on bile composition

J. R. THORNTON AND K. W. HEATON

INTRODUCTION

It has been suggested that increased return of secondary bile acids to the liver favours the secretion of bile supersaturated with cholesterol[1]. In support of this theory, feeding small amounts of deoxycholic acid (DCA) to normal subjects raised biliary cholesterol saturation[1] (though feeding larger amounts failed to produce any change)[2,3]. In addition, the administration to normal volunteers of metronidazole, an antimicrobial agent active against many anaerobic colonic bacteria, reduced the proportion of DCA in bile, raised that of chenodeoxycholic acid (CDCA), and lowered bile cholesterol saturation[4].

The conversion of primary to secondary bile acids by 7α-dehydroxylation is a pH-dependent reaction which is inhibited below pH 6.5[5,6]. Lactulose is a non-absorbable carbohydrate which is metabolized to organic acids by colonic bacteria and has been shown to reduce the pH in the right colon of normal subjects to less than 5.0[7]. We predicted, therefore, that lactulose would inhibit 7α-dehydroxylation. To test this hypothesis, and to look for possible improvement in bile cholesterol saturation, we have carried out a preliminary study in which we have analysed bile before and after administration of lactulose for 6 weeks.

SUBJECTS AND METHODS

Ten healthy female volunteers gave informed consent to be studied. None was taking any medication, including oral contraceptives. All had normal standard liver function tests. Oral cholecystograms were not performed on ethical grounds, but no subject had symptoms suggestive of gallbladder disease. Their mean age was 46 years (range 42–51) and mean body weight was 118% of ideal (range 104–135). The subjects maintained their usual diet throughout the duration of the study.

The subjects were asked to take lactulose syrup 15 ml (10 g) t.d.s. with meals for 1 week and then increase the dosage to 30 ml (20 g) t.d.s. for a further 5 weeks. After an overnight fast, duodenal bile was sampled following gallbladder stimulation with cholecystokinin. Bile was collected before and immediately after the 6 weeks of lactulose administration.

Both bile samples from each subject were analysed in the same batch. The concentrations of total bile salts, phospholipids and cholesterol were measured[8] and used to calculate a cholesterol saturation index using the criteria of Hegardt and Dam[9]. Individual bile acid composition was determined by gas–liquid chromatography. The statistical significance of differences was calculated by Student's *t* test.

RESULTS

Lactulose increased mean bowel frequency from 8 ± 2 to 14 ± 3 per week. No subject dropped out of the study because of diarrhoea, though two subjects were only able to tolerate a maximum dose of 20 ml (13 g) t.d.s. of lactulose. There was no significant change in the subjects' body weight.

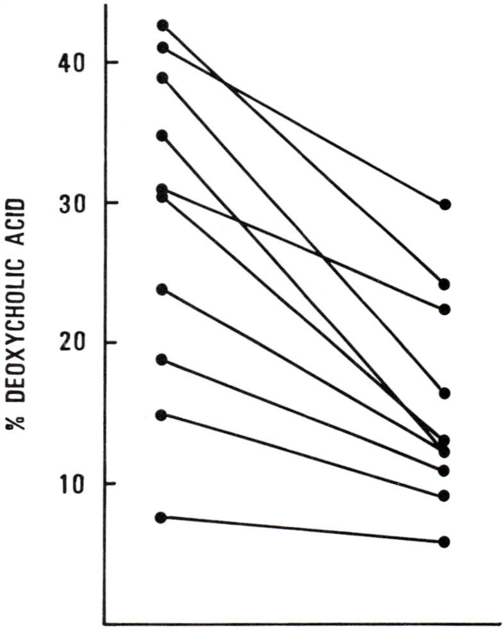

Figure 1 Effect of lactulose on percentage biliary deoxycholic acid

There was a highly significant reduction in the percentage of DCA in bile from 28.4 ± 3.7 to 15.6 ± 2.4 ($p < 0.002$). Figure 1 shows that this fall occurred in all ten subjects. Conversely, as shown in Figure 2, all subjects showed a rise in the percentage of biliary CDCA after lactulose (33.2 ± 3.2 to 42.9 ± 2.9; $p < 0.001$). There was a rise in the percentage of cholic acid (CA) in eight of the ten subjects but the mean value only rose from 36.0 ± 1.4 to 39.0 ± 1.3 and this change was not statistically significant (Figure 3). The small percentage of biliary lithocholic acid did not change (2.5 ± 0.2 to 2.5 ± 0.2). Concurrently, lactulose lowered bile cholesterol saturation in nine of the ten subjects (Figure 4) with a fall in the mean saturation index from 1.40 ± 0.11 to 1.19 ± 0.07 ($p<0.005$).

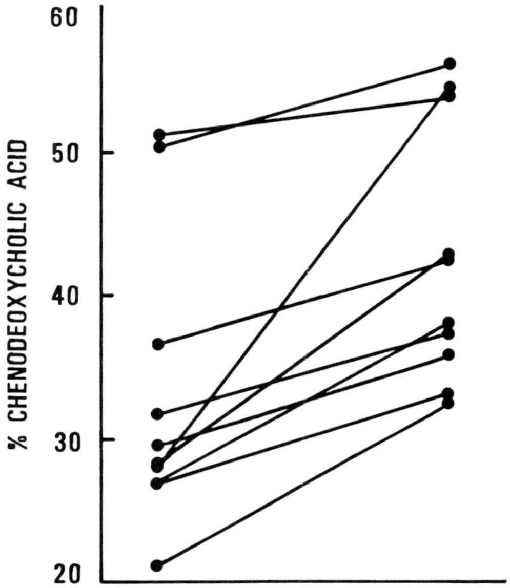

Figure 2 Effect of lactulose on percentage biliary chenodeoxycholic acid

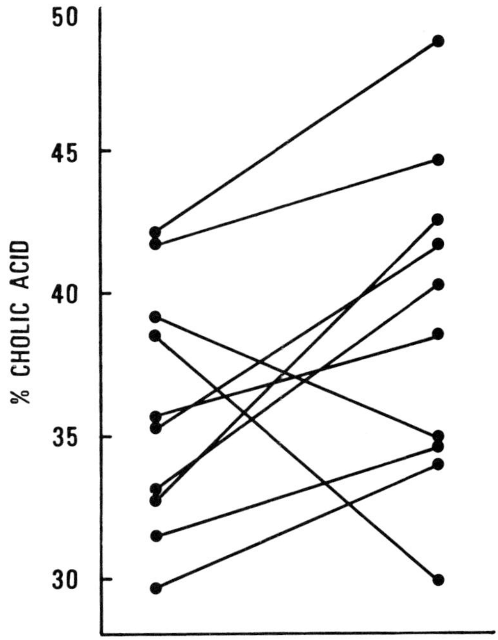

Figure 3 Effect of lactulose on percentage biliary cholic acid

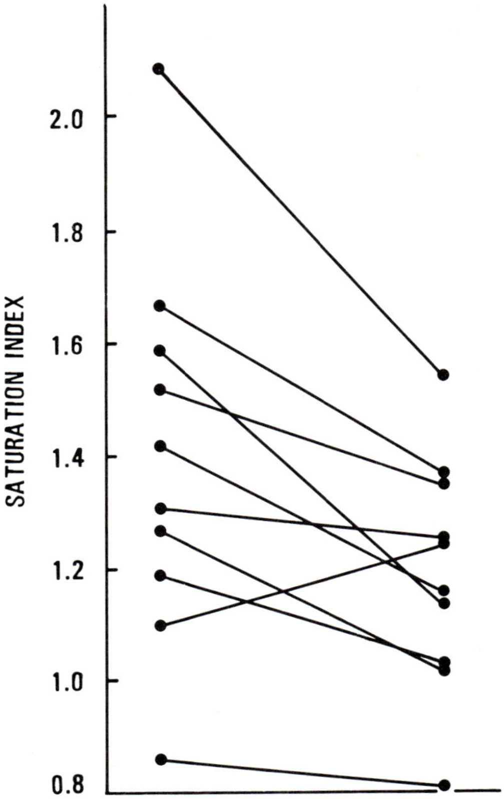

Figure 4 Effect of lactulose on bile cholesterol saturation index

DISCUSSION

This preliminary study shows that lactulose lowers bile cholesterol saturation. This change is associated with a significant fall in the percentage of biliary DCA and a significant rise in that of CDCA.

The reduction in the proportion of DCA is consistent with the idea that lactulose inhibits bacterial 7α-dehydroxylation of bile acids. However, other explanations of our findings must be considered. Lactulose might accelerate colonic transit, so reducing the time available for formation or absorption of secondary bile acids. Alternatively, acidification of the colon by lactulose might increase bile acid excretion, either by precipitation[10] or by promoting binding to components of dietary fibre[11]. The scanty data available suggest that lactulose does not decrease colonic transit time or increase faecal bile acid excretion[12]. However, further work is indicated including the determination of rates of 7α-dehydroxylation and of primary bile acid synthesis, in addition to measurement of faecal bile acids, during lactulose administration.

Acknowledgments

We are grateful to Duphar Laboratories Limited for providing lactulose.

References

1. Low-Beer, T. S. and Pomare, E. W. (1975). Can colonic bacterial metabolites predispose to cholesterol gallstones? *Br. Med. J.*, **1**, 438
2. LaRusso, N. F., Szczepanik, P. A. and Hofmann, A. F. (1977). Effect of deoxycholic acid ingestion on bile acid metabolism and biliary lipid secretion in normal subjects. *Gastroenterology*, **72**, 132
3. Ahlberg, J., Angelin, B., Einarsson, K., Hellström, K. and Leijd, B. (1977). Influence of deoxycholic acid on biliary lipids in man. *Clin. Sci. Mol. Med.*, **53**, 249
4. Low-Beer, T. S. and Nutter, S. (1978). Colonic bacterial activity, biliary cholesterol saturation and pathogenesis of gallstones. *Lancet*, **2**, 1063
5. Midtvedt, T. and Norman, A. (1968). Parameters in 7α-dehydroxylation of bile acids by anaerobic lactobacilli. *Acta Pathol. Microbiol. Scand.*, **72**, 313
6. Aries, V. and Hill, M. J. (1970). Degradation of steroids by intestinal bacteria II. *Biochim. Biophys. Acta*, **202**, 535
7. Bown, R. L., Gibson, J. A., Sladen, G. E., Hicks, B. and Dawson, A. M. (1974). Effects of lactulose and other laxatives on ileal and colonic pH as measured by a radiotelemetry device. *Gut*, **15**, 999
8. Bolton, C. H., Low-Beer, T. S., Pomare, E. W., Wicks, A. C. B., Yeates, J. and Heaton K. W. (1974). A simplified procedure for the analysis of cholesterol, phospholipids and bile salts in human bile. *Clin. Chim. Acta*, **83**, 177
9. Hegardt, F. G. and Dam, H. (1971). The solubility of cholesterol in aqueous solutions of bile salts and lecithin. *Z. Ernahrung*, **10**, 223
10. Igimi, H. and Carey, M. C. (1980). pH-solubility relations of chenodeoxycholic and ursodeoxycholic acids: physical–chemical basis for dissimilar solution and membrane phenomena. *J. Lipid Res.*, **21**, 72
11. Kay, R. M., Wayman, M. and Strasberg, S. M. (1979). Effect of autohydrolysed lignin and lactulose on gallbladder bile composition in the hamster. *Gastroenterology*, **76**, 1167 (abstr.)
12. Eastwood, M. A., Smith, A. N., Brydon, W. G. and Pritchard, J. (1978). Comparison of bran, ispaghula and lactulose on colon function in diverticular disease. *Gut*, **19**, 1144

27
Immediate effects of individual primary bile acid conjugates on biliary phospholipid and cholesterol secretion in man

I. T. GILMORE, K. STOKES, A. F. HOFMANN AND D. GURANTZ

In all animals studied, acute infusions of chenodeoxycholyl or ursodeoxycholyl conjugates cause either no change or, more commonly, an increase in biliary cholesterol and lecithin secretion when compared to cholyl conjugates. In man, however, these dihydroxy bile acids, when administered chronically in unconjugated form, reduce cholesterol secretion and bile saturation. Further, unconjugated chenodeoxycholic or ursodeoxycholic acid, when given acutely to patients with T-tubes after cholecystectomy, is reported to reduce cholesterol secretion and bile saturation[1,2]. The aim of the present study was to define the effect of individual conjugated bile acids on biliary secretion and to test whether man is indeed different from all animal species studied to date.

The experiment comprised three consecutive 72 h periods during which the bile acid pool was largely replaced with either synthetically prepared chenodeoxycholyl, ursodeoxycholyl or cholyl conjugates (glycine : taurine, 3 : 1) in random order. Studies were completed in two healthy subjects, two post-cholecystectomy patients, and two with cholesterol gallstones. A triple-lumen orojejunal tube was passed and bile aspirated at the level of the ampulla while a solution of the conjugated bile acid, 2 mmol/h, was infused beyond the duodenojejunal flexure for 8 h; for up to 28 h thereafter bile was sampled hourly and analysed enzymatically for bile acids, lecithin and cholesterol.

Using this design, replacement of the bile acid pool by the infused species was usually greater than 80% within 8 h. Preliminary results suggest that, under these conditions, ursodeoxycholyl but not chenodeoxycholyl or cholyl conjugates reduce cholesterol and lecithin secretion and lower bile saturation acutely in patients with gallstones. These immediate effects may contribute to the efficacy of ursodeoxycholic acid during chronic treatment for gallstone dissolution.

Acknowledgment

This work was supported by NIH Grant AM 21506.

References

1. Lindblad, L., Lundholm, K. and Scherstén, T. (1977). Influence of cholic and chenodeoxycholic acid on biliary cholesterol secretion in man. *Eur. J. Clin. Invest.*, **7,** 383
2. Marteau, C., Reynier, M. O., Mathieu, S., Salasc, B., Mule, A., Montet, J. C. and Gerolami, A. (1980). L'état de la circulation entérohépatique influence-t'il l'action immédiate de différents sels bilaires sur la saturation de la bile en cholestérol. *Gastroenterol. Clin. Biol.*, **4,** 70 A (Abstr.)

28
Effect of chenodeoxycholic and ursodeoxycholic acid administration on biliary lipid secretion in normal-weight and obese gallstone patients

E. RODA, G. MAZZELLA, A. RODA, R. ALDINI, D. FESTI, F. BAZZOLI, E. MESSALE, A. M. MORSELLI AND L. BARBARA

INTRODUCTION

The long-term administration of chenodeoxycholic acid (CDCA) and ursodeoxycholic acid (UDCA) inhibits cholesterol secretion in man[1,2].

Recent studies[3–5] pointed out that different mechanisms are responsible for cholesterol gallstone formation in obese and non-obese patients.

In obese patients a disturbance in cholesterol metabolism may lead to an increased cholesterol secretion in bile[6,7], whereas in non-obese patients with gallstones, the basic defect is a decreased bile acid secretion, probably related to an alteration in their enterohepatic circulation dynamics[7].

It is still unknown whether these differences may influence the response to the CDCA and UDCA treatment for cholesterol gallstone dissolution in obese and non-obese patients. Differences, if any, in the response to therapy, may provide further information on the mechanisms of cholesterol gallstone formation in the two different series of patients. Moreover, clinical and biochemical studies suggest that obese patients with gallstones may be resistant to CDCA treatment[8].

Our study was carried out to further clarify the mechanisms by which CDCA and UDCA desaturate bile in cholesterol, as well as to compare the effects of CDCA and UDCA feeding on the secretion of biliary lipids.

MATERIALS AND METHODS

Patients

Four normal-weight patients (two men and two women; mean weight 95% ideal weight; age range 33–59 years) and four obese patients (two men and two women, mean weight 131% ideal weight; age range 32–55 years) with radiolucent gallstones in normal functioning gallbladder were admitted to the study.

No patient presented liver disease or intestinal or metabolic disorders. The patients gave informed consent.

EXPERIMENTAL DESIGN

Two patients of each group were first treated with CDCA (12.5 mg kg b.w.$^{-1}$ day^{-1}, over 1 month) and then with UDCA (7.5 mg kg b.w.$^{-1}$ day^{-1} over 1 month). In two patients first UDCA and then CDCA were administered. CDCA (125 mg capsules) and UDCA (150 mg capsules) were purchased from Giuliani, Milan. Bile lipid secretion was investigated before and after each bile acid feeding period. CDCA and UDCA administration was stopped the day before the study of biliary lipid secretion was started. Liver function tests remained normal throughout the study in all the patients; two patients on CDCA developed diarrhoea.

BILIARY LIPID COMPOSITION AND SECRETION STUDY

Biliary lipid secretion was carried out according to Grundy and Metzger[9], Gordon *et al.*[10] and Schaffer and Small[7].

The fasting subjects were intubated with a triple-lumen polyvinyl tube. The proximal outlets were positioned fluoroscopically in the duodenum at the level of the ampulla of Vater and a more distal port was situated 10 cm further along, at the ligament of Treitz.

Through one of the proximal outlets, an essential amino-acid solution[11] was constantly infused at a constant rate (1.8 ml/min) via a Harvard peristaltic pump (Harvard Apparatus Co., Inc. Millis, Mass.), to tonically contract the gallbladder and to provide a source of calories.

BSP[7,12] (5 mg%) or PEG 4000[13] (5 g/l) were used as non-absorbable markers.

Duodenal contents were continuously aspirated in hourly aliquots (8–10 ml). The quantity collected represented less than 5% of duodenal output.

Bile was diluted 1 : 5 with isopropanol; cholesterol[14] (XOL), phospholipids (PL) (A. Roda, data to be published), and bile acids (BA) (3α-Stevognost, Nieegard) were assayed. BSP and PEG 4000 were measured in the undiluted bile[12,13]. The hourly rate of XOL secretion was determined from the sample withdrawn distally by means of the marker dilution principle[9]:

$$\text{XOL secretion (mg/h)} = \text{XOL concentration (mg/ml) in the distal aspirate} \times \frac{\text{[BSP or PEG infused (mg/h)]}}{\text{BSP or PEG concentration in distal aspirate (mg/ml)}}$$

From the ratios of bile acid (or PL) to XOL which are determined on the duodenal samples collected from the proximal aspirating site, bile acid and PL secretion were calculated:

$$\text{BA (or PL) secretion (mg/h)} = \text{XOL secretion (mg/h)} \times \frac{\text{BA (or PL).}}{\text{XOL}}$$

Table 1 Biliary secretion before and after CDCA and UDCA treatment

	XOL output (mg/h)			*BA output* (mg/h)			*PL output* (mg/h)		
	Before	*After*		*Before*	*After*		*Before*	*After*	
		CDCA	*UDCA*		*CDCA*	*UDCA*		*CDCA*	*UDCA*
Obese (No. 4)	85 ± 32	62 ± 15.4	54 ± 11*	882 ± 202	1108 ± 360	1172 ± 472	500 ± 134	490 ± 98	558 ± 226
Normal weight (No. 4)	36 ± 7	31 ± 11.5	26.5 ± 6.5	$562 + 187$	696 ± 348	720 ± 280	226 ± 93	249 ± 68	271 ± 105
	$p < 0.05$	$p < 0.05$	$p < 0.01$	p NS	p NS	p NS	$p < 0.05$	$p < 0.01$	$p < 0.05$

* $p < 0.05$ vs. values before treatment

BILE ACID POOL SIZE AND BILIARY ACID COMPOSITION

[24-^{14}C]CDA (chenodeoxycholic acid) (New England Nuclear, Boston, Mass.) was administered intravenously before the biliary lipid secretion study. The specific activity (i.e. the ratio of the isotope to total bile acid mass) became constant 3 h after the beginning of the study.

The total bile acid pool was calculated by dividing the dose of radioactivity given by the specific activity in each sample. Biliary bile acid composition was evaluated by gas–liquid chromatography.

RESULTS

Biliary lipid outputs are shown in Table 1. Mean XOL secretion in bile was twice as high in obese patients as in normal-weight patients, before treatment.

Similarly, PL secretion was higher in obese than in non-obese patients, while bile acid outputs were only slightly higher in obese than in non-obese patients.

The administration of CDCA decreased cholesterol secretion in obese and in non-obese patients, but not significantly. In obese patients, XOL secretion remained still higher than in normal weight patients. The administration of ursodeoxycholic acid (UDCA) decreased cholesterol secretion in the obese patients ($p < 0.05$).

UDCA is effective in lowering XOL output in bile, also in normal-weight patients, but not at a statistically significant extent.

In obese patients, UDCA decreased XOL secretion more than CDCA did. Neither CDCA nor UDCA induced any significant modification in PL and bile acid outputs in all the groups. Similarly, total bile acid pool size remained unchanged (Table 2).

Table 2 Bile acid pool size (mg) before and after CDCA and UDCA in obese and in non-obese cholesterol gallstone patients

	Total bile acid pool size (mg) m.v. ± SD	
	Obese	*Non-obese*
Before	2200 ± 1300	1560 ± 800
CDCA	2120 ± 360	1840 ± 760
UDCA	2040 ± 1400	1640 ± 800

After CDCA treatment, CDCA became the predominant bile acid in bile (75% of total bile acid in obese and non-obese patients), whereas after UDCA therapy, UDCA accounts for about 25% of total bile acids.

DISCUSSION

These data show that in all the patients bile acid pool size does not change after CDCA and UDCA treatment. CDCA and UDCA become the predominant bile acids in bile after CDCA and UDCA respectively.

Both CDCA and UDCA desaturate bile in cholesterol by significantly decreasing the hepatic secretion of cholesterol, mainly in obese patients. Hepatic secretion of cholesterol is significantly lower during UDCA than during CDCA administration in obese patients. In conclusion, the present investigation shows that both UDCA (7.5 mg kg b.w.$^{-1}$ day^{-1}) and CDCA (12.5 mg kg b.w.$^{-1}$ day^{-1}) inhibit cholesterol secretion. This is more evident for UDCA, mainly in obese patients. Moreover, this effect is not related to large changes in the rate of entry of cholesterol into its metabolically active pool (obese and non-obese patients seem to be different as far as cholesterol metabolism is concerned). Therefore, the desaturating effect of CDCA and UDCA might be due to the degree of coupling cholesterol and PL, mainly at lower bile acid excretion, but to confirm this, biliary secretion studies in the fasting state are necessary using UDCA.

References

1. Northfield, T. C., LaRusso, N. F. and Hofmann, A. F. (1975). Biliary lipid output during three meals and an overnight fast. II: Effect of chenodeoxycholic acid treatment in gallstone subjects. *Gut*, **16,** 12
2. Von Bergmann, K., Gustsfeld, M. and Schulze-Hagen, K. (1978). Comparison of urso- versus chenodeoxycholic acid on biliary lipid secretion in man. *Gastroenterology*, **75,** 955
3. Grundy, S. M., Metzeger, A. L. and Adler, R. D. (1972). Mechanisms of lithogenic bile formation in American Indian women with cholesterol gallstones. *J. Clin. Invest.*, **51,** 3026
4. Grundy, S. M., Duane, W. C., Adler, R. D., Aron, J. M. and Metzeger, A. L. (1974). Biliary lipid outputs in young women with cholesterol gallstones. *Metab. Clin. Exp.*, **23,** 67
5. Northfield, T. C. and Hofmann, A. F. (1975). Biliary lipid outputs during three meals and an overnight fast. I: Relationship to bile acid pool size and cholesterol saturation of bile in gallstone and control subjects. *Gut*, **16,** 1
6. Bennion, L. J. and Grundy, S. M. (1975). Effect of obesity and caloric intake on biliary lipid metabolism in man. *J. Clin. Invest.*, **56,** 966
7. Shaffer, E. A. and Small, D. M. (1977). Biliary lipid secretion in cholesterol gallstone disease. The effect of cholecystectomy and obesity. *J. Clin. Invest.*, **59,** 828
8. Mok, M. Y. I., Von Bergmann, K., Crause, J. R. and Grundy, S. M. (1979). Biliary lipid metabolism in obesity. Effects of bile acid feeding before and during weight reduction. *Gastroenterology*, **76,** 556
9. Grundy, S. M. and Metzger, A. L. (1972). A physiological method for estimation of hepatic secretion of biliary lipids in man. *Gastroenterology*, **62,** 1200
10. Gordon, E. R., Shaffer, E. A. and Sass-Kortsak, A. (1976). Bilirubin secretion and conjugation in the Crigler–Najjar syndrome type II. *Gastroenterology*, **70,** 761
11. Go, V. L. W., Hofmann, A. F. and Summerskill, W. H. J. (1970). Pancreozymin bioassay in man based on pancreatic enzyme secretion: potency of specific amino acids and other digestive products. *J. Clin. Invest.*, **49,** 1558
12. Seligson, D., Marino, J. and Dodson, E. (1957). Determination of sulfobromophtalein in serum. *Clin. Chem.*, **3,** 638
13. Hyden, S. (1957). Polyethylene glycols in biological materials. *K. Lautbrukshoegsk. Ann.*, **22**
14. Roda, A., Roda, E., Festi, D., Sama, C., Mazzella, G., Aldini, R. and Barbara, L. (1975). Enzymatic determination of cholesterol in bile. *Clin. Chim. Acta*, **64,** 337

29
Increased glycine conjugation of biliary bile acids during treatment of gallstone patients with chenodeoxycholic acid or ursodeoxy-cholic acid: effects on biliary cholesterol saturation

R. RAEDSCH, A. STIEHL, P. CZYGAN, R. GÖTZ, Ch. MÄNNER, S. WALKER AND B. KOMMERELL

INTRODUCTION

Formation of cholesterol gallstones is related to supersaturation of bile with cholesterol[1]. Chenodeoxycholic acid (CDCA) and ursodeoxycholic acid (UDCA) are both efficient in conservative cholesterol gallstone therapy by decreasing biliary cholesterol saturation[2–18]. Several studies indicate that UDCA treatment decreases biliary cholesterol more markedly than CDCA treatment[16–18]. Side-effects such as elevated serum transaminases and diarrhoea are noted during CDCA treatment but are at present unknown during UDCA treatment[2–13,15,16,18–21]. These apparent advantages of UDCA led to an increased use of this bile acid in the treatment of cholesterol gallstones in man.

Recently it has been demonstrated that glyco-UDCA has only a very low solubilizing capacity for cholesterol crystals *in vitro* compared to the CDCA conjugate[1,22]. UDCA-formed micelles, however, are possibly smaller in size than CDCA-formed micelles[23] which may effect larger diffusion coefficients. Furthermore UDCA-rich solutions have a tendency for increased solubility of cholesterol by mesophase formation[24]. Both factors might accelerate gallstone dissolution. Therefore in a first study we determined the kinetics of cholesterol gallstone dissolution in aqueous solutions of 100 mmol/l glyco-CDCA, 100 mmol/l glyco-UDCA, and mixtures of both consisting of 40 mmol/l glyco-UDCA plus 60 mmol/l glyco-CDCA and 80 mmol/l glyco-UDCA plus 20 mmol/l glyco-CDCA *in vitro*. Increased amounts of UDCA metabolites in bile of patients during UDCA treatment have to be considered in calculations of cholesterol saturation indices[23,25,26] and could influence treatment efficacy. Thus we designed a second study to compare the effects of CDCA, UDCA, and CDCA + UDCA treatment in a controlled prospective cross-over study. During each treatment period biliary lipid composition and conjugation of bile acids with glycine and taurine were determined.

METHODS

In vitro study

In each experiment four cholesterol gallstones comparable in weight and size were incubated each in 4 ml bile acid solution in a shaking waterbath at 37 °C. Incubations were carried out up to 4 months, or until complete stone dissolution. We tested aqueous solutions of 100 mmol/l glyco-CDCA, 100 mmol/l glyco-UDCA, and mixtures of both consisting of 40 mmol/l glyco-UDCA plus 60 mmol/l glyco-CDCA and 80 mmol/l glyco-UDCA plus 20 mmol/l glyco-CDCA. The incubation medium was renewed daily and assayed enzymatically for cholesterol[27]. Weight and diameter of the gallstones were daily controlled.

Patients study

Ten patients with radiolucent gallstones and functioning gallbladders (seven women and three men) were included in the study. Each patient was studied before and during treatment with UDCA, CDCA, and CDCA+UDCA. During treatment with CDCA or UDCA daily doses of 11.9–15.6 mg/kg were administered orally while during treatment with CDCA+UDCA each bile acid was administered at one-half of the dose. Each of the treatment periods lasted for 3 months. The following sequences of treatment were chosen to exclude any order effect.

Five patients were first treated with CDCA+UDCA followed by UDCA and CDCA, and five patients were first treated with CDCA and subsequently with UDCA and CDCA+UDCA.

Plasma for routine laboratory tests was obtained in the control period and after 4, 8 and 12 weeks of each test period. Concentrated bile was obtained after overnight fasting by a duodenal tube following cholecystokinin-induced gallbladder contraction and was analysed in the control period and after 12 weeks of each treatment period.

Analytical methods

Glycine and taurine conjugates of CDCA and UDCA were separated by thin-layer chromatography and analysed by gas–liquid chromatography. Details of the methods have been described previously in detail[16,28]. For determination of cholesterol, saturation of bile cholesterol and bile acids were measured enzymatically[16]. Phospholipids were extracted and measured colorimetrically[6]. Cholesterol saturation was calculated by the method of Thomas and Hofmann[29] according to the limits of cholesterol saturation defined by Hegardt and Dam[30] and Holzbach *et al.*[31]. Correction of the saturation indices for the biliary content of glyco-UDCA and tauro-UDCA was performed according to Carey *et al.*[25].

Statistical methods

Non-parametrical variance analysis was performed for comparison of the control period and the three treatment periods[32–34].

Table 1 Cholesterol gallstone dissolution in 100 mmol/l aqueous solutions of glyco-CDCA, glyco-UDCA, and mixtures of both *in vitro* ($n=4$ in each experiment; data expressed as mean ± SEM)

	Glyco-CDCA, 100 *mmol/l*	*Glyco-UDCA*, 40 *mmol/l* *Glyco-CDCA*, 60 *mmol/l*	*Glyco-UDCA*, 80 *mmol/l* *Glyco-CDCA*, 20 *mmol/l*	*Glyco-UDCA*, 100 *mmol/l*
Dissolved cholesterol (mg/day)	0.87 ± 0.1	0.28 ± 0.003	0.07 ± 0.002	0.07 ± 0.03
Weight decrease of the gallstones (mg/day)	1.2 ± 0.1	0.3 ± 0.009	0.11 ± 0.02	0.1 ± 0.002
Complete dissolution of the gallstones (weeks)	12.8 ± 3.3	—	—	—

RESULTS

In vitro study

The dissolution rates of the cholesterol gallstones achieved by the tested bile acid solutions are shown in Table 1. 100 mmol/l glyco-CDCA had the highest dissolution rate, whereas increasing concentrations of glyco-UDCA resulted in lower dissolution rates. Correspondingly the weight decreases of the gallstones were the highest by 100 mmol/l glyco-CDCA and minimal by 100 mmol/l glyco-UDCA. Complete gallstone dissolution occurred during observation time only by 100 mmol/l glyco-CDCA by which all four gallstones were dissolved in 12 $\pm$ 3.3 weeks (mean $\pm$ SEM).

Patients study

Treatment of patients with cholesterol gallstones with CDCA, UDCA, or CDCA+UDCA led to marked increases of these bile acids in bile. During all three treatment periods the relative amount of glycine conjugates of the administered bile acid in bile rose significantly ($p=0.05$) from about 70 to 90%. Only trace amounts of unconjugated bile acids were detected. During treatment with UDCA, glyco-UDCA in bile was positively correlated to the UDCA dose administered ($p=0.05$), while no correlation was found between tauro-UDCA in bile and the dose of UDCA. During UDCA therapy glyco-UDCA became dose-dependent, and the predominant bile acid conjugate in bile, with up to 70% at a dose of 15 mg/kg.

Analysis of biliary bile acids and bile lipids revealed a significantly greater decrease of biliary cholesterol during treatment with UDCA than during

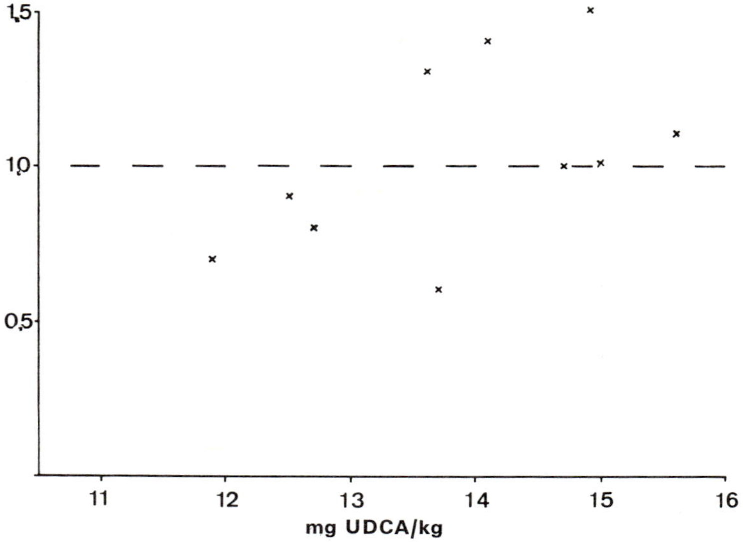

Figure 1 Cholesterol saturation indices during UDCA treatment at varying doses corrected for glyco-UDCA and tauro-UDCA in bile. At doses higher than 13 mg/kg six of seven patients had supersaturated bile

treatment with CDCA. Biliary cholesterol during UDCA and CDCA+UDCA treatment was not significantly different.

Saturation indices corrected for the biliary content of glyco-UDCA and tauro-UDCA were significantly lower during treatment with CDCA (0.8 ± 0.1 mean ± SEM) and CDCA+UDCA (0.7 ± 0.1) than during treatment with UDCA alone (1.0 ± 0.1) ($p = 0.05$). At doses of UDCA greater than 13 mg/kg in six of seven patients saturation indices corrected for glyco-UDCA and tauro-UDCA in bile were greater than 1.0, while at doses lower than 13 mg/kg all patients had saturation indices below 1.0 (Figure 1). Side-effects were only observed during treatment with CDCA. Three patients had slightly elevated serum transaminases and four patients had occasional diarrhoea.

DISCUSSION

In the *in vitro* experiments we tested the efficacy of the glycine conjugate of UDCA for gallstone dissolution compared to the CDCA conjugate. The unconjugated UDCA could not be tested since the solubility of free UDCA in aqueous solutions is minimal at physiological pH values[35]. Complete gallstone dissolution occurred only in the 100 mmol/l glyco-CDCA incubates within the observation time of 4 months. The dissolution rates decreased gradually with increasing concentrations of glyco-UDCA. 100 mmol/l glyco-UDCA achieved only about 10% of the dissolution rates of 100 mmol/l glyco-CDCA. These results are in good agreement with findings of Carey who showed that the solubilizing capacity for cholesterol crystals of UDCA and its conjugates is far inferior to that of CDCA[1,22]. It was suggested that the smaller size of UDCA-formed micelles may effect larger diffusion coefficients[23] and the ability of UDCA of mesophase formation[24] may accelerate gallstone dissolution. Our data show that the smaller micelle size of glyco-UDCA and its tendency for mesophase formation have no advantage in cholesterol gallstone dissolution compared to glyco-CDCA. Whereas the cholesterol-solubilizing capacity of UDCA is very limited, UDCA feeding is more effective than CDCA in reducing cholesterol excretion into bile. Oral CDCA administration decreases biliary cholesterol excretion less than UDCA, but as our studies show it is a good solubilizer for cholesterol and high concentrations of CDCA conjugates in bile enhance gallstone dissolution.

This gave the rationale to compare the effects of oral administration of CDCA, UDCA, and CDCA+UDCA on biliary bile acids and bile lipids in gallstone patients.

During the control period in our patients 73% of CDCA was glycine-conjugated and 27% was taurine-conjugated. The glycine : taurine ratio was quite similar to the conjugation pattern in healthy men. During treatment with CDCA, UDCA, and CDCA+UDCA conjugation with glycine increased in all patients. The amounts of glyco-UDCA in bile during UDCA treatment were considerably greater than previously anticipated[25]. The increase in glycine conjugation of bile acids during CDCA, UDCA, and CDCA+UDCA feeding is in agreement with previous observations during administration of

CDCA and cholic acid (CA)[36,37]. In a situation of constant dietary intake of taurine and increased intake of bile acids taurine conjugation remains constant, and with the increase of conjugating requirements conjugation with glycine increases.

A previous study on the effects of CDCA and UDCA had indicated that UDCA decreases biliary cholesterol more markedly than CDCA[16]. In our patients cholesterol saturation indices not corrected for the biliary content of glyco-UDCA and tauro-UDCA were lower during treatment with UDCA than during treatment with CDCA. The increase of glycine and taurine conjugates of UDCA in bile requires correction of the saturation indices. Equimolar amounts of glyco-UDCA depress cholesterol solubility about twice as much as tauro-UDCA[25]. The present study indicates that the glyco-UDCA content of bile increases markedly during UDCA feeding and that therefore saturation indices during this treatment are higher than previously anticipated. During treatment with CDCA at doses of 5–20 mg/kg biliary cholesterol saturation is negatively correlated to the dose administered[38,39]. Similar results were obtained during treatment with UDCA at doses of 5–15 mg/kg when the saturation indices were not corrected for the biliary content of glyco-UDCA and tauro-UDCA. The present study indicates that during treatment with UDCA at doses above 13 mg/kg cholesterol saturation indices corrected for UDCA conjugates in bile may increase. It is evident from these data that no negative correlation exists between UDCA dose and cholesterol desaturation. During treatment with UDCA, five of 10 patients had corrected saturation indices greater than 1.0. All these patients had doses of UDCA above 13 mg/kg and therefore a high biliary content of glyco-UDCA. It seems possible that in these patients no gallstone dissolution can be achieved with this high dose of UDCA, and better results could be obtained with a lower dose of UDCA.

During treatment with CDCA+UDCA, glyco-UDCA and tauro-UDCA concentrations in bile and cholesterol saturation indices corrected for the biliary content of glyco-UDCA and tauro-UDCA were significantly lower than during treatment with UDCA. Our study periods of 3 months were too short to allow any conclusions on the clinical efficacy of the three different treatment regimens. But from the low saturation indices during treatment with CDCA+UDCA fast stone dissolution may be expected.

CDCA+UDCA treatment could be the treatment of choice on patients with cholesterol gallstones as it combines the advantages of having the lowest biliary cholesterol, the lowest saturation indices and no side-effects.

References

1. Carey, M. C. and Small, D. (1978). The physical chemistry of cholesterol solubility in bile: relationship to gallstone formation and dissolution in man. *J. Clin. Invest.*, **61,** 998
2. Danzinger, R. G., Hofmann, A. F., Schoenfield, L. S. *et al.* (1972). Dissolution of cholesterol gallstones by chenodeoxycholic acid. *N. Engl. J. Med.*, **289,** 1
3. Bell, C. D., Whitney, B. and Dowling, R. H. (1972). Gallstone dissolution in man using chenodeoxycholic acid. *Lancet*, **2,** 1213
4. Thistle, J. L. and Hofmann, A. F. (1973). Efficacy and specificity of chenodeoxycholic acid therapy for dissolving gallstones. *N. Engl. J. Med.*, **289,** 655
5. Iser, J. H., Dowling, R. H., Mok, H. Y. I. *et al.* (1975). Chenodeoxycholic acid treat-

ment of gallstones: a follow up report and analysis of factors influencing response to therapy. *N. Engl. J. Med.*, **293,** 378
6. Barbara, L., Roda, E., Roda, A. *et al.* (1976). The medical treatment of cholesterol gallstones: experience with chenodeoxycholic acid. *Digestion*, **14,** 209
7. Makino, J., Shinozaki, K., Yoshino, K. *et al.* (1975). Dissolution of cholesterol gallstones by ursodeoxycholic acid. *Jpn. J. Gastroenterol.*, **72,** 690
8. Nakagawa, S., Makino, I. and Ishizaki, T. (1977). Dissolution of cholesterol gallstones by ursodeoxycholic acid. *Lancet*, **2,** 367
9. Maton, P. N., Murphy, G. M. and Dowling, R. H. (1977). Ursodeoxycholic acid treatment of gallstones. Dose-response study and possible mechanism of action. *Lancet*, **2,** 1297
10. Fedorowski, T., Salen, G., Colallilo, A. *et al.* (1977). Metabolism of ursodeoxycholic acid in man. *Gastroenterology*, **73,** 1131.
11. Makino, I. and Nakagawa, S. (1978). Changes in biliary lipid and biliary bile acid composition in patients after administration of ursodeoxycholic acid. *J. Lipid Res.*, **19,** 723
12. Attili, A. F., Angelico, M., Cantafora, A. *et al.* (1978). Effect of low doses of ursodeoxycholic acid on biliary lipid composition in non-obese gallstone patients. *Ital. J. Gastroenterol.*, **10,** 119.
13. Thistle, L. J., Carlson, G. L., LaRusso, N. F. *et al.* (1979). Comparison of the effects of 5 and 10 mg/kg/day of ursodeoxycholic acid and chenodeoxycholic acid on cholesterol saturation of bile in patients with gallstones. In Paumgartner, G., Stiehl, A. and Gerok, W. (eds.) *Biological Effects of Bile Acids*, p. 67. (Lancaster: MTP Press)
14. Von Bergmann, K., Gutsfeld, M., Schulze-Hagen, K. *et al.* (1979). Effects of ursodeoxycholic acid on biliary lipid secretion in patients with radiolucent gallstones. In Paumgartner, G., Stiehl, A. and Gerok, W. (eds.) *Biological Effects of Bile Acids*, p. 61. (Lancaster: MTP Press)
15. Weis, H. J., Holtermüller, K. H., Stiehl, A. *et al.* (1979). Clinical experience and bile composition in patients taking ursodeoxycholic acid for gallstone dissolution. In Paumgartner, G., Stiehl, A. and Gerok, W. (eds.) *Biological Effects of Bile Acids*, p. 99. (Lancaster: MTP Press)
16. Stiehl, A., Czygan, P., Kommerell, B. *et al.* (1978) Ursodeoxycholic acid versus chenodeoxycholic acid. Comparison of their effects on bile acids and bile lipid composition in patients with cholesterol gallstones. *Gastroenterology*, **75,** 1016
17. Scherstén, T. and Lindblad, L. (1979). Biliary cholesterol output during ursodeoxycholic acid secretion in man. In Paumgartner, G., Stiehl, A. and Gerok, W. (eds.) *Biological Effects of Bile Acids*, p. 53. (Lancaster: MTP Press)
18. Salvioli, G. and Salati, R. (1979). Faecal bile acid loss and bile acid pool size during short-term treatment with ursodeoxycholic and chenodeoxycholic acid in patients with radiolucent gallstones. *Gut*, **20,** 698
19. Menghini, G. and Pallotta, B. (1976). Marked increase in serum levels of liver enzymes in patients receiving chenic acid and phenobarbital for gallstone dissolution. *Digestion*, **14,** 163
20. Stiehl, A., Ast, E., Czygan, P. *et al.* (1976). Elevated serum transaminases following treatment of patients with cholesterol gallstones with chenodeoxycholic acid. *Inn. Med.*, **3,** 75
21. Volpi, C., Ciravegna, G., Canepa, A. *et al.* (1979). A cross-over double blind trial comparing the effects of ursodeoxycholic acid and chenodeoxycholic acid on bowel habit in man. *Curr. Ther. Res.*, **26,** 225
22. Carey, M. C. (1978). Critical tables for calculating the cholesterol saturation in native bile. *J. Lipid Res.*, **19,** 945
23. Carey, M. C., Mazer, N. A. and Benedek, G. B. (1977). Novel physical–chemical properties of ursodeoxycholic acid and its conjugates: relevance to gallstone dissolution in man. *Gastroenterology*, **72,** 1036 (Abstr.)
24. Corrigan, O. I., Su, C. C. and Alkan, M. H. (1980). Cholesterol dissolution in ursodeoxycholate-lecithin containing media: involvement of mesophase formation *in vitro*. *VIth Bile Acid Meeting*, Freiburg, Germany. (Abstr.)
25. Carey, M. C. and Grace, K. O. (1979). The importance of total lipid concentration

in determining cholesterol solubility in bile and the development of critical table for calculating percent cholesterol saturation with a correction factor for ursodeoxycholate-rich bile. In Paumgartner, G., Stiehl, A. and Gerok, W. (eds.) *Biological Effects of Bile Acids*, p. 299. (Lancaster: MTP Press)
26. Stiehl, A., Raedsch, R., Czygan, P., Götz, R., Männer, Ch., Walker, S. and Kommerell, B. (1980). Effects of biliary bile acid composition on biliary cholesterol saturation in gallstone patients treated with chenodeoxycholic acid and/or ursodeoxycholic acid. *Gastroenterology*, **79,** 1192
27. Fausa, O. and Skalhegg, B. A. (1974). *Scand. J. Gastroenterol.*, **9,** 249
28. Fröhling, W. and Stiehl, A. (1976). Bile salt glucuronides: identification and quantitative analysis in the urine of patients with cholestasis, *Eur. J. Clin. Invest.*, **6,** 67
29. Thomas, P. J. and Hofmann, A. F. (1973). A simple calculation of the lithogenic index of bile: expressing biliary lipid composition on rectangular coordinates. *Gastroenterology*, **65,** 898
30. Hegardt, F. and Dam, H. (1971). The solubility of cholesterol in aqueous solutions of bile salts and lecithin. *Z. Ernährungswiss*, **10,** 223
31. Holzbach, R. T., Marsh, M., Olszewski, M. *et al.* (1973). Cholesterol solubility in bile. Evidence that supersaturated bile is frequent in healthy man. *J. Clin. Invest.*, **52,** 1467
32. Friedman, M. (1937). The use of ranks to avoid the assumption of normality implicit in the analysis of variance. *J. Am. Stat. Assoc.*, **32,** 657
33. Wilcoxon, F. and Wilcox, R. A. (1964). Some rapid approximate statistical procedures. (Pearl River, NY: Lederle Laboratories)
34. Sachs, L. (1974). *Angewandte Statistik*. (Heidelberg, NY: Springer)
35. Igimi, H. and Carey, M. C. (1980). pH-solubility relations of chenodeoxycholic and ursodeoxycholic acids: physical-chemical basis for dissimilar solution and membrane phenomena. *J. Lipid Res.*, **21,** 72
36. Danzinger, R. G., Hofmann, A. F., Schoenfield, L. J. *et al.* (1973). Effect of oral chenodeoxycholic acid feeding on bile acid kinetics and biliary lipid composition in women with cholelithiasis. *J. Clin. Invest.*, **52,** 2809
37. Von Bergmann, K., Schultheiss, H. R., Paumgartner, G. *et al.* (1975). Die Konjugation von Chenodesoxycholsäure und Cholsäure während einer Leberpassage. *Schweiz. Med. Wochenschr.*, **105,** 413
38. Mok, H. Y. I., Bell, G. D. and Dowling, R. H. (1974). Effect of different doses of chenodeoxycholic acid on bile-lipid composition and on frequency of side-effects in patients with gallstones. *Lancet*, **2,** 253
39. Thistle, J. L., Hofmann, A. F., Yu, P. Y. S. *et al.* (1977). Effect of varying doses of chenodeoxycholic acid on bile lipid and biliary bile acid composition in gallstone patients: a dose-response study. *Dig. Dis.*, **22,** 1

30
Cholesterol synthesis and biliary cholesterol secretion in obesity

A. REUBEN, P. N. MATON, G. M. MURPHY
AND R. H. DOWLING

INTRODUCTION

The increased prevalence of cholesterol gallstones in obesity[1–4] has been linked to the high degree of biliary cholesterol supersaturation known to occur in the majority of overweight individuals[5–7]. However, although supersaturated bile is important in the formation of cholesterol gallstones[8,9] measurement of fasting duodenal bile lipid composition can only tell us whether or not the bile is supersaturated with cholesterol. It cannot tell us why the bile is supersaturated in obese patients nor whether the supersaturation is due to excess biliary cholesterol secretion, reduced bile acid or phospholipid secretion (or both) or some combined secretory defect. Fortunately, direct measurement of bile lipid secretion is now possible in intact man using duodenal marker perfusion techniques[6,10,11] and in the few studies reported to date, biliary cholesterol hypersecretion appears to be common in obesity[5,6,12]. However, the results are less clear-cut when obesity and gallstones are combined[13,14]. Therefore, we not only measured biliary cholesterol saturation indices in fasting duodenal bile but also measured bile lipid secretion rates in four groups of patients: obese and non-obese, with and without gallstones.

The results of cholesterol balance and isotope kinetic studies[15–17] have shown that total body cholesterol production is increased in obesity. However the contribution of hepatic cholesterol synthesis to total body cholesterol production is unknown. Furthermore, the role of hepatic cholesterogenesis in biliary cholesterol secretion is also unknown. What is clear, however, is that untreated cholesterol gallstone patients have increased hepatic cholesterol synthesis, at least as judged by raised activity of the enzyme 3-hydroxy, 3-methylglutaryl coenzyme A reductase[18,19] (HMG-CoAR-rate limiting for cholesterogenesis[20]). Therefore as an index of hepatic cholesterol synthesis, HMG-CoAR activities were measured in operative liver biopsies from the same four patient categories described above.

Key and colleagues[21], reported a significant linear correlation between HMG-CoAR activity and biliary cholesterol secretion measured in individual untreated gallstone patients. To study this further, we too examined the relationship between the two variables in those patients who underwent both investigations, to see whether or not hepatic cholesterol synthesis determines the cholesterol content of bile.

PATIENTS STUDIED AND METHODS

Saturation indices (SIs) of fasting duodenal bile, bile lipid secretion and hepatic cholesterol synthesis rates (HMG-CoAR activity) were measured in the four groups of individuals already described – obese and non-obese without gallstones and obese and non-obese with cholesterol gallstones, obesity being defined arbitrarily as $>130\%$ ideal body weight (IBW).

Cholesterol SI in fasting duodenal bile

For the SI studies in bile-rich duodenal fluid, there were 15 non-obese individuals without gallstones who served as controls, 24 obese patients without stones, 29 non-obese with stones and 15 who had a combination of obesity and gallstones. After an overnight fast, the duodenum was intubated under fluoroscopic control, gallbladder contraction stimulated with an intravenous injection of 70–100 IU cholecystokinin (Boots 'Pancreozymin', Nottingham, England), the bile acid, phospholipid and cholesterol concentrations measured using standard techniques and the resultant SIs calculated using the polynomial equation of Thomas and Hofmann and the cholesterol solubility criteria of Holzbach *et al.*, and Hegardt and Dam.

Steady-state bile lipid secretion

Bile lipid secretion rates were measured using a modification of the technique of Shaffer and Small[6]. There were 17 patients without gallstones (10 women and 7 men), 7 of whom were obese and 10 of whom were non-obese (as defined above) and 13 with cholesterol gallstone disease (11 women and 2 men), 7 of whom were obese and 6 non-obese.

In brief, the duodenum of fasting patients was again intubated – this time with a three-lumen tube – under fluoroscopic control so that the proximal aspiration site and the infusion port lay in the second part of the duodenum, whilst the distal aspiration site lay 14 cm downstream at the ligament of Trietz. Before starting the infusion, gallbladder contraction was again stimulated by intravenous cholecystokinin as described above. The hourly secretion rates of the three major biliary lipids were then measured during a 10 h continuous infusion of an isotonic, essential amino acid solution containing bromsulphthalein (BSP – Hynson, Westcott & Dunning Inc., Baltimore, Maryland, USA) as a poorly absorbable marker. After a 2–4 h equilibration period, samples were collected over a 6–8 h period and the bile acid, phospholipid and cholesterol secretion rates calculated as previously described, the results being expressed as mean outputs of the three lipids in μmol/h.

Hepatic cholesterol synthesis

Hepatic HMG-CoAR activity was measured in the microsomal fractions of homogenates from operative liver biopsies, using a modification of the method of Nicolau *et al.*[22]. Thirteen patients without gallstones (10 non-obese and 3 grossly obese; $>200\%$ IBW) and 14 patients with cholesterol gallstones (4 non-obese and 3 grossly obese; $>175\%$ IBW) were studied. Enzyme activity was expressed conventionally as picomoles of mevalonate formed mg microsomal protein^{-1} min^{-1}. However, because of the possibility of a different microsomal yield/unit weight of liver in obese and non-obese individuals, the amount of microsomal protein/g wet weight liver was recorded in 42 non-obese and 8 obese patients.

To study the relationship between hepatic cholesterol synthesis and biliary cholesterol secretion, in 9 patients bile lipid secretion rates were measured on the day prior to the laparotomy at which the liver biopsy (for measurement of HMG-CoAR activity) was taken.

Statistical methods

The statistical significance of differences in mean SI values and in bile lipid secretion results between the four patient groups was tested by analysis of variance. Student's *t* tests were used to compare hepatic HMG-CoAR activity in the four patient groups and product–moment correlation coefficients between enzyme activity and cholesterol secretion calculated.

RESULTS

Cholesterol SIs in fasting duodenal bile

The mean SI in the non-obese 'controls' was $0.89 \pm$ SEM 0.06, 40% of the individuals in this group having supersaturated bile. The mean SI in the obese patients without stones of 1.14 ± 0.07 was significantly greater than that in the controls ($p < 0.01$) but was not significantly different from that in non-obese patients with radiolucent, presumed cholesterol-rich gallstones (1.30 ± 0.05). However, the greatest SI values were seen in obese patients with gallstone disease, all of whom had SIs > 1.0 (mean 1.55 ± 0.06). The results in this group were significantly greater than those in all the other groups ($p < 0.01$–0.001).

Steady-state bile lipid secretion

An analysis of the overall results of bile lipid secretion showed two major findings:

(1) hypersecretion of cholesterol by the obese, whether or not gallstones were present; and
(2) hyposecretion of bile acids in the non-obese gallstone patients.

The mean hourly secretion rates of cholesterol were 51 ± 7 μmol/h in the controls, 81 ± 15 in the obese patients without stones ($p < 0.002$) and 107 ± 7

in the obese with stones ($p<0.001$). In contrast, biliary cholesterol secretion in non-obese patients with gallstones (42 ± 4) was not significantly different from the controls.

The mean bile acid output in the non-obese controls of 1078 ± 210 μmol/h was not significantly different from that in the obese gallstone patients (1138 ± 84) but it was significantly greater than that in the non-obese gallstone group (563 ± 70; $P<0.05$). In general, the pattern of phospholipid secretion closely followed that of bile acid output in non-obese patients and of cholesterol output in the obese.

Hepatic cholesterol synthesis

Hepatic HMG-CoAR activity was markedly increased in non-obese patients with gallstones ($32.2\pm$SEM 2.0 pmol mg^{-1} min^{-1}) compared with controls (14.6 ± 1.7; $p<0.001$). Mean activity was also slightly, but significantly, raised in gross obesity (21.8–28.5; $p<0.05$) but was not significantly different from normal in the three grossly obese gallstone patients.

The microsomal yield in hepatic biopsies from obese individuals of 8.7 ± 0.8 mg/g fresh liver was only half that of the non-obese group (16.7 ± 1.1) and this difference was statistically significant ($p<0.001$). Expressed per unit weight of liver, therefore, the mean amounts of HMG-CoAR were actually *less* in both obese subgroups than in the non-obese controls.

Despite a four-fold range in hepatic HMG-CoAR levels (9.2–40.3 pmol mg^{-1} min^{-1}) and a comparable range in biliary cholesterol secretion, there was no correlation between biliary cholesterol output and enzyme activity in the 9 patients in whom both variables were measured ($r=0.18$; $p>0.05$).

DISCUSSION

The present results emphasize the importance of obesity as a factor influencing the cholesterol saturation of fasting duodenal bile, biliary cholesterol secretion and hepatic cholesterol synthesis. They clearly show that the mean biliary cholesterol SIs are higher in the obese than in the non-obese – whether or not gallstones are present – but that still higher SIs are found in fasting duodenal bile when obesity and gallstones are combined.

These varying degrees of biliary cholesterol supersaturation are associated with quite different patterns of bile lipid secretion in the various patient groups. The finding that obese patients secrete excess biliary cholesterol confirms and extends the results of others[5,6,12] as does the observation that in non-obese patients with cholesterol gallstones, bile acid secretion is reduced. However, the present results differ from previous reports in two respects. First, Grundy and colleagues[13,14] suggested that obese gallstone patients not only secrete excess biliary cholesterol but that they also had hyposecretion of bile acids. In the 7 gallstone patients in this study, mean bile acid secretion was clearly normal. Secondly, although both groups of obese patients (with and without gallstones) showed cholesterol hypersecretion, the levels of biliary cholesterol output were even higher when obesity and gallstones were combined (the group which also showed the greatest degree of saturation of fasting duodenal bile) than in obesity alone.

In theory, the differences between the present results and those of previous studies could be related to the type of infusion medium used to stimulate bile flow. We chose an isotonic amino acid infusion similar to that used by Shaffer and Small[6] and obtained comparable overall secretion results. In contrast, the use of liquid formula infusions generally yields higher absolute secretion rates – particularly for cholesterol[5,12–14] – but this does not necessarily mean that liquid formula infusions are better or that they give more physiological results. It does mean, however, that while it may be valid to compare *patterns* of results from different studies, one cannot, with validity, compare secretion rates when different infusion methods are being used.

The reason why the pattern of results in the present study should be different from those reported previously is not known, but may be due to different genetic and environmental factors in the various centres. Bile acid pool sizes were not measured in the present study but small bile acid pools are known to occur both in gallstone patients[23] and when bile acid secretion is low[12]. It is tempting to speculate, therefore, that a small bile acid pool, cycling with a normal frequency, could explain the low bile acid secretion rate seen in the present group of non-obese gallstone patients and in some obese gallstone patients reported in other studies[13,14].

If a small bile acid pool and a low bile acid secretion rate might explain the underlying defect leading to supersaturated bile in non-obese gallstone patients, what is the mechanism for the supersaturated bile and the increased biliary cholesterol output in the obese? One obvious possibility is that hepatic cholesterol synthesis is increased. Indeed in the present study, hepatic HMG-CoAR activity (expressed/mg microsomal protein) was modestly raised in the obese individuals without stones, though it was higher still in the non-obese gallstone group. However, in the small number of obese gallstone patients studied here, mean HMG-CoAR activity was not significantly different from that seen in our controls[24].

This pattern of enzyme results may well not reflect total hepatic cholesterol synthesis since the microsomal yield in liver biopsies from obese individuals was only half that in the non-obese group. It is not known whether the resultant slight reduction in the amount of HMG-CoAR/g of liver is offset by a larger than normal total mass of liver in the obese, but the results of post-mortem studies suggest that this may indeed be so.

With all these caveats, increased hepatic cholesterol synthesis (at least as judged by the activity of HMG-CoAR/mg microsomal protein in operative liver biopsies) cannot explain the biliary cholesterol hypersecretion seen in the obese gallstone group. Indeed, although hepatic cholesterogenesis contributes significantly to total body cholesterol synthesis[25], hepatic cholesterol production, both in man and in other species[26], does not seem to be the major determinant of biliary cholesterol secretion. This dissociation between hepatic cholesterogenesis and biliary cholesterol secretion suggests that the two variables cannot be related and indeed when both measurements were made in the same individuals, we found no correlation between hepatic HMG-CoAR activity and biliary cholesterol output. Our results, therefore, do not support the observation made originally by Key and colleagues[21] who showed a significant linear correlation between hepatic HMG-CoAR levels and biliary cholesterol secretion in untreated gallstone patients – a finding which the authors themselves could not confirm in gallstone patients treated with chenodeoxycholic acid.

Acknowledgments

We wish to thank Miss Julia Ellis and Mr Y. Qureshi for technical assistance, Sister and Staff of the Metabolic Ward, Guy's Hospital for their co-operation in patient care, Professor I. McColl of the Department of Surgery, Guy's Hospital Medical School for his help in obtaining operative liver biopsies, and Mrs S. Das who kindly typed the manuscript. A.R. was supported by a grant from Organon Laboratories Ltd., and P.N.M. by a grant from Weddel Pharmaceuticals[27].

References

1. Gross, D. M. B. (1929). A statistical study of cholelithiasis. *J. Pathol. Bacteriol.*, **32,** 503
2. Friedman, G. D., Kannel, W. B. and Dawber, T. R. (1966). The epidemiology of gallbladder disease: observations in the Framingham Study. *J. Chron. Dis.*, **19,** 273
3. Wheeler, M., Loftus-Hills, L. and Laby, B. (1970). Cholelithiasis: a clinical and dietary survey. *Gut*, **11,** 430
4. Sturdevant, R. A. L., Pearce, M. L. and Dayton, S. (1973). Increased prevalence of cholelithiasis in men ingesting a serum-cholesterol-lowering diet. *N. Engl. J. Med.*, **288,** 24
5. Bennion, L. J. and Grundy, S. M. (1975). Effect of obesity and caloric intake on biliary lipid metabolism in man. *J. Clin. Invest.*, **56,** 996
6. Shaffer, E. A. and Small, D. M. (1977). Biliary lipid secretion in cholesterol gallstone disease: the effect of cholecystectomy and obesity. *J. Clin. Invest.*, **59,** 828
7. Reuben, A. and Dowling, R. H. (1978). Does obesity complicate chenodeoxycholic acid (CDCA) treatment of gallstones? *Gut*, **19,** A452
8. Admirand, W. H. and Small, D. M. (1968). The physico-chemical basis of cholesterol gallstone formation in man. *J. Clin. Invest.*, **61,** 716
9. Carey, M. C. and Small, D. M. (1978). The physical chemistry of cholesterol solubility in bile: relating to gallstone formation and dissolution in man. *J. Clin. Invest.*, **61,** 998
10. Go, V. L. W., Hofmann, A. F. and Summerskill, W. H. J. (1970). Simultaneous measurements of total pancreatic, biliary and gastric outputs in man using a perfusion technique. *Gastroenterology*, **58,** 321
11. Grundy, S. M. and Metzger, A. L. (1972). A physiologic method for estimation of hepatic secretion of biliary lipids in man. *Gastroenterology*, **62,** 1200
12. Mabee, T. M., Meyer, P., Denbesten, L. and Mason, E. E. (1976). The mechanism of increased gallstone formation in obese human subjects. *Surgery*, **79,** 460
13. Grundy, S. M., Metzger, A. L. and Adler, R. D. (1972). Mechanisms of lithogenic bile formation in American Indian women with cholesterol gallstones. *J. Clin. Invest.*, **51,** 3026
14. Grundy, S. M., Duane, W. C., Adler, R. D., Aron, J. M. and Metzger, A. L. (1974). Biliary lipid outputs in young women with cholesterol gallstones. *Metabolism*, **23,** 67
15. Nestel, P. J., Whyte, H. M. and Goodman, D. S. (1969). Distribution and turnover of cholesterol in humans. *J. Clin. Invest.*, **48,** 982
16. Nestel, P. J., Schreibman, P. H. and Ahrens, E. H. Jr (1973). Cholesterol metabolism in human obesity. *J. Clin. Invest.*, **52,** 2389
17. Leijd, B. (1980). Cholesterol and bile acid metabolism in obesity. *Clin. Sci.*, **59,** 203
18. Salen, G., Nicolau, G., Shefer, S. and Mosbach, E. H. (1975). Hepatic cholesterol metabolism in patients with gallstones. *Gastroenterology*, **69,** 676

19. Coyne, M. J., Bonorris, G. G., Goldstein, L. I. and Schoenfield, L. J. (1975). Effect of chenodeoxycholic acid and phenobarbital on the rate-limiting enzymes of hepatic cholesterol and bile acid synthesis in patients with gallstones. *J. Lab. Clin. Med.*, **87,** 281
20. Rodwell, V. W., Nordstrom, J. L. and Mitschelen, J. J. (1976). Regulation of HMGCoA reductase. *Adv. Lipid Res.*, **14,** 1
21. Key, P. H., Bonorris, G. G., Coyne, M. J., Taub, M. and Schoenfield, L. J. (1977). Hepatic cholesterol synthesis: a determinant of cholesterol secretion in gallstone patients. *Gastroenterology*, **72,** 1182 (abstr.)
22. Nicolau, G., Shefer, S., Salen, G. and Mosbach, E. H. (1974). Determination of hepatic 3-hydroxy, 3-methylglutaryl CoA reductase activity in man. *J. Lipid Res.*, **15,** 94
23. Vlahcevic, Z. R., Bell, C. C. Jr, Buhac, I., Farrar, J. T. and Swell, L. (1970). Diminished bile acid pool size in patients with gallstones. *Gastroenterology*, **59,** 165
24. Maton, P. N., Ellis, H. J., Higgins, M. J. P. and Dowling, R. H., (1980). Hepatic HMGCoA reductase in human cholelithiasis: effects of chenodeoxycholic and ursodeoxycholic acids. *Eur. J. Clin. Invest.*, **10,** 325
25. Angel, A. and Bray, G. A. (1979). Synthesis of fatty acids and cholesterol by liver, adipose tissue and intestinal mucosa from obese and control patients. *Eur. J. Clin. Invest.*, **9,** 355
26. Turley, S. D. and Dietschy, J. M. (1979). Regulation of biliary cholesterol output in the rat: dissociation from the rate of hepatic cholesterol synthesis, the size of the hepatic cholesteryl ester pool and the hepatic uptake of chylomicron cholesterol. *J. Lipid Res.*, **20,** 923
27. Key, P. H., Bonorris, G. G., Marks, J. W., Chung, A. and Schoenfield, L. J. (1980). Biliary lipid synthesis and secretion in gallstone patients before and during treatment with chenodeoxycholic acid. *J. Lab. Clin. Med.*, **95,** 816

31 Mechanism of the lithogenic effects of oral contraceptives

L. J. BENNION, D. M. MOTT AND B. V. HOWARD

In a series of related studies[1,2] we have searched for the mechanisms by which contraceptive steroid hormones cause cholesterol gallstones[3–5]. We assumed that the mechanisms would involve either an alteration of gallbladder motility favouring stone retention and growth, or a change in bile composition promoting nucleation or precipitation of cholesterol. The former possibility was studied in Denver by Kern's group, who found no effect of oral contraceptive usage on gallbladder size or motility[6]. Our own studies have focused instead on the effects of oral contraceptives on bile lipid composition and secretion rates.

Preliminary data in animals and in cholecystectomized humans had suggested that exogenous oestrogens and progestins might increase the degree of cholesterol saturation of bile by interfering with bile acid secretion[7–13]. These studies, however, involved much larger doses of hormone, relative to body weight, than those used for human contraception, and in some instances the models studied lacked a gallbladder or an intact enterohepatic circulation.

Our own studies in intact Pima Indians had also suggested a lithogenic effect of female sex hormones, mediated perhaps by an interference with bile acid production and secretion. For example, we studied a 36-year-old Pima woman before and after her castration for early endometrial carcinoma[14]. Her bile was more highly saturated, and her bile acid pool smaller, while she had functioning ovaries, than after their removal. Moreover, the onset of ovarian function during puberty is accompanied by a rise in bile saturation, and a decline in bile acid pool size relative to body weight[15]. For these reasons we thought it quite likely that exogenous oestrogens and progestins in the form of oral contraceptives might raise bile saturation, and that the most likely mechanism for this effect would be an interference with bile acid secretion. As our results will show, we were partially mistaken in these expectations.

We studied a total of 27 healthy young women[1,2] of child-bearing age, two of whom were American Indian and the rest of whom were white. Their ages ranged from 19 to 39 years. Each woman who entered these studies was either planning to start using oral contraceptives, or was already using them but planning to stop soon. The decision to start or stop their use was entirely independent of these studies. The indication for starting oral contraceptives in each case was a desire for contraception, rather than any hormonal deficiency or disorder. The indication for stopping them was a termination of the need or desire for contraception, rather than any adverse effect. None of the women reported any adverse symptoms or side-effects of oral contraceptive usage. Thus, this was routine clinical usage of a variety of commercially available oral contraceptives, as practised by millions of women world-wide.

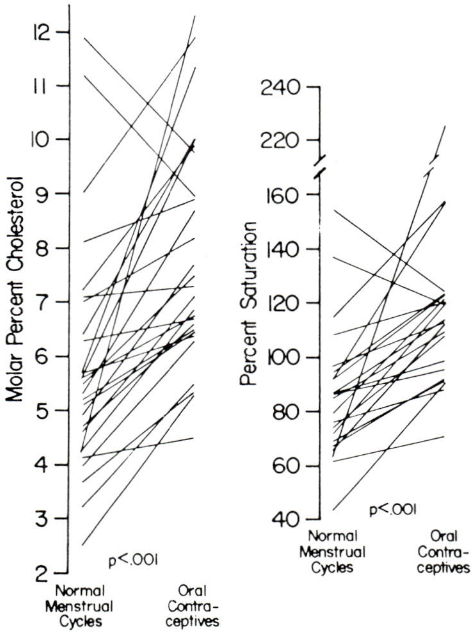

Figure 1 Effects of oral contraceptive use on gallbladder bile saturation in 27 healthy young women

Each woman was studied twice: once while taking oral contraceptives, and once during normal menstrual cycles on no medication. All our data are therefore paired, each woman serving as her own control. Bile samples during contraceptive usage were taken during the third week of consecutive daily pill ingestion. Bile samples during normal menstrual cycles were taken without regard to the day of the cycle in 22 of the 27 women. In the other five women – the five in whom bile acid pool size and lipid secretion studies were done in addition to gallbladder bile sampling – specimens were collected within the first 6 days after the onset of normal menstrual bleeding, the subject having had at least two normal menstrual cycles immediately prior to the cycle during which sampling was done.

In Figure 1 we have combined the gallbladder bile composition data from our studies. The data are expressed both as molar percentage cholesterol and as saturation computed according to Carey and Small[16], assuming a total lipid concentration of 10 g/dl. Gallbladder bile was significantly more saturated with cholesterol during oral contraceptive usage than during normal menstrual cycles on no medication.

Figure 2 shows the composition of hepatic bile, obtained during prolonged infusion of 40% fat liquid formula into the duodenum. Each point is the mean of eight 1 h samples collected during constant formula infusion after gall-bladder emptying was complete. In each instance this stimulated hepatic bile was more highly saturated during routine oral contraceptive usage than during normal menstrual cycles. The lithogenic effects of oral contraceptives are thus detectable both during feeding, when bile acid secretion rates are high, and during the postprandial and fasting periods when the gallbladder is filling and bile acid flux is lower.

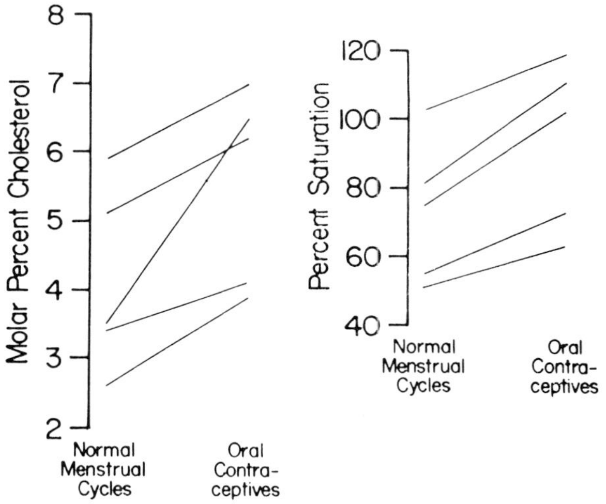

Figure 2 Effects of oral contraceptive use on hepatic bile saturation in five healthy young women

We measured biliary lipid secretion rates in these five subjects, using the Grundy method of intestinal perfusion with a triple-lumen duodenal tube[17]. Beta-sitosterol was infused as a dilution marker through the most proximal lumen, along with a 40% fat liquid formula to stimulate bile flow. Samples were taken by slow continuous aspiration 12 cm distal for determination of cholesterol secretion rates. Bile acid and phospholipid secretion rates were calculated from bile lipid composition, as determined from bile collected more proximally, adjacent to the ampulla of Vater. Sampling was not begun until 4 h of continuous perfusion had elapsed, to allow time for stabilization of lipid flow rates following initial emptying of the gallbladder. Eight hourly samples were collected, and the results were averaged. The entire process was

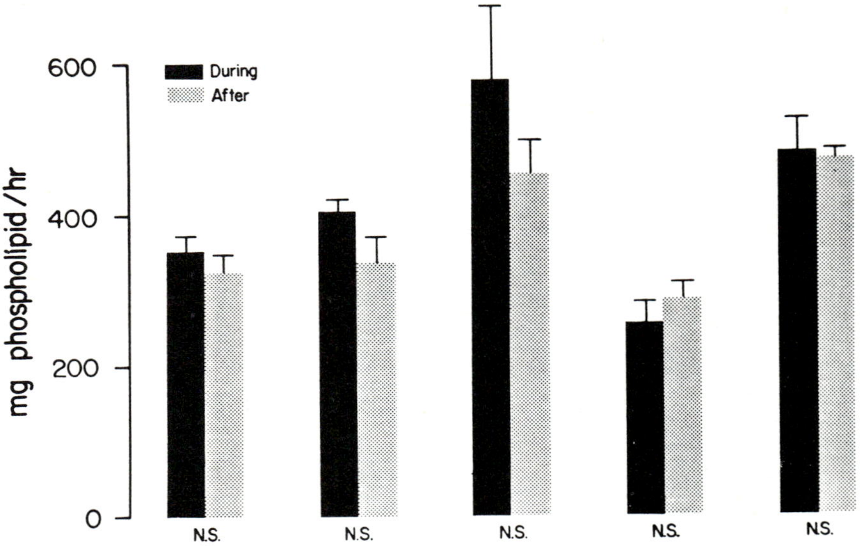

Figure 3 Effects of oral contraceptives on biliary phospholipid secretion in five healthy young women

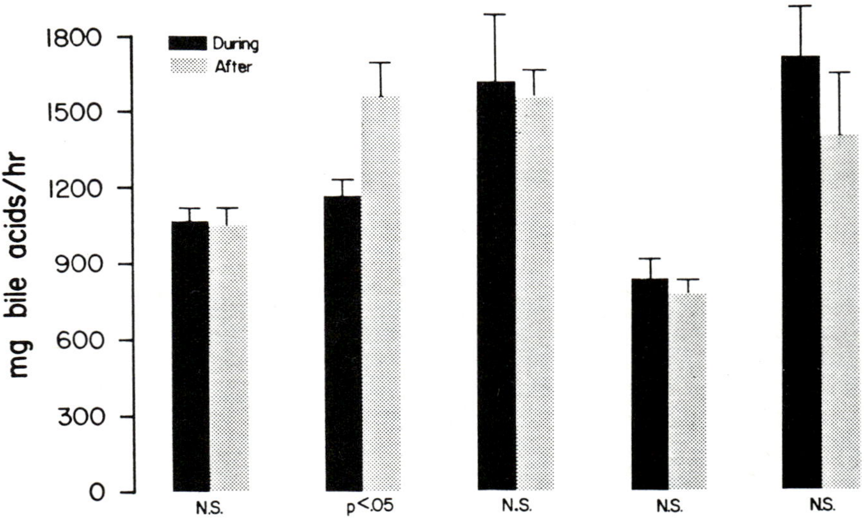

Figure 4 Effects of oral contraceptives on biliary secretion of bile acids in five healthy young women

repeated after oral contraceptives had been stopped and menstrual function had returned to normal. The results of phospholipid secretion measurements are shown in Figure 3. Oral contraceptive medication did not appear to have any significant impact on the rate of biliary phospholipid secretion.

Figure 4 shows bile acid output, which changed significantly in only one of the five subjects studied. This subject, who demonstrated a significant diminution in bile acid secretion on oral contraceptives, behaved as we had expected, on the basis of animal data cited above, that all our human subjects would. Nevertheless, four of our five subjects showed no significant effect of oral contraceptive usage on bile acid output.

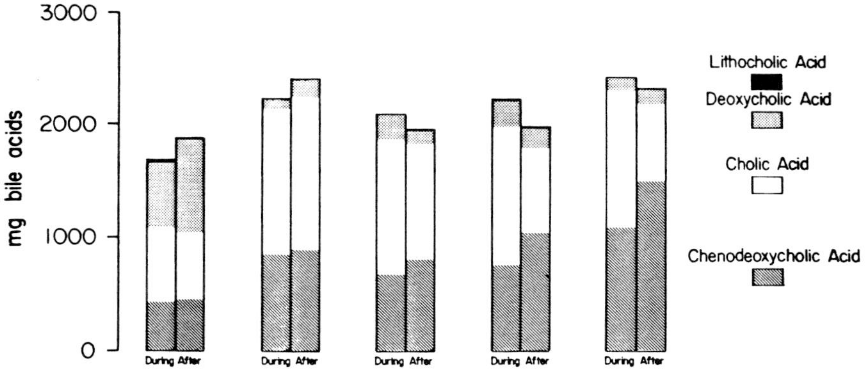

Figure 5 Effects of oral contraceptives on biliary cholesterol secretion in five healthy young women. Each subject had a significantly higher rate of cholesterol secretion during oral contraceptive usage than during normal menstrual cycles on no medication

Cholesterol secretion, on the other hand, was significantly enhanced in every subject while taking oral contraceptives, as shown in Figure 5. This hypersecretion of cholesterol appears to be the predominant mechanism responsible for the increased saturation of bile, and therefore the increased incidence of gallstones, which accompany oral contraceptive usage.

In these same five subjects we measured total bile acid pool size by the single sample method of Duane *et al.*[18]. Oral contraceptive usage did not appreciably alter total bile acid pool size, as shown in Figure 6. We interpret these data as further evidence that oral contraceptives cause lithogenic bile not through a total bile acid deficiency, but through cholesterol excess. Although total bile acid pool sizes were not significantly altered by oral contraceptive usage, these medications did have a significant effect on the composition of the bile acid pool.

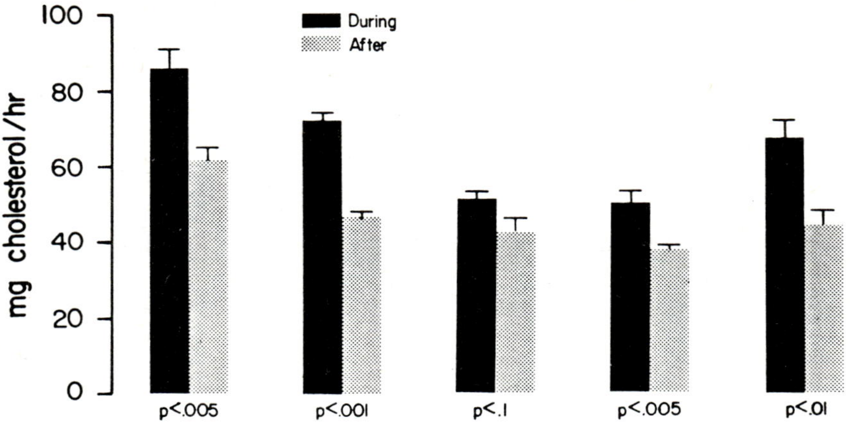

Figure 6 Bile acid pool size and composition in five healthy women during oral contraceptive usage, and again during normal menstrual cycles

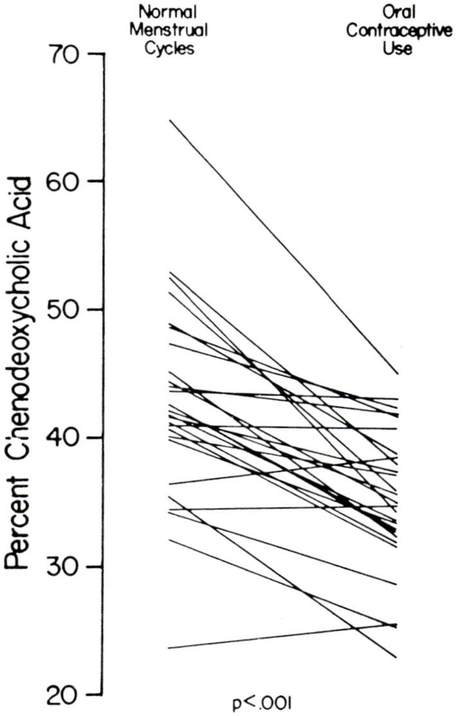

Figure 7 Effects of oral contraceptive usage on the CDCA content, as a percentage of total bile acids, in the gallbladder bile of healthy women. Oral contraceptive usage was accompanied by a significant reduction in percentage of CDCA

Figures 7 and 8 combine bile acid composition data from all our studies on the effects of oral contraceptive usage on the bile of normal humans. The percentage of chenodeoxycholic acid (CDCA) is significantly decreased, and that of cholic acid (CA) significantly increased, by oral contraceptive usage. This finding raises the possibility that the effects of contraceptive steroids on biliary cholesterol secretion and saturation may be mediated via the change in CDCA levels, in a manner converse to the feeding of CDCA. Several of the effects of using oral contraceptives are directly opposite to those of feeding CDCA; namely, an increase in the percentage of CA and a decrease in the percentage of CDCA in bile, an increase in biliary cholesterol secretion and saturation and in the likelihood of cholesterol cholelithiasis, and an increase in plasma triglyceride levels.

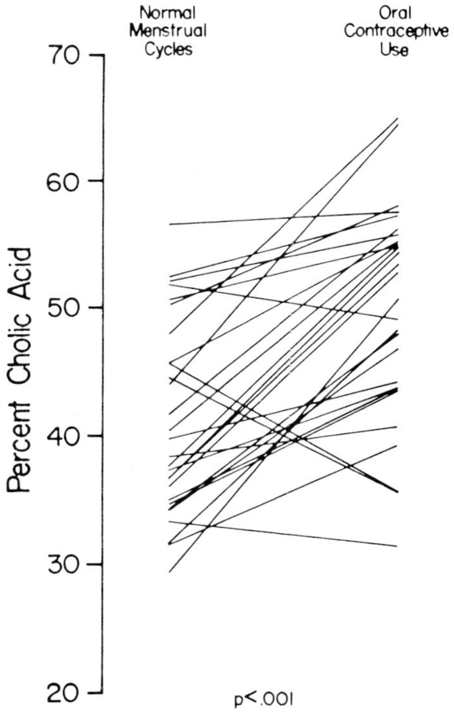

Figure 8 Cholic acid (CA) content, as a percentage of total bile acids, in the gallbladder bile of healthy women taking oral contraceptives, and also during normal menstrual cycles on no medication. Oral contraceptive usage was accompanied by a significant increase in percentage of CA

We examined plasma lipoprotein levels on and off oral contraceptives, and noted changes similar to those already described by other investigators. Very low-density lipoprotein (VLDL) and total triglyceride levels were increased, as were total and low-density lipoprotein cholesterol levels, during oral contraceptive usage as compared to normal menstrual cycles. We were looking for some correlation between high-density lipoprotein cholesterol levels and biliary cholesterol secretion rates, but we found none. We also wondered whether alterations in VLDL triglyceride levels might be mirrored by corresponding changes in bile acid secretion rates. No such correlations between plasma lipoprotein levels and biliary lipid secretion rates were evident in our small series. It did appear, however, that oral contraceptive usage may induce a generalized augmentation of lipid secretion from the liver, into blood as well as bile.

The main conclusions reached from these studies are that the increased risk of gallstones associated with routine usage of oral contraceptives appears to be due to increased cholesterol saturation of bile, and that this results from enhanced cholesterol secretion rather than from bile acid deficiency. The changes in bile acid composition which characterize oral contraceptive usage suggest that the concomitant administration of CDCA or ursodeoxycholic acid in low doses might provide a physiological reversal of those processes leading to cholesterol hypersecretion, supersaturation, and stone formation.

References

1. Bennion, L. J., Ginsberg, R. L., Garnick, M. B. and Bennett, P. H. (1976). Effects of oral contraceptives on the gallbladder bile of normal women. *N. Engl. J. Med.*, **294**, 189
2. Bennion, L. J., Mott, D. M. and Howard, B. V. (1980). Oral contraceptives raise the cholesterol saturation of bile by increasing biliary cholesterol secretion. *Metabolism*, **29,** 18
3. Boston Collaborative Drug Surveillance Program (1973). Oral contraceptives and venous thromboembolic disease, surgically confirmed gallbladder disease, and breast tumours, *Lancet*. **1,** 1404
4. The Royal College of General Practitioners (1974). *Oral Contraceptives and Health*, pp. 57–59 (Tunbridge Wells: Pitman Medical)
5. Stolley, P. D., Tonascia, J. A., Tockman, M. S., Sartwell, P. E., Rutledge, A. H. and Jacobs, M. P. (1975). Thrombosis with low-estrogen oral contraceptives. *Am. J. Epidemiol.*, **102,** 197
6. Braverman, D. Z., Johnson, M. L. and Kern, F. Jr. (1980). Effects of pregnancy and contraceptive steroids on gallbladder function. *N. Engl. J. Med.*, **302,** 362
7. Lynn, J., Williams, L., O'Brien, J., Wittenberg, J. and Egdahl, R. H. (1973). Effects of estrogen upon bile. Implications with respect to gallstone formation. *Ann. Surg.*, **178,** 514
8. Tritapepe, R., Cesana, A., Gandini, R. and Trivellini, G. (1969). Experimental research into the aetiopathogenesis of biliary calculosis. *Panminerva Med.*, **11,** 410
9. Davis, R. A. and Kern, F. Jr. (1976). Effects of ethinyl estradiol and phenobarbital on bile acid synthesis and biliary bile acid excretion. *Gastroenterology*, **70,** 1130
10. Kern, F. Jr., Eriksson, H., Curstedt, T. and Sjövall, J. (1977). Effect of ethynylestradiol on biliary excretion of bile acids, phosphatidylcolines, and cholesterol in the bile fistula rat. *J. Lipid Res.*, **18,** 623
11. Coyne, M. J., Bonorris, G. G., Chung, A., Winchester, R. and Schoenfield, L. J. (1978). Estrogen enhances dietary cholesterol induction of saturated bile in the hamster. *Gastroenterology*, **75,** 76
12. Barth, A., Bergmann, R., Saumseil, J. and Klinger, W. (1978). Influence of drugs on bile acid excretion. *Arch. Toxicol.* (Suppl. 1), 359
13. Pertsemlidis, D., Panveliwalla, D. and Ahrens, E. H. (1974). Effects of clofibrate and of an estrogen-progestin combination on fasting biliary lipids and cholic acid kinetics in man. *Gastroenterology*, **66,** 565
14. Bennion, L. J. (1977). Changes in bile lipids accompanying oophorectomy in a premenopausal woman. *N. Engl. J. Med.*, **297,** 709
15. Bennion, L. J., Knowler, W. C., Mott, D. M., Spagnola, A. M. and Bennett, P. H. (1979). Development of lithogenic bile during puberty in Pima Indians. *N. Engl. J. Med.*, **300,** 873

16. Carey, M. C. and Small, D. M. (1978). The physical chemistry of cholesterol solubility in bile. Relationship to gallstone formation and dissolution in man. *J. Clin. Invest.*, **61,** 998
17. Grundy, S. M. and Metzger, A. L. (1972). A physiologic method for estimation of hepatic secretion of biliary lipids in man. *Gastroenterology*, **62,** 1200
18. Duane, W. C., Adler, R. A., Bennion, L. J. and Grundy, S. M. (1975). Determination of bile acid pool size in man: a simplified method with advantages of increased precision, shortened analysis time, and decreased isotope exposure. *J. Lipid Res.*, **16,** 155

SECTION 4
Bile Acids, Lipids and Lipoproteins

32
An overview of lipid transport and lipoprotein metabolism

D. M. SMALL

The intestine and the liver are the primary sources of lipoproteins in higher animals. These organs primarily produce triglyceride-rich lipoproteins, the chylomicrons from the intestine and very low-density lipoproteins (VLDL) from the liver, small amounts of more dense smaller lipoproteins are also produced under normal circumstances by each organ. The subsequent physical and metabolic modifications of these primary triglyceride-rich particles produce a variety of secondary particles such as chylomicron remnants, intermediate density lipoproteins (IDL), low-density lipoproteins (LDL), and some of the high-density lipoproteins (HDL). The fate of the different lipoproteins depends largely on the apoproteins associated with the particle. Some apoproteins may act as cofactors for enzymes which further modify the lipoproteins and other apoproteins act as specific ligands for cellular uptake of lipoproteins.

Chylomicrons are triglyceride-rich emulsion particles of 1000–5000 Å diameter whose core contains triglycerides and small amounts of free and esterified cholesterol. Their surface contains phospholipids, free cholesterol and specific apolipoproteins. The apoliproproteins synthesized in the intestine and secreted on the nascent chylomicrons include intestinal apolipoprotein B (molecular weight about 125 000), apolipoproteins A–I, A–II and A–IV. Once the chylomicron enters the plasma free cholesterol and other apoproteins absorb to its surface resulting in a net increase in apoprotein and cholesterol and a net decrease in phospholipid concentration. Specifically, C apoproteins and E apoproteins are adsorbed from the plasma onto the chylomicron and A–II and A–IV are lost into the plasma. The chylomicron then attaches to the capillary endothelium where lipoprotein lipase assisted by its cofactor apoprotein C–II promotes triglyceride hydrolysis to fatty acids and partial glycerides. As triglyceride is lost the core shrinks and finally gives rise to a 400–500 Å core remnant particle which is partially depleted of triglyceride, certain apoproteins (specifically apoprotein A–I) and phospholipids. The apoprotein A–I and phospholipid leave the surface of the chylomicron as redundant folds (bilayers) which rapidly enter the high-density lipoprotein fraction where they become substrates for lecithin cholesterol acyl transferase (LCAT) and are converted into more conventional cholesterol ester containing HDL particles. These remnants also lose C peptides and gain some E. Apoprotein E is a specific ligand for a receptor site on hepatic parenchymal cells so that chylomicron remnants rich in E are rapidly taken up by the liver delivering their contents to the hepatocyte.

VLDL are smaller emulsion particles secreted from the liver with apoprotein B of molecular weight ~250 000 (different from apoprotein B of the intestine). Apoprotein E, C and A–I are also present. VLDL are metabolized by lipoprotein lipase in a similar fashion but their core remnants vary depending on the species. In the human the final remnant is LDL and it contains essentially all apoprotein B originally secreted on VLDL. In the rat the VLDL remnant is taken up by the liver like the chylomicron remnant. LDL supplies cholesterol to cells which have a need for it through the LDL receptor of Brown and Goldstein.

Surface remnants of apoprotein E, C and phospholipid are generated during VLDL lipolysis and enter the HDL fraction. In certain species on HDL containing a high concentration of apoprotein E (HDL-E) is readily taken up by the liver by the chylomicron remnant receptor thus delivering its contents to the hepatic parenchymal cell.

Finally in some species cholesterol ester produced by the LCAT reaction may be transferred by a specific apoprotein (probably apoprotein D) from HDL to LDL, VLDL and chylomicron remnants so that a fraction of the cholesterol esters formed by the LCAT reaction are distributed to the liver and to peripheral tissues.

33
Bile acids and triglyceride metabolism in man

B. ANGELIN, K. EINARSSON AND B. LEIJD

INTRODUCTION

Several lines of evidence suggest an interrelationship between bile acid and plasma triglyceride metabolism in man. Thus, bile acid synthesis is frequently increased in endogenous hypertriglyceridaemia (type IV hyperlipoproteinaemia)[1–4]. Feeding with chenodeoxycholic acid (CDCA), which inhibits bile acid production, has been reported to reduce plasma triglyceride levels[5–7]. Induction of an enhanced bile acid biosynthesis with cholestyramine treatment or biliary drainage, on the other hand, is often linked to an increase of plasma triglyceride levels[8–11].

These observations have initiated a series of investigations, aimed at characterizing the possible influence of bile acids on the metabolism of plasma triglycerides in man. The present work summarizes and discusses some recent studies concerning this question performed in our laboratories.

PATIENTS STUDIED

We have mainly studied patients with various types of primary hyperlipoproteinaemia, characterized according to WHO recommendations[12]. It is important to remember that a certain lipoprotein pattern (phenotype) may be the result of several underlying genetic disorders[13]. Our patient series thus includes subjects with familial hypercholesterolaemia (type IIa pattern), with familial combined hyperlipidaemia (who may have either type IIa, type IIb, or type IV pattern), and with familial hypertriglyceridaemia (type IV pattern). In many cases the genetic origin of the hyperlipidaemia cannot be adequately determined, and each 'group' of lipoprotein phenotypes is therefore probably heterogeneous with regard to its metabolic 'defect'.

In order to avoid variation due to environmental influences, patients have been hospitalized and fed a weight-maintaining, standardized diet of natural type[14].

METHODS

Plasma triglyceride production rate

In our evaluation of plasma triglyceride transport we have used the method originally developed by Reaven and co-workers[15] as described by Nikkilä and Kekki[16–18]. After a pulse injection of [2-^{3}H]glycerol, the specific activity of plasma total or very low-density lipoprotein (VLDL) triglyceride is determined during a 10 h fast[14,19–21]. The fractional catabolic rate is calculated, assuming first-order kinetics, and the production rate is obtained as the product of pool size and fractional catabolic rate. Although the fractional catabolic rate of VLDL triglycerides is faster than that of total plasma triglycerides, the production rates of VLDL and total triglycerides generally agree well[18,20].

The method employed in the present studies gives values in good agreement with those obtained by other techniques for measuring plasma (VLDL) triglyceride turnover[18,22–24]. It should be emphasized that there exists today no perfect method for determining true plasma (VLDL) triglyceride production rate[25]. However, for the comparative purposes of the present investigations, the methodology employed should be considered as adequate.

Bile acid production

For determination of bile acid synthesis 24-^{14}C-labelled cholic acid (CA) and chenodeoxycholic acid (CDCA) have been given perorally. Fasting duodenal bile samples have been obtained on four or five occasions, and the specific activity of the individual bile acids have been determined[14,21]. Pool size, fractional catabolic rate, and production rate have been calculated for CA and CDCA as outlined by Lindstedt[26].

CHARACTERIZATION OF PATIENTS WITH TYPE IV HYPERLIPOPROTEINAEMIA AND DISTURBED BILE ACID METABOLISM

Type IV hyperlipoproteinaemia is obviously of heterogeneous origin, and the elevated VLDL triglyceride levels may be the consequence of an increased production rate and/or a delayed clearance of the lipoprotein particle or some of its constituents. Also with respect to bile acid metabolism, there is marked heterogeneity in this lipoprotein abnormality[1–4]. In order to characterize metabolically the group of patients with an increased production rate of bile acids, we performed simultaneous measurements of bile acid turnover and plasma triglyceride metabolism in 22 patients with primary type IV hyperlipoproteinaemia[14]. As demonstrated in Figure 1, there was a positive relationship between bile acid biosynthesis and plasma triglyceride turnover ($r = +0.71$, $p < 0.001$). All the patients who had an enhanced bile acid formation also displayed an increased production rate of plasma triglycerides. Later studies on the genetic origin of the hypertriglyceridaemia suggest that many of these patients have familial hypertriglyceridaemia, an entity of

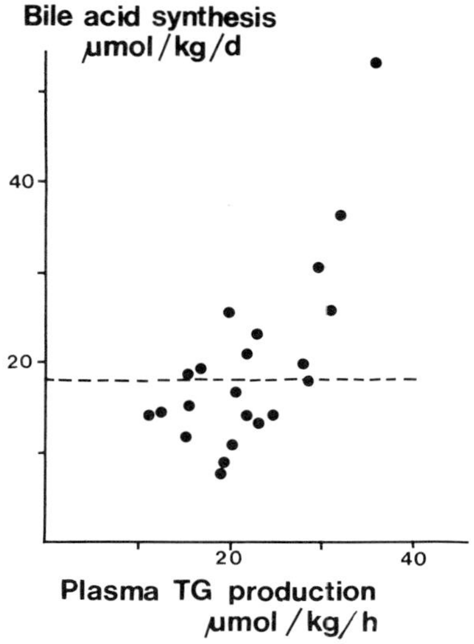

Figure 1 Bile acid synthesis (µmol kg^{-1} day^{-1}) as a function of endogenous plasma triglyceride production rate (µmol kg^{-1} h^{-1}) in patients with type IV hyperlipoproteinaemia. The dotted line indicates the upper normal range for bile acid synthesis. Data from ref. 14

disease that seems to be linked to an enhanced production of triglyceride-rich VLDL[27].

It may also be mentioned that later studies in which VLDL triglyceride kinetics were specifically determined have confirmed the presence of this relationship in patients with type IV hyperlipoproteinaemia[21].

INDUCED CHANGES IN BILE ACID METABOLISM: INFLUENCE ON PLASMA TRIGLYCERIDE KINETICS

In order to test the hypothesis that disturbances of bile acid metabolism may directly influence plasma triglyceride turnover, we have performed perturbations of the system in two ways. First, we have studied the effect on plasma triglyceride turnover in patients with normal bile acid and triglyceride synthesis when treated with cholestyramine. Second, we have studied the effects of treating patients with primary hyperlipoproteinaemia with different bile acids.

Cholestyramine treatment and plasma triglyceride metabolism

When given to patients with hyperlipoproteinaemia type IIa, cholestyramine increased the production rate of endogenous plasma triglycerides by over 30%[19]. Due to the fact that the fractional catabolic rate was also increased, the effects on total plasma triglyceride concentration were generally more modest. Treatment of patients with type IV hyperlipoproteinaemia does not generally increase bile acid production to the same extent[28]; in such patients treatment also had no effect on plasma triglyceride turnover[19].

The results of the original report concerning total plasma triglyceride kinetics[19] have recently been confirmed for specific measurements of VLDL triglyceride turnover and fractional catabolic rate in patients with heterozygous familial hypercholesterolaemia.

Bile acid treatment and plasma triglyceride metabolism

Figure 2 summarizes our current experience of the effects on plasma triglyceride turnover during treatment with different bile acids in hyperlipoproteinaemia type IIa and type IV[19,20,29]. CDCA treatment was associated with a 40% reduction of triglyceride production rate both in type IIa and type IV hyperlipoproteinaemia[19]. Generally, a reduced fractional catabolic rate of plasma triglycerides was also seen[19]. CA was not linked to any significant changes in the turnover of plasma triglycerides, although patients with type IV lipoprotein phenotype and an initially increased triglyceride synthesis clearly reduced their triglyceride production[20]. Treatment with ursodeoxycholic acid (UDCA) was not associated with any consistent change in plasma triglyceride turnover in a more limited series of patients[29]. The fasting concentration of VLDL triglycerides was lowered during CDCA therapy but not significantly so during treatment with CA or UDCA[19,20,29].

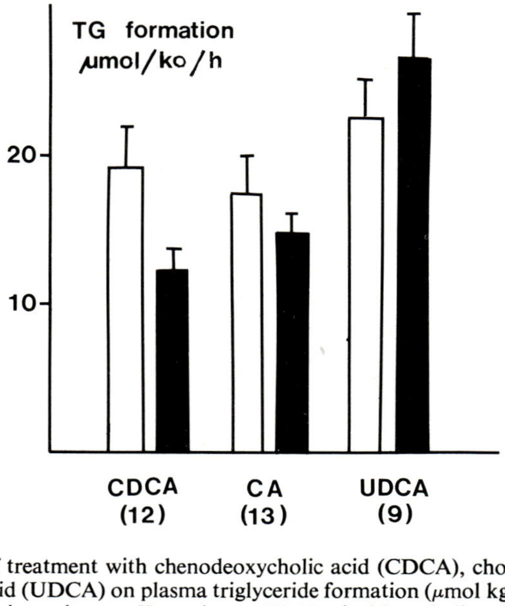

Figure 2 Effect of treatment with chenodeoxycholic acid (CDCA), cholic acid (CA), and ursodeoxycholic acid (UDCA) on plasma triglyceride formation (μmol kg^{-1} h^{-1}) in patients with hyperlipoproteinaemia type IIa and type IV. Vertical bars indicate SEM. Number of subjects within parentheses. Data from refs. 19, 20 and 29

DISCUSSION

The major conclusions of the studies summarized here are:

(a) that patients with primary type IV hyperlipoproteinaemia due to overproduction of VLDL triglycerides often display an increased biosynthesis of bile acids; and
(b) that experimental conditions primarily aimed at changing bile acid metabolism are associated with corresponding changes in the metabolism of plasma VLDL triglycerides.

When discussing possible mechanisms responsible for these findings it may be helpful to consider at which sites the metabolism of bile acids/cholesterol and triglycerides may interact. In Figure 3 a highly simplified schedule of human cholesterol and lipoprotein metabolism is outlined.

In the fasting state triglycerides and cholesterol, together with phospholipids and various apoproteins, are secreted into plasma as VLDL from the liver (pool I) and the intestine (pool IV). Triglycerides are hydrolysed and taken up in peripheral tissues, and cholesterol is esterified under the influence of plasma lecithin : cholesterol acyl transferase (LCAT). Cholesterol is presently believed to reach the liver in VLDL remnants (IDL, intermediate-density lipoproteins) or via the high-density lipoproteins (HDL); the importance of low-density lipoprotein (LDL) contribution to hepatic cholesterol is less clear. This 'catabolized' cholesterol (pool II) may either be re-utilized for lipoprotein formation or secreted into the bile as free cholesterol

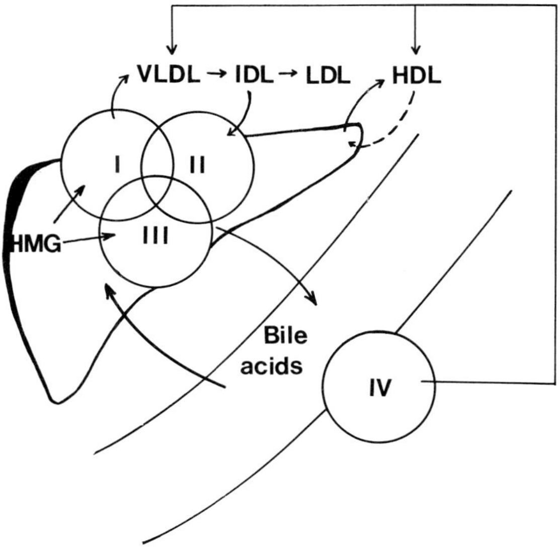

Figure 3 Simplified schedule of cholesterol/bile acid and lipoprotein triglyceride metabolic pathways. HDL, high-density lipoproteins; HMG, hydroxymethylglutaryl coenzyme A reductase; IDL, intermediate-density lipoproteins; LDL, low-density lipoproteins; VLDL, very low-density lipoproteins. I–IV indicate 'subpools' of cholesterol (see text)

or after conversion to bile acids (pool III). Newly synthesized cholesterol may contribute to 'pools' I and III (Figure 3).

The findings on bile acid metabolism in type IV hyperlipoproteinaemia may either reflect a generalized relationship between bile acid and triglyceride metabolic pathways, or it may be the result of the inclusion of several forms of hypertriglyceridaemia with different metabolic abnormalities. Studies of genetically well-defined patients will be necessary to resolve this question. Furthermore, the increased bile acid production in some of these patients may be a primary or a secondary phenomenon. In the latter case, an enhanced flux of VLDL (due to overproduction) would supply the liver with an increased load of lipoprotein cholesterol, thereby increasing the need for cholesterol breakdown and elimination. In some agreement with this view may be the finding of an increased turnover of plasma cholesterol esters in patients with type IV lipoprotein pattern and bile acid overproduction[21].

The findings of changes in lipoprotein metabolism during perturbations of bile acid turnover would, however, suggest a more direct effect. Such an influence of bile acids on triglyceride metabolism may be hypothesized to take place in several ways. First, an increased need for cholesterol aimed for bile acid synthesis in the liver (pool III of Figure 3) could increase the uptake of cholesterol-rich lipoproteins by the liver into pool II, resulting in an increased flux through the lipoprotein breakdown pathway, indirectly resulting in VLDL overproduction. A reverse effect could take place during a reduced need for bile acid synthesis, e.g. during CDCA treatment. Second, changes in hepatic cholesterol production might influence both VLDL formation and bile acid biosynthesis in parallel. In some support for this contention, CDCA, but not CA, has been found to have an inhibitory effect on hepatic hydroxymethylglutaryl CoA reductase, the rate-limiting step in cholesterol biosynthesis[30]. Third, bile acids returning to the liver may exert a direct influence on triglyceride synthesis in the liver. Finally, the possible importance of bile acid-mediated regulation of intestinal lipoprotein synthesis (cholesterol pool IV in Figure 3) should not be forgotten.

Preliminary studies in the rat liver suggest that the supposedly rate-limiting enzymatic step in hepatic triglyceride biosynthesis, phosphatidic acid phosphatase, may be influenced by disturbances of bile acid enterohepatic circulation[31]. Thus, cholestyramine treatment and biliary drainage increased enzymatic activity, whereas bile acid treatment – especially CDCA – decreased enzymatic activity considerably[31].

Thus, our clinical studies suggest that changes in bile acid metabolism may induce changes in plasma VLDL triglyceride turnover. More detailed studies are needed, however, to elucidate the mechanisms behind this relationship and its possible importance for the development of hypertriglyceridaemia.

Acknowledgments

The skilful technical assistance of Mrs Ruth Detlofsson, Miss Helene Saranius, Miss Anna-Maija Suontaka, and Mrs Margret Wahlström in the performance of these studies is gratefully acknowledged. The work summarized here has been supported by grants from the Swedish Medical

Research Council (19X-04793), the Swedish National Association against Heart and Chest Diseases, Karolinska Institutets Fonder, and the Tore Nilson Foundation. Dr Angelin is the recipient of a fellowship from the Ernst Klenk Foundation.

References

1. Kottke, B. A. (1969). Differences in bile acid excretion. Primary hypercholesterolemia compared to combined hypercholesterolemia and hypertriglyceridemia. *Circulation*, **40,** 13
2. Einarsson, K. and Hellström, K. (1972). The formation of bile acids in patients with three types of hyperlipoproteinaemia. *Eur. J. Clin. Invest.*, **2,** 225
3. Wollenweber, J. and Stiehl, A. (1972). Grösse des Pools und Turnover der primären Gallensäuren bei Hyperlipoproteinämien: Unterschiedliche Befunde bei Typ II und Typ IV Hyperlipoproteinämie. *Klin. Wochenschr.*, **50,** 33
4. Einarsson, K., Hellström, K. and Kallner, M. (1974). Bile acid kinetics in relation to sex, serum lipids, body weights, and gallbladder disease in patients with various types of hyperlipoproteinemia. *J. Clin. Invest.*, **54,** 1301
5. Bell, G. D., Lewis, B., Petrie, A. ana Dowling, R. H. (1973). Serum lipids in cholelithiasis: effect of chenodeoxycholic acid therapy. *Br. Med. J.*, **3,** 520
6. Miller, N. E. and Nestel, P. J. (1974). Triglyceride-lowering effect of chenodeoxycholic acid in patients with endogenous hypertriglyceridaemia. *Lancet*, **2,** 929
7. Angelin, B., Einarsson, K. and Leijd, B. (1978). Effect of chenodeoxycholic acid on serum and biliary lipids in patients with hyperlipoproteinaemia. *Clin. Sci. Mol. Med.*, **54,** 451
8. Jones, R. J. and Dobrilovic, L. (1970). Lipoprotein lipid alterations with cholestyramine administration. *J. Lab. Clin. Med.*, **75,** 953
9. Carlson, L. A., Olsson, A. G., Orö, L., Rössner, S. and Walldius, G. (1974). Effects of hypolipidaemic regimes on serum lipoproteins. In Schettler, G. and Weizel, A. (eds.). *Proceedings of the III International Symposium on Atherosclerosis*, pp. 768–781. (Berlin: Springer-Verlag)
10. Miller, N. E. and Nestel, P. J. (1975). Differences among hyperlipoproteinaemic subjects in the response of lipoprotein lipids to resin therapy. *Eur. J. Clin. Invest.*, **5,** 241
11. Nestel, P. J. and Grundy, S. M. (1976). Changes in plasma triglyceride metabolism during withdrawal of bile. *Metabolism*, **25,** 1259
12. Beaumont, J. L., Carlson, L. A., Cooper, G. R., Fejfar, Z., Fredrickson, D. S. and Strasser, T. (1970). Classification of hyperlipidaemias and hyperlipoproteinaemias. *Bull. WHO*, **43,** 891
13. Goldstein, J. L., Schrott, H. B., Hazzard, W. R., Bierman, E. L. and Motulsky, A. G. (1973). Hyperlipidemia in coronary heart disease. II. Genetic analysis of lipid levels in 176 families and delineation of a new inherited disorder, combined hyperlipidemia. *J. Clin. Invest.*, **52,** 1544
14. Angelin, B., Einarsson, K., Hellström, K. and Leijd, B. (1978). Bile acid kinetics in relation to endogenous triglyceride metabolism in various types of hyperlipoproteinemia. *J. Lipid Res.*, **19,** 1004
15. Farquhar, J. W., Gross, R. C., Wagner, R. M. and Reaven, G. M. (1965). Validation of an incompletely coupled two-compartment nonrecycling catenary model for turnover of liver and plasma triglyceride in man. *J. Lipid Res.*, **6,** 119
16. Nikkilä, E. A. and Kekki, M. (1971). Polymorphism of plasma triglyceride kinetics in normal human adult subjects. *Acta Med. Scand.*, **190,** 49
17. Nikkilä, E. A. and Kekki, M. (1972). Plasma endogenous triglyceride transport in hypertriglyceridaemia and effect of a hypolipidaemic drug (SU-13437). *Eur. J. Clin. Invest.*, **2,** 231
18. Kekki, M. and Nikkilä, E. A. (1975). Turnover of plasma total and very low density lipoprotein triglyceride in man. *Scand. J. Clin. Lab. Invest.*, **35,** 171
19. Angelin, B., Einarsson, K., Hellström, K. and Leijd, B. (1978). Effects of cholestyramine

and chenodeoxycholic acid on the metabolism of endogenous triglyceride in hyperlipoproteinemia. *J. Lipid Res.*, **19,** 1017
20. Angelin, B. and Leijd, B. (1980). Effects of cholic acid on the metabolism of endogenous plasma triglyceride and on biliary lipid composition in hyperlipoproteinemia. *J. Lipid Res.*, **21,** 1
21. Angelin, B., Einarsson, K., Leijd, B. and Wallentin, L. (1981). Plasma cholesterol esterification rate in type IV hyperlipoproteinaemia: relation to bile acid kinetics and triglyceride metabolism. *J. Lab. Clin. Med.* (In press)
22. Steiner, G. and Murase, T. (1975). Triglyceride turnover: a comparison of simultaneous determinations using the radioglyceride and the lipolytic rate procedures. *Fed. Proc.*, **34,** 2258
23. Chait, A., Albers, J. J. and Brunzell, J. D. (1977). Comparison of methods of plasma triglyceride turnover. In Schettler, G., Goto, Y., Hata, Y. and Klose, G. (eds.). *Atherosclerosis IV*, pp. 132–137. (Berlin: Springer-Verlag)
24. Zech, L. A., Grundy, S. M., Steinberg, D. and Berman, M. (1979). Kinetic model for production and metabolism of very low density lipoprotein triglycerides. *J. Clin. Invest.*, **63,** 1262
25. Carlson, L. A. (1980). Regulation of endogenous plasma triglyceride concentration: can we measure the rate of production or of removal of endogenous plasma triglycerides in man? *Eur. J. Clin. Invest.*, **10,** 5
26. Lindstedt, S. (1957). Turnover of cholic acid in man. *Acta Physiol. Scand.*, **40,** 1
27. Chait, A., Albers, J. J. and Brunzell, J. D. (1980). Very low density lipoprotein overproduction in genetic forms of hypertriglyceridaemia. *Eur. J. Clin. Invest.*, **10,** 17
28. Einarsson, K., Hellström, K. and Kallner, M. (1974). The effect of cholestyramine on the elimination of cholesterol as bile acids in patients with hyperlipoproteinaemia type II and IV. *Eur. J. Clin. Invest.*, **4,** 405
29. Angelin, B., Einarsson, K. and Leijd, B. (1981). Effects of ursodeoxycholic acid on plasma and biliary lipid metabolism in hyperlipoproteinaemia. (In preparation)
30. Ahlberg, J., Angelin, B. and Einarsson, K. (1981). Hepatic 3-hydroxy-3-methylglutaryl coenzyme A reductase activity and biliary lipid composition in man: Relation to cholesterol gallstone disease and effects of cholic acid and chenodeoxycholic acid treatment. *J. Lipid Res.* (In press)
31. Angelin, B., Björkhem, I. and Einarsson, K. (1981). Influence of bile acids on the rate-limiting step in biosynthesis of triglycerides in rat liver. (In preparation)

34
Transport of bile acids: lipoproteins, membrane polypeptides and cytosolic proteins as carriers

H. ABBERGER, U. BICKEL, H.–P. BUSCHER, K. FUCHTE, W. GEROK, W. KRAMER AND G. KURZ

INTRODUCTION

Bile salts are amphiphilic molecules and most likely transported in intimate association with carrier molecules. In order to identify all potential carriers for bile salts in

(1) their transport in plasma
(2) their uptake by hepatocytes
(3) their intracellular translocation
(4) their secretion into bile canaliculi

these processes were investigated by photoaffinity labelling. 3β-Azido-7α,12α-dihydroxy-5β-cholan-24-oic acid, 7,7-azo-3α,12α-dihydroxy-5β-cholan-24-oic acid, 11ξ-azido-12-oxo-3α,7α-dihydroxy-5β-cholan-24-oic acid and the corresponding taurine conjugates (Figure 1) were used as photolabile derivatives of cholate and taurocholate. Each of the photolabile derivatives carries the photoreactive group at a different position of the steroid nucleus and leaves two of the three hydroxyl groups of cholic acid (CA) unchanged. The unconjugated derivatives were tritium-labelled at carbon 7 or 12 with a specific radioactivity of 2.3 Ci/mmol, whereas the conjugated derivatives we used were tritium-labelled in the taurine residue with a specific radioactivity of 20–40 Ci/mmol. These photolabile derivatives of bile salts are chemically as similar as possible to the physiological molecules and behave as analogues of the natural bile salts. They all are completely secreted into the bile, the unconjugated derivatives as conjugated bile salts and the taurine-conjugated derivatives absolutely unchanged.

BILE ACID BINDING COMPONENTS IN SERUM

Photoaffinity labelling of whole human serum with 3β-azido-7α,12α-dihydroxy-5β-cholan-24-oic acid revealed that in addition to albumin two further polypeptides were modified, as demonstrated by SDS-disc poly-

3β-Azido Derivative

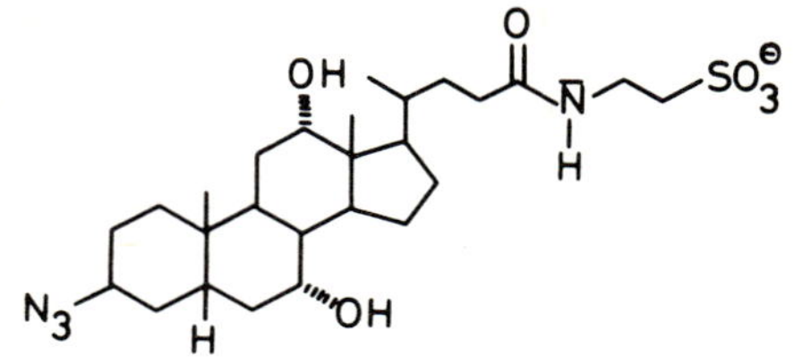

(3β-azido-7α,12α-dihydroxy-5β-cholan-24-oyl)-2-aminoethanesulfonate

7,7-Azo Derivative

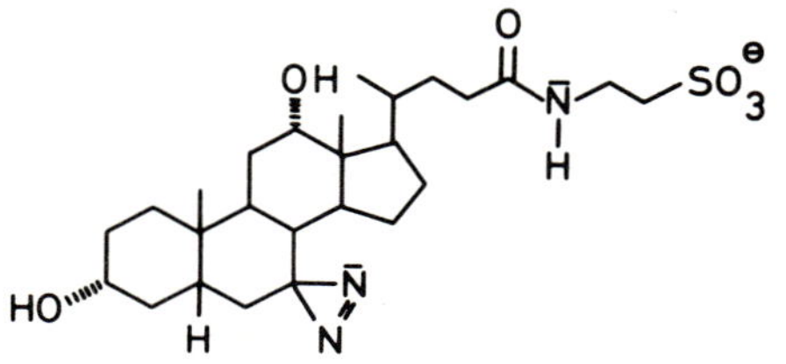

(7,7-azo-3α,12α-dihydroxy-5β-cholan-24-oyl)-2-aminoethanesulfonate

11-Azido-12-oxo Derivative

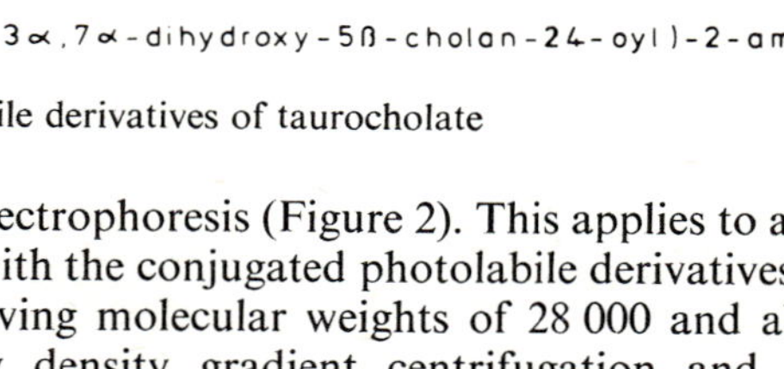

(11-azido-12-oxo-3α,7α-dihydroxy-5β-cholan-24-oyl)-2-aminoethanesulfonate

Figure 1 Photolabile derivatives of taurocholate

acrylamide gel electrophoresis (Figure 2). This applies to all three photolabile derivatives. As with the conjugated photolabile derivatives of bile salts[1] these polypeptides, having molecular weights of 28 000 and about 10 000, could be identified by density gradient centrifugation and by immunological characterization (Figure 3) as apolipoproteins A–I, A–II and C of high-density lipoprotein (HDL). After immunoprecipitation with anti-HDL they are

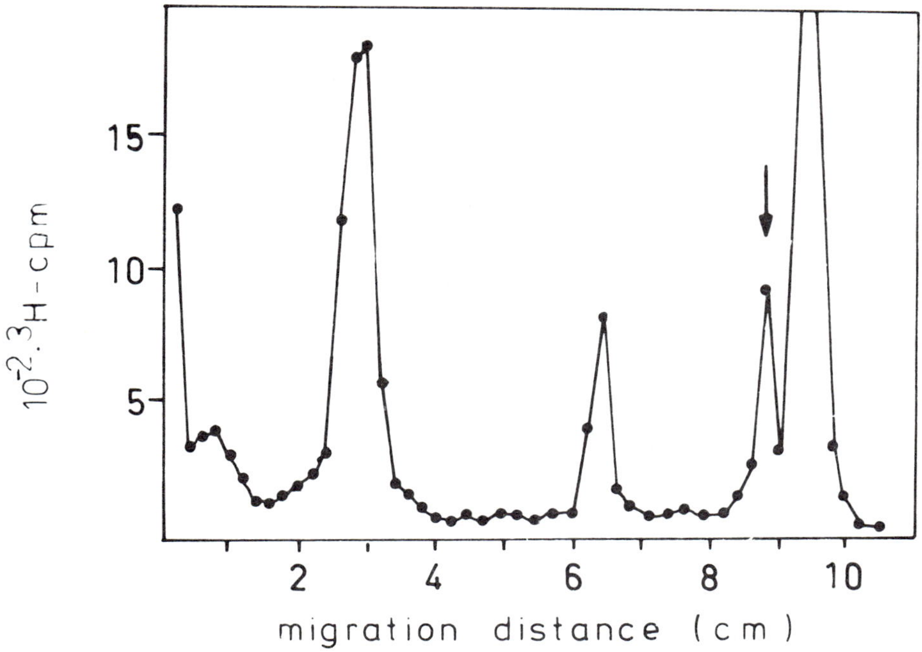

Figure 2 Distribution of radioactivity after SDS-disc polyacrylamide gel electrophoresis of whole human serum after photoaffinity labelling with 3β-azido-7α,12α-dihydroxy-5β-cholan-24-oic acid. 200 μl serum were incubated with 60.5 μM (23 μCi) [12-^{3}H]3β-azido-7α,12α-dihydroxy-5β-cholan-24-oic acid for 7 h at 25 °C in the dark. Subsequently photolysis was performed at 320 nm for 30 min at 30 °C in a cylindrical cuvette[1]. After electrodialysis discontinuous SDS-polyacrylamide gel electrophoresis was performed in cylindrical gels (6 mm dia. × 170 mm length). The temperature during electrophoresis was maintained at 10 °C; the current was kept constant at 4 mA/gel tube (about 200 V) during separation. The total acrylamide concentration was 10.5% at a ratio of acrylamide : bisacrylamide of 97.2 : 2.8. The gel was loaded with 430 μg protein. After electrophoresis the gel was cut into discs of 2 mm thickness and radioactivity of each gel fraction was determined. The arrow indicates the position of bromophenol blue

missing in the supernatant (Figure 3A) and clearly detectable in the precipitate (Figure 3B).

The distribution of bile salts between albumin and the lipoproteins was checked by density gradient centrifugation[1]. Dependent upon the chemical structure 15–50% of the respective bile salt is incorporated into HDL, whereas only minor amounts could be detected in other lipoproteins (Table 1). The relative incorporation of bile salts into HDL rises with the number of hydroxyl groups and is higher for the conjugated than for the unconjugated derivatives. Comparable results were obtained with fasting and with post-prandial serum.

BILE ACID BINDING POLYPEPTIDES IN MEMBRANES

Photoaffinity labelling of plasma membrane subfractions from rat liver was

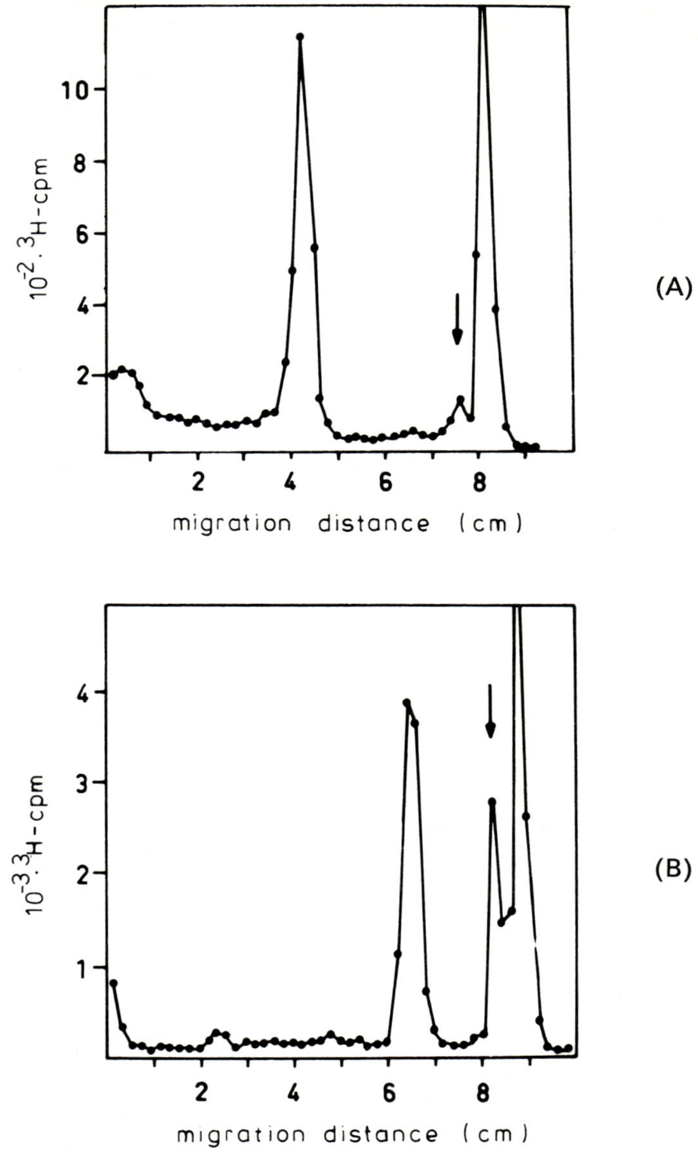

Figure 3 Distribution of radioactivity after SDS-disc polyacrylamide gel electrophoresis of the supernatant and the precipitate obtained on treatment of serum with anti-HDL after photoaffinity labelling with 3β-azido-7α,12α-dihydroxy-5β-cholan-24-oic acid. 200 μl serum were incubated with 50 μM (28 μCi) [12-^{3}H]3β-azido-7α,12α-dihydroxy-5β-cholan-24-oic acid for 7 h at 25 °C in the dark. After photoaffinity labelling the serum was treated with anti-HDL and the precipitate collected by centrifugation. All other conditions were as described in the legend to Figure 2. (A) Supernatant of immunoprecipitation. The gel was loaded with 160 μg protein. (B) Precipitate obtained with anti-HDL. The gel was loaded with 70 μg protein. The arrow indicates in each case the position of bromophenol blue

Table 1 Relative distribution of bile salts among serum proteins

Bile acid derivative	*Fasting state* ($n = 6$)				*Postprandial state* ($n = 5$)			
	Albumin	*HDL*	*LDL*	*VLDL*	*Albumin*	*HDL*	*LDL*	*VLDL*
Cholic acid	71	25	0–4	—	70	30	—	—
Chenodeoxycholic acid	85	15	—	—	85	15	—	—
Lithocholic acid	87.5	11	1.5	—	88	11	1	—
3β-Azido-derivative	50.5	45	4	0.5	53.5	41	5	0.5
11ξ-Azido-12-oxo-derivative	78	18	3	0.2	74	22	2	2
Taurocholic acid	66	34	—	—	61	39	—	—
Chenodeoxytaurocholic acid	n.d.	n.d.	n.d.	n.d.	68	25	7	—
3β-Azido-taurine-conjugate	50	45	5	—	39	53	8	0.2
7,7-Azo-taurine-conjugate	92	8	—	—	84	16	—	—
11ξ-Azido-12-oxo-taurine-conjugate	77	23	—	—	67	33	—	—

Human serum was incubated with the different bile acids at 25 °C for 1 h and submitted to density gradient centrifugation either directly or after photoaffinity labelling. The concentration of the unconjugated bile acids was in the range of 15–80 μmol/l, that of the conjugated in the range of 0.5–20 μmoll. All other conditions were as described[1]
n.d. = no data

performed to reveal all membrane polypeptides involved in the binding of conjugated and unconjugated bile salts during their hepatobiliary transport. The plasma membrane subfractions used have been characterized morphologically by electron microscopy, enzymatically by the specific activities of characterizing enzymes (Table 2) and by their polypeptide pattern (Figure 4). In order to identify the polypeptides interacting with conjugated bile salts

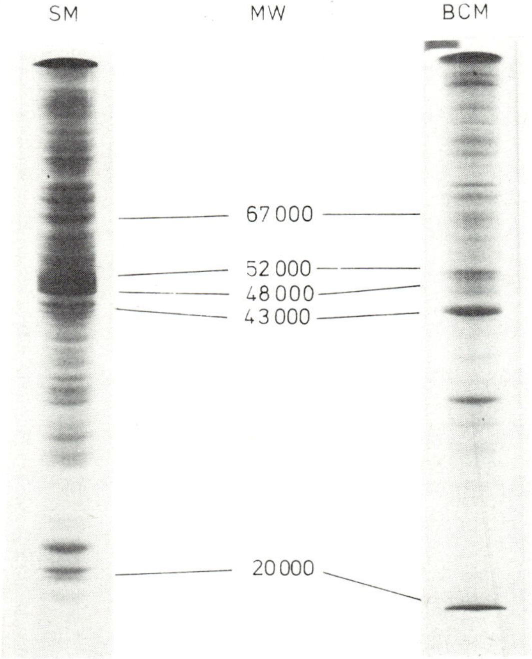

Figure 4 Comparison of the polypeptide pattern of subfractions of liver cell membranes. Bile canalicular membranes (BCM) and the subfraction enriched with sinusoidal surfaces (SM) were prepared according to Kramer, W., Bickel, U., Buscher, H.-P., Gerok, W. and Kurz, G., manuscript in preparation. Approximately 400 μg of protein were applied to each gel. The molecular weights (MW) of the polypeptides modified by photoaffinity labelling are indicated between the gels

during uptake by hepatocytes photoaffinity labelling of subfractions enriched with sinusoidal surfaces was carried out with the 3β-azido derivative of taurocholate at a concentration of 1 μmol/l. Following the labelling of the membrane subfraction SDS-disc polyacrylamide gel electrophoresis was performed (Figure 5). A clear photogenerated incorporation of radioactivity was found only in four or perhaps five polypeptides, the molecular weights of which are 67 000, 52 000, 48 000, 43 000 and about 20 000. The same labelling pattern has been obtained with the other photolabile derivatives of taurocholate, the extent of incorporation and radioactivity, however, being different for the different photoaffinity labels[11].

Photoaffinity labelling of another plasma membrane subfraction, predominantly composed of bile canaliculi, resulted in the modification of

Table 2 Comparison of specific activities of enzymes in subfractions of plasma membranes from rat liver

	Ref.	Bile canalicular membranes		Sinusoidal membranes	
		Specific activity (mU/mg)	*Membrane/homogenate ratio*	*Specific activity* (mU/mg)	*Membrane/homogenate ratio*
5′-Nucleotidase	(2)	1095	51.5	685	28.5
Mg^{2+}-ATPase	(3)	634	10.5	404	7.5
Na^+, K^+-ATPase	(3)	36.3	5.6	169	28.2
Nucleotide pyrophosphatase	(4)	3697	75.5	3078	38.8
Alkaline phosphatase	(5)	103	54.5	73.5	51.0
Leucine aminopeptidase	(6)	373	11.0	234	8.3
D-Glucose-6-phosphatase	(7)	21	1.7	24.9	1.6
Succinate dehydrogenase	(8)	4	0.35	0.3	0.05
Acid phosphatase	(9)	38	1.9	63	4.2
Galactosyl transferase	(10)	0.604	7	1.087	18.7

Enzyme activities were determined at 30 °C and are expressed as nmol of product liberated min^{-1} mg $protein^{-1}$

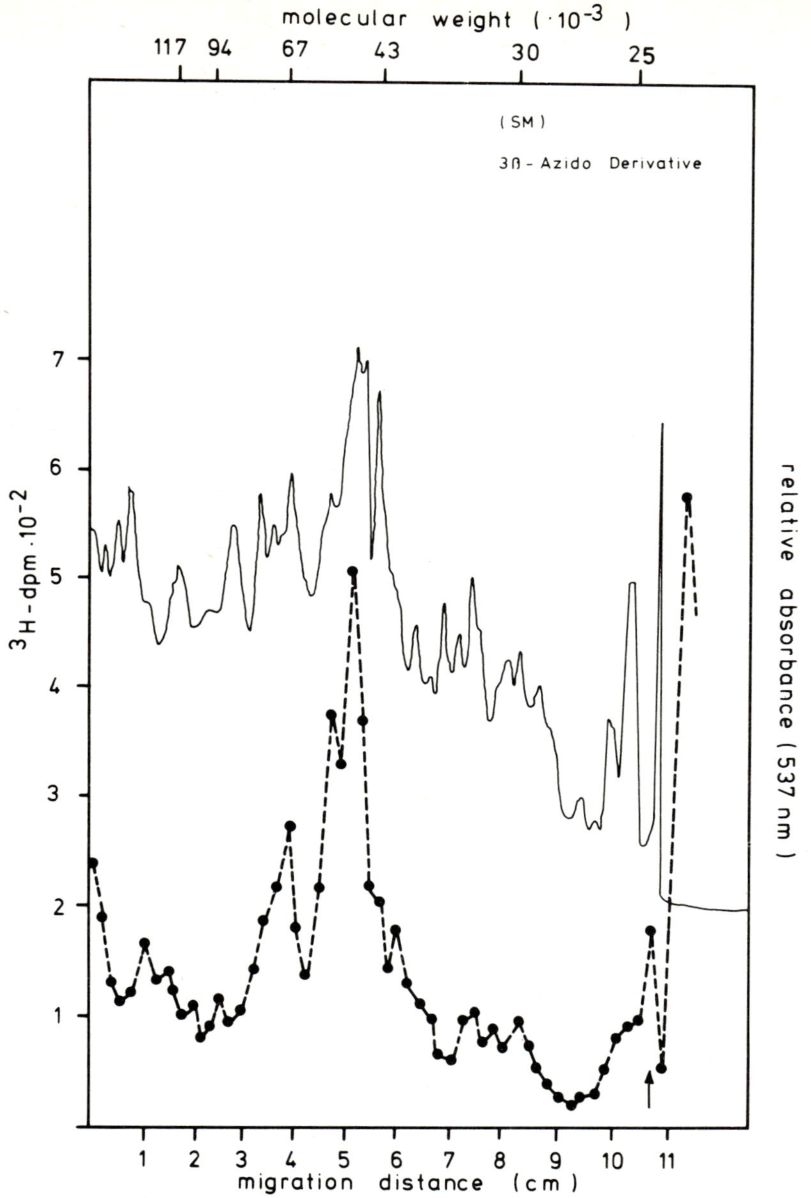

Figure 5 Distribution of radioactivity after SDS-polyacrylamide gel electrophoresis of plasma membrane subfractions of hepatocytes enriched in sinusoidal surfaces after photo-affinity labelling. 1.23 mg of sinusoidal membranes were incubated in the dark with 1.91 μM (13.12 μCi) [3β-azido-7α,12α-dihydroxy-5β-cholan-24-oyl]-2-amino[2-^{3}H(N)]ethane-sulphonic acid for 4 min. Photolysis was carried out at 320 nm for 30 min at 30 °C. Discontinuous SDS-polyacrylamide gel electrophoresis was performed with a total acrylamide concentration of 9% at a ratio of acrylamide : bisacrylamide 97.2 : 2.8. All other conditions were as described in the legend to Figure 2. The gel was loaded with 500 μg protein. The arrow indicates the position of bromophenol blue

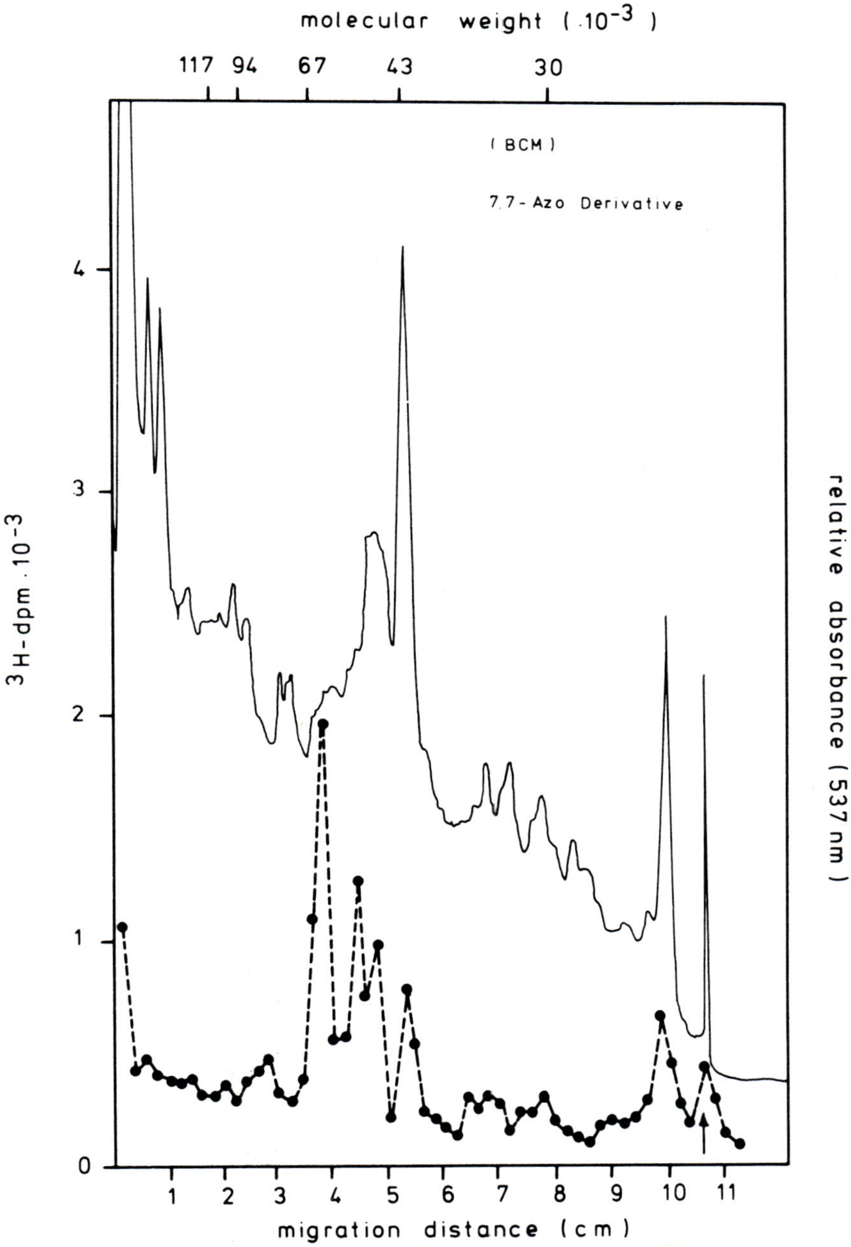

Figure 6 Distribution of radioactivity after SDS-polyacrylamide gel electrophoresis of bile canalicular membranes of hepatocytes after photoaffinity labelling. 1.15 mg of bile canalicular membranes were incubated in the dark with 1.13 μM (14.3 μCi) [7,7-azo-3α,12α-dihydroxy-5β-cholan-24-oyl]-2-amino[2-^{3}H(N)]ethanesulphonic acid for 4 min. Photolysis was carried out at 350 nm for 10 min. All other conditions were as described in the legend to Figure 5. The arrow indicates the position of bromophenol blue

polypeptides with the same molecular weights only. This result, demonstrated in Figure 6 with the 7,7-azo derivative of taurocholate, has been confirmed with all three photolabile derivatives of taurocholate.

Despite the fact that the two membrane subfractions of hepatocytes, the bile canalicular membranes and the fraction enriched with sinusoidal surfaces, differ in their morphological and enzymatical characterization and clearly show a different polypeptide pattern (Figure 4), the application of all three photoaffinity labels resulted in the modification of the same polypeptides.

Photoaffinity labelling of both membrane subfractions with the photolabile derivatives of unconjugated bile salts was performed to see whether different membrane polypeptides are involved in the binding of conjugated and unconjugated bile salts. As shown in Figure 7 photoaffinity labelling of the subfraction predominantly composed of bile canalicular membranes with 3β-azido-7α,12α-dihydroxy-5β-cholan-24-oic acid resulted once more in the incorporation of radioactivity in polypeptides with the same molecular weights only. The polypeptide with the molecular weight of 67 000 exhibits immunological cross-reactivity with serum albumin, but is – according to its chemical properties – not identical with it. Thus we assume that the polypeptides with the molecular weights of 67 000, 52 000, 48 000 and 43 000 are components of a carrier system for all bile salts, whether conjugated or unconjugated.

In order to get an insight into the specificity of the binding of bile salts photoaffinity labelling was performed in the presence of organic anions to study their protective effect. Bile salts, dehydrocholate, sulphobromophthalein, bilirubin, probenecide, 4,4′-diisothiocyano-2,2′-stilbenedisulphonate, as well as phalloidin at a concentration of 100 μmol/l, exert a clear protective effect when the photoaffinity labels are used at a concentration of 1 μmol/l, whereas indocyanine green, palmitate and organic cations have no influence. At present we cannot decide whether one of the polypeptides revealed by photoaffinity labelling with the photolabile derivatives of bile salts is identical with one of the organic anion binding polypeptides characterized recently[12–15].

BILE ACID BINDING PROTEINS IN CYTOPLASMA

The detection of potential intracellular carriers for bile salts presupposes a clear conception about the intracellular behaviour of conjugated and unconjugated derivatives. For this reason we have primarily investigated the properties and the localization of the conjugating enzymes. Whereas the microsomal hydroxycholanoate : CoA ligase (AMP) (EC6.2.1.7) has been purified only partially, the hydroxycholanoyl-CoA : acceptor *N*-hydroxycholanoyl transferase (EC 2.3.1.?) has been isolated from rat liver[16]. The homogeneous enzyme has a molecular weight of 86 000 and is composed of two subunits of the molecular weight of 43 000. It exhibits a clear product inhibition by taurocholate (K_i = 0.7 mM), competitive for the leading substrate cholyl-CoA (K_M = 1 mM). The enzyme was localized intracellularly by immunofluorescence microscopy in distinct particular structures, which

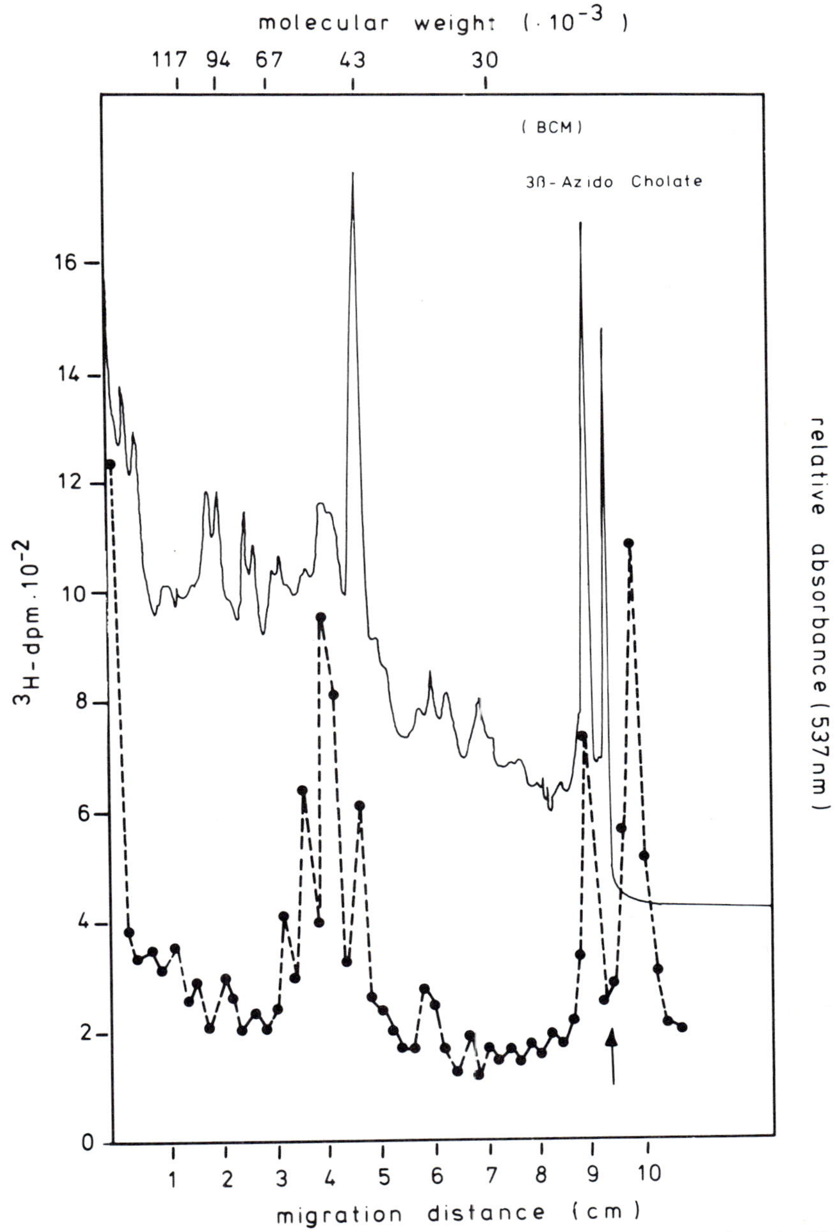

Figure 7 Distribution of radioactivity after SDS-polyacrylamide gel electrophoresis of bile canalicular membranes of hepatocytes after photoaffinity labelling. 1.15 mg of bile canalicular membranes were incubated in the dark with 32 μM (14 μCi) [12-^{3}H]3β-azido-7α,12α-dihydroxy-5β-cholan-24-oic acid for 4 min. Photolysis was carried out at 320 nm for 30 min. SDS gel electrophoresis was performed in 9% gels. All other conditions were as described in the legend to Figure 5. The arrow indicates the position of bromophenol blue

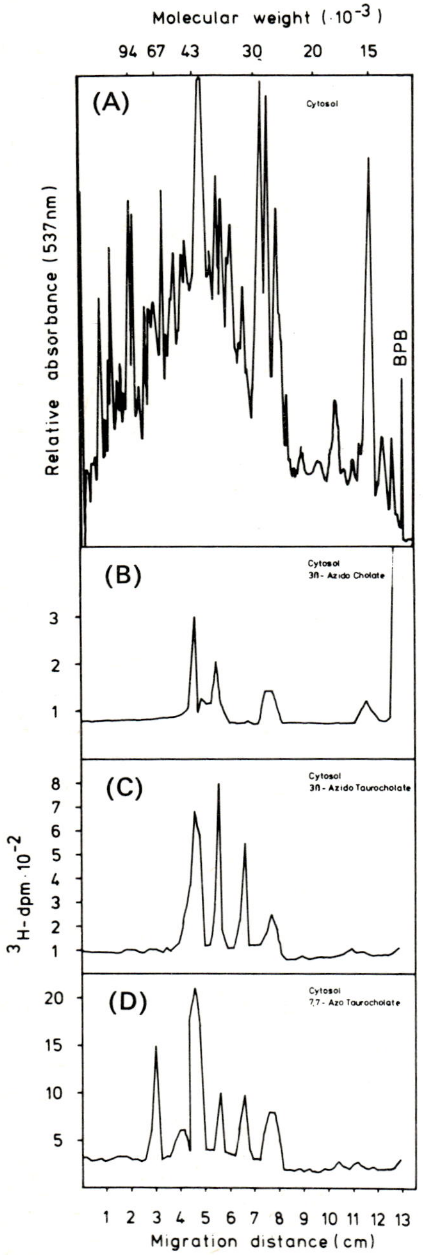

Figure 8 Distribution of radioactivity after SDS-disc polyacrylamide gel electrophoresis of photoaffinity labelled cytosol from rat liver. The protein concentration of cytosol has been adjusted to 10 mg/ml; the gels were loaded with about 700 μg protein. All other conditions were as described in the legend to Figure 5. (A) Densitometer scanning of the polypeptides of rat liver cytosol after staining with Coomassie blue at 575 nm. (B) Cytosol was incubated in the dark with 11 μM (13 μCi) [12-^{3}H]3β-azido-7α, 12α-dihydroxy-5β-cholan-24-oic acid for 1 h. Photolysis was carried out at 320 nm for 30 min. (C) Cytosol was incubated in the dark with 1 μM (10,5 μCi) of [3β-azido-7α, 12α-dihydroxy-5β-cholan-24-oyl]-2-aminol[2-^{3}H(N)]ethanesulphonic acid for 1 h. Photolysis was carried out at 320 nm for 30 min. (D) Cytosol was incubated in the dark with 1 μM (10μCi) [7.7-azo-3α, 12α-dihydroxy-5β-cholan-24-oyl] -2-aminol [2-^{3}H (N)]ethanesulphonic acid for 1 h. Photolysis was carried out at 350 nm for 10 min.

are found throughout the hepatocyte in a slightly polar distribution. The localization of the conjugating enzymes and the inhibition of the hydroxycholanoyl transferase by the end-products, the conjugated bile salts, are suggestive for a branching off for the unconjugated derivatives in the intracellular transport of bile salts.

Photoaffinity labelling of the cytosolic fraction resulted in a different labelling pattern for conjugated and unconjugated derivatives[16]. Figure 8 demonstrates the densitometer tracing of the polypeptides of cytosol stained with Coomassie blue after SDS-disc polyacrylamide gel electrophoresis and the distribution of radioactivity after photoaffinity labelling with different derivatives. With the conjugated derivatives radioactivity is predominantly incorporated into five, perhaps six polypeptides, the molecular weights of which are 67 000, 43 000, 39 000, 32 000 and 23 000. With the unconjugated derivative the decisive difference lies in the modification of a further polypeptide with a molecular weight of about 15 000. The polypeptide with the molecular weight of 67 000 may be one of the membrane polypeptides and/or albumin, the one with the molecular weight of 43 000 has been identified as the subunit of hydroxycholanoyl transferase and that with a molecular weight of 23 000 as the subunit of a glutathione S-transferase. The polypeptide with the molecular weight of 32 000, only occasionally modified, is derived from an oligomeric protein, probably an enzyme with a function unknown to us at present. Thus, we may consider only the glutathione S-transferase as carrier, in accordance with the work of Hayes *et al.*[17,18], as well as the two polypeptides with the molecular weights of 39 000 and about 15 000, which are monomeric proteins. Of these three only the smallest polypeptide is labelled by the unconjugated photolabile derivatives and we assume that this polypeptide is specifically involved in the intracellular transport of unconjugated bile salts.

CONCLUSIONS

With regard to the different potential carriers for bile salts on their way from blood to bile the following conclusions can be drawn:

(1) albumin and HDL act as carriers for unconjugated and conjugated bile salts in blood;
(2) polypeptides with the molecular weights of 67 000, 52 000, 48 000 and 43 000 are components of a transport system for bile salts in their membrane transport by hepatocytes;
(3) an intracellular transport working differently for unconjugated and conjugated bile salts is plausible.

Acknowledgments

This investigation was supported by the Fonds der Chemischen Industrie, the Freiburger Wissenschaftliche Gesellschaft, the Fritz-Thyssen-Stiftung and in a decisive way by Giulini Pharma GmbH, Hannover, FRG.

References

1. Kramer, W., Buscher, H.-P., Gerok, W. and Kurz, G. (1979). Bile salt binding to serum components. Taurocholate incorporation into high-density lipoprotein revealed by photoaffinity labelling. *Eur. J. Biochem.*, **102,** 1
2. Widnell, C. C. and Unkeless, J. C. (1968). Partial purification of a lipoprotein with 5′-nucleotidase activity from membranes of rat liver. *Proc. Natl. Acad. Sci. USA*, **61,** 1050
3. Reichen, J. and Paumgartner, G. (1977). Relationship between bileflow and Na^+, K^+-adenosinetriphosphatase in liver plasma membranes enriched in bile canaliculi. *J. Clin. Invest.*, **60,** 429
4. Bischoff, E., Tran-Thi, T.-A. and Decker, K. F. A. (1975). Nucleotide pyrophosphatase of rat liver. A comparative study on the enzymes solubilized and purified from plasma membrane and endoplasmic reticulum. *Eur. J. Biochem.*, **51,** 353
5. Khattab, M. and Pfleiderer, G. (1976). Alkaline phosphatase of human and calf small intestine. Purification and immunochemical characterization. *Hoppe-Seyler's Z. Physiol. Chem.*, **357,** 377
6. Goldbarg, J. A. and Rutenburg, A. M. (1958). The colormetric determination of leucine aminopeptidase in urine and serum of normal subjects and patients with cancer and other diseases. *Cancer*, **11,** 283
7. Hübscher, G. and West, G. R. (1965). Specific assays of some phosphatases in subcellular fractions of small intestinal mucosa. *Nature* (*Lond*), **205,** 799
8. Brown, A. E., Lok, M. P. and Elovson, J. (1976). Improved method for the isolation of rat liver plasma membrane. *Biochim. Biophys. Acta*, **426,** 418
9. Trouet, A. (1974). Isolation of modified liver lysosomes. *Methods Enzymol.*, **31,** 323
10. Bergeron, J. J. M., Ehrenreich, J. H., Siekevitz, P. and Palade, G. E. (1973). Golgi fractions prepared from rat liver homogenates. II. Biochemical characterization. *J. Cell. Biol.*, **59,** 73
11. Kramer, W., Bickel, U., Buscher, H.-P., Gerok, W. and Kurz, G. (1980). Binding proteins for bile acids in membranes of hepatocytes revealed by photoaffinity labelling. *Hoppe-Seyler's Z. Physiol. Chem.*, **361,** 1307
12. Wolkoff, A. W. and Chung, C. T. (1980). Identification, purification and partial characterization of an organic anion binding protein from rat liver cell plasma membrane. *J. Clin. Invest.*, **65,** 1152
13. Cheng, S. and Levy, D. (1980). Characterization of the anion transport system in hepatocyte plasma membranes. *J. Biol. Chem.*, **255,** 2637
14. Levy, D. and Cheng, S. (1980). Photoaffinity labelling of anion transport components in hepatocyte plasma membranes. *Ann. N.Y. Acad. Sci.*, **346,** 232
15. Reichen, J. and Berk, P. D. (1979). Isolation of an organic anion binding protein from rat liver plasma membrane fraction by affinity chromatography. *Biochem. Biophys. Res. Commun.*, **91,** 484
16. Abberger, H., Fuchte, K., Buscher, H.-P., Gerok, W. and Kurz, G. (1980). Localization of hydroxycholanoyl-transferase in rat liver hepatocytes and the transport of bile acids. *Hoppe-Seyler's Z. Physiol. Chem.*, **361,** 1261
17. Hayes, J. D., Strange, R. C. and Percy-Robb, I. W. (1979). Identification of two lithocholic acid-binding proteins. *Biochem. J.*, **181,** 699
18. Hayes, J. D., Strange, R. C. and Percy-Robb, I. W. (1980). Cholic acid binding by glutathione S-transferase from rat liver cytosol. *Biochem. J.*, **185,** 23

35
Effects of bile acid feeding on lipoprotein concentration, change in cholesterol synthesis and biliary lipid secretion in patients with radiolucent gallstones

O. LEISS, T. BOSCH AND K. VON BERGMANN

INTRODUCTION

Oral administration of either chenodeoxycholic acid (CDCA) or its 7β-hydroxy epimer, ursodeoxycholic acid (UDCA), lowers cholesterol saturation of bile and promotes cholesterol gallstone dissolution[1,2].

Measurements of the rate-limiting enzyme of cholesterol synthesis, hydroxymethyl glutaryl CoA reductase (HMG-CoAR), in liver microsomes of patients treated with CDCA or UDCA revealed a reduction of the activity of this enzyme[3,4]. Therefore it was postulated that the decreased hepatic secretion of cholesterol during therapy of gallstone dissolution is due to a reduction in cholesterol synthesis.

However, serum cholesterol levels, cholesterol pool size or turnover rates were unaffected[5–7]. On the other hand, during treatment with CDCA, a decrease in serum triglycerides in patients with gallstones[8,9] and hyperlipaemic subjects could be detected[10–12].

Since the effect of UDCA on serum lipids and lipoproteins is less well known, the influence of both CDCA and UDCA on biliary lipid secretion, serum lipoprotein concentration, and change of cholesterol synthesis were studied in eight subjects with radiolucent gallstones under steady-state conditions of the enterohepatic circulation.

The results of the present study indicate that both bile acids decrease cholesterol saturation of bile by decreasing cholesterol secretion and increasing the biliary output of bile acids and phospholipids. As a result of decreased biliary secretion of cholesterol and decreased bile acid production, synthesis of cholesterol was reduced by both bile acids to the same extent. However, their effects on serum lipoprotein concentrations are quite different: CDCA increases the ratio of LDL/HDL-cholesterol (atherogenic index) whereas UDCA decreases this ratio by 8%.

MATERIALS AND METHODS

Patients

Four non-obese women and four non-obese men referred to the department of medicine for gallstone dissolution therapy participated in this study. Their age ranged from 31 to 69 years (mean 51 years) and their actual weights were 100–120% of their ideal weight and remained constant throughout the study. All patients had normal routine liver function tests and no signs of renal disease, intestinal or thyroid dysfunction and none had diabetes. Peroral cholecystograms were performed in all patients and all had radiolucent gallstones in a functioning gallbladder. None of the subjects received any drug known to influence biliary lipid or serum lipoprotein metabolism, except the bile acids prescribed. The aims of the study were explained to all subjects and all gave their informed consent.

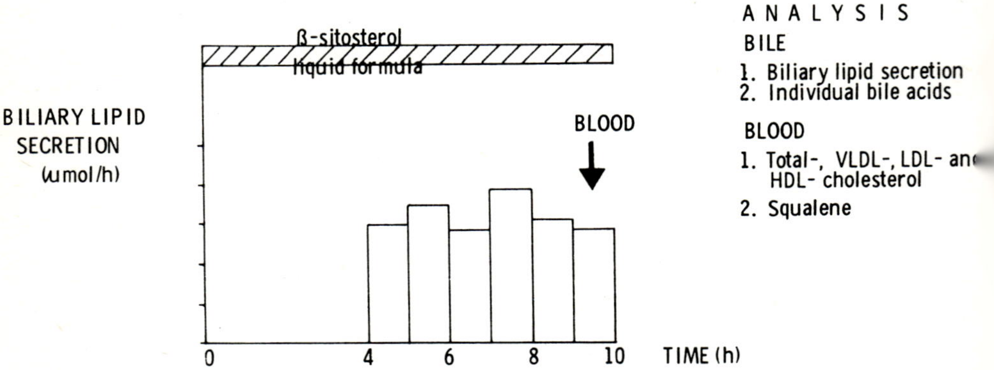

Figure 1 Experimental design

Experimental design (Figure 1)

Serum lipoprotein, squalene analysis, and measurements of biliary lipid secretion were performed after an overnight fast at the beginning of the study. Thereafter every patient received each bile acid (CDCA, UDCA; 1 g/day) during two consecutive, randomized 4-week periods. At the end of each period analysis of serum lipoproteins, squalene, and measurements of biliary lipid secretion were repeated. During the time of the study subjects were allowed to continue their usual eating habits and during the measurements of biliary lipid secretion patients received a liquid formula diet (Nutrison®; B. Braun, Melsungen; West Germany) containing 37% of calories as fat, 16% as protein, and 46% as carbohydrate. The fat of the diet comprised 70% of lard and 30% of soy oil.

Lipoprotein analysis

VLDL-, LDL-, and HDL-cholesterol analysis were performed according to a micromethod[13] using 100 μl serum. In order to test recovery from lipoprotein cholesterol quantification, lipid analyses of total plasma were performed in parallel according to the method of Egge *et al.*[14].

Squalene analysis

Plasma squalene concentrations were measured by a modification of the method of Liu *et al.*[15].

Biliary lipid secretion

Lipid composition of stimulated hepatic bile was obtained during measurements of biliary lipid secretion by the intestinal perfusion technique described by Grundy and Metzger[16]. After an overnight fast a triple lumen tube was positioned with two proximal outlets adjacent to ampulla of Vater and a third outlet 10 cm distally, just beyond the ligamentum of Treitz. Liquid formula (1.4 kcal kg^{-1} h^{-1}) together with β-sitosterol (22.5 mg/h) as non-absorbable marker were infused constantly through one proximal outlet. After allowing 4 h for stabilization of hepatic bile secretion, hourly samples were obtained for the following 6 h from the distal and the other proximal lumens by continuous aspiration. Less than 5% of passing bile was withdrawn.

Measurements of total bile acids, cholesterol, and phospholipids were carried out on every proximal sample. Individual bile acids were analysed by GLC[17]. Cholesterol and β-sitosterol were measured by GLC as trimethylsilylethers. Bile acids were determined enzymatically[18], and phospholipids were measured by the method of Bartlett[19]. Bile lipid composition was expressed as molar percentage (mol%) for each lipid component according to Admirand and Small[20].

Statistic analysis

The results are given as mean±SD, statistical evaluations were performed by paired *t*-test analysis.

RESULTS

Administration of either CDCA or UDCA reduced mol% of cholesterol of hepatic bile from 6.0% during the control period to 4.9% and 3.6%, respectively. This reduction was highly significant ($p < 0.05$ or better). In all patients reduction of mol% of cholesterol during UDCA treatment was more pronounced than during CDCA administration ($p < 0.005$).

The reduction during both bile acid treatment periods was due to a triple mechanism. Mean biliary reduction of cholesterol was reduced from 130 μmol/h to 120 μmol/h during CDCA administration (9%). Although this decrease in biliary secretion of cholesterol was not significant, it contributes to the overall reduction of saturation of hepatic bile. The decrease of biliary secretion of cholesterol during UDCA administration was highly significant when compared to control values (130 μmol/h *v.* 90 μmol/h (31 %); $p < 0.005$) and when compared to CDCA period ($p < 0.005$).

In addition to this effect on biliary secretion of cholesterol, both bile acids increase the secretion rates of bile acids. During the control period bile acid secretion averaged 1800 μmol/h. The mean bile acid secretion during CDCA and UDCA was 2050 μmol/h and 2240 μmol/h, respectively. Again, the change in biliary secretion of bile acids during CDCA was not significant when compared to control values. However, the increase of bile acid secretion during UDCA administration was significant ($p < 0.005$), but not different from the CDCA period.

The increased bile acid secretion during the feeding of CDCA and UDCA was followed by a significant increase of phospholipid secretion during both treatment periods. During the control period biliary secretion of phospholipids averaged 385 μmol/h. During treatment with CDCA and UDCA biliary secretion of phospholipids averaged 570 μmol/h and 510 μmol/h, respectively. This increase was highly significant ($p < 0.005$).

The reduction of biliary secretion of cholesterol, together with the suppression of endogenous bile acid synthesis during feeding of CDCA and UDCA, was followed by a change in cholesterol synthesis. Squalene concentration in plasma, a marker of changes of cholesterol synthesis, was reduced by CDCA and UDCA from 0.30 μg/ml (control period) to 0.21 μg/ml and 0.22 μg/ml, respectively.

Total, LDL, and VLDL cholesterol were not different during either treatment period. In contrast, HDL cholesterol was significantly reduced by CDCA treatment. During the control period HDL cholesterol concentration during the duodenal perfusion averaged 42 mg/dl. CDCA treatment decreased HDL-cholesterol by 48 % to 22 mg/dl. This reduction was highly significant ($p < 0.001$). In contrast, UDCA did not reduce HDL-cholesterol (44 mg/dl).

Why CDCA and not UDCA exhibit this effect remains unclear but might be due to the flux of different bile acids through the liver. Indeed, a good positive correlation between the ratio of LDL- to HDL-cholesterol and biliary secretion of CDCA ($\mu mol\ kg^{-1}\ h^{-1}$) could be found. During all three periods this correlation was highly significant ($r = 0.843$; $p < 0.001$) and even during the CDCA treatment period a significant correlation between the ratio of LDL- to HDL-cholesterol and CDCA secretion could be demonstrated ($r = 0.901$; $p < 0.01$).

DISCUSSION

A decrease in lithogenicity of bile could be achieved through an increase in hepatic secretion of bile acids and/or phospholipids or by a reduction of biliary cholesterol secretion or by both mechanisms[21,22]. The present results indicate that CDCA and UDCA decrease hepatic secretion of cholesterol and increase bile acid and phospholipid secretion. These findings are in agreement with previous studies concerning the effects of CDCA[22,23] and UDCA[24,25] on biliary lipid secretion. The results further show that UDCA lowers biliary secretion of cholesterol significantly more than an equimolar dose of CDCA.

The mechanism whereby CDCA and UDCA lowers biliary cholesterol secretion might be due to a reduction in hepatic cholesterol synthesis. Indeed, the activity of the rate-limiting enzyme of cholesterogenesis, HMG-CoA reductase, was reduced during CDCA treatment[26,27] as well as during UDCA treatment[4,9].

In the present study plasma squalene concentration was used as an indirect marker of cholesterol synthesis[28]. As shown above during both bile acid treatment periods, plasma squalene concentration was significantly reduced, 30% during CDCA and 27% during UDCA, respectively, indicating reduced cholesterol synthesis.

This change of cholesterol synthesis was not associated with change of total cholesterol concentration in plasma. However, HDL-cholesterol was quite differently influenced by CDCA and UDCA treatment. During CDCA administration HDL-cholesterol was significantly reduced compared to the control as well as to the UDCA treatment period. This decrease in HDL-cholesterol was more pronounced than in a study of Bateson and Igbal[12], whereas Miller and Nestel[9] and Thistle *et al.*[29] found a slight increase in HDL-cholesterol during CDCA treatment. However, the experimental conditions in the present study were quite different.

Since HDL-cholesterol is one of the most powerful predictors for atherosclerosis[30], the decrease in HDL-cholesterol to values in the same range as for patients with myocardial infarction[31] or high coronary risk patients[32] may indicate increased risk for atherosclerosis during long-term treatment with CDCA. HDL-cholesterol is inversely correlated with total body cholesterol[33]. Therefore the present findings may support an earlier suggestion of Small that CDCA administration may increase body cholesterol pool size[34]. Why UDCA does not exhibit this effcct is not clear, but might be due to the flux of different bile acids through the liver.

One may speculate that during UDCA treatment hepatic bile acid synthesis is not as far suppressed as during CDCA treatment and since cholesterol synthesis as shown by squalene concentration is suppressed to the same extent by both bile acids, the cholesterol used for bile acid synthesis (other than UDCA plus CDCA) may derive from HDL-cholesterol.

CONCLUSIONS

It is concluded that UDCA might be a better and safer agent for cholesterol gallstone dissolution.

Acknowledgments

This work was supported by the Minister für Wirtschaft und Forschung des Landes Nordrhein-Westfalen and the Sandoz-Stiftung. The technical assistance of Mrs G. Westphal and Mr S. Weiner is gratefully acknowledged.

References

1. Danzinger, R. G., Hofmann, A. F., Schoenfield, L. J. and Thistle, J. L. (1972). Dissolution of cholesterol gallstones by chenodeoxycholic acid. *N. Engl. J. Med.*, **268,** 1

2. Bell, G. D., Whitney, B. and Dowling, R. H. (1972). Gallstone dissolution in man using chenodeoxycholic acid. *Lancet*, **2,** 1213
3. Maton, P. N., Murphy, G. M. and Dowling, R. H. (1977). Ursodeoxycholic acid treatment of gallstones. Dose–response and possible mechanism of action. *Lancet*, **2,** 1297
4. Salen, G., Colalillo, A., Tint, G. S. *et al.* (1978). Comparative effects of high and low dose ursodeoxycholic acid on gallstones dissolution and biliary lipid composition. (abstr.) *Gastroenterology*, **75,** 986
5. Bell, G. D., Lewis, B., Petrie, A. and Dowling, R. H. (1973). Serum lipids in cholelithiasis: effect of chenodeoxycholic acid therapy. *Br. Med. J.*, **3,** 520
6. Hoffman, N. E., Hofmann, A. F. and Thistle, J. L. (1974). Effect of bile acid feeding on cholesterol metabolism in gallstone patients. *Mayo Clin. Proc.*, **49,** 236
7. Pederson, L., Arnfred, T. and Thaysen, H. E. (1974). Cholesterol kinetics in patients with cholesterol gallstones before and during chenodeoxycholic acid treatment. *Scand. J. Gastroenterol.*, **9,** 787
8. Begemann, F. (1978). Influence of chenodeoxycholic acid on the kinetics of endogenous triglyceride transport in man. *Eur. J. Clin. Invest.*, **8,** 283
9. Miller, N. E. and Nestel, P. J. (1974). Triglyceride-lowering effect of chenodeoxycholic acid in patients with endogenous hypertriglyceridaemia. *Lancet*, **2,** 929
10. Angelin, B., Einarsson, K. and Leijd, B. (1978). Effect of chenodeoxycholic acid on serum and biliary lipids in patients with hyperlipoproteinaemia. *Clin. Sci. Mol. Med.*, **54,** 451
11. Camarri, E., Marcolongo, R., Zaccherotti, L. and Marini, G. (1978). The hypotriglyceridaemic effect of chenodeoxycholic acid in type IV hyperlipidaemia. *Biomedicine*, **29,** 193
12. Bateson, M. C. and Iqbal, J. (1979). Chenodeoxycholic acid, postprandial serum-triglycerides, and HDL cholesterol. *Lancet*, **1,** 930
13. Leiss, O., Murawski, U. and Egge, H. (1979). Mikrobestimmung von Lipoproteinlipiden im Serum. *J. Clin. Chem. Clin. Biochem.*, **17,** 619
14. Egge, H., Murawski, U., Müller, J. and Zilliken, F. (1970). Mikrolipidanalysen aus Serum mit dem Eppendorfsystem 3000. *Z. klin. Chem. u. klin. Biochem.*, **8,** 488
15. Liu, G. C. K., Ahrens, E. H. Jr., Schreibman, P. H. and Crouse, J. R. (1976). Measurement of squalene in human tissues and plasma: validation and application. *J. Lipid Res.*, **17,** 38
16. Grundy, S. M. and Metzger, A. L. (1972). A physiologic method for estimation of hepatic secretion of biliary lipids in man. *Gastroenterology*, **62,** 1200
17. Von Bergmann, J., Von Bergmann, K., Hadorn, B. and Paumgartner, G. (1975). Biliary lipid composition in early childhood. *Clin. Chim. Acta*, **64,** 241
18. Paumgartner, G., Horak, W., Probst, P. and Grabner, G. (1971). Effect of phenobarbital on bile flow and bile salt excretion in the rat. *Naunyn-Schmiedeberg's Arch. Pharmakol.*, **270,** 98
19. Bartlett, G. R. (1959). Phosphorus assay in column chromatography. *J. Biol. Chem.*, **234,** 466
20. Admirand, W. H. and Small, D. M. (1968). The physicochemical basis of cholesterol gallstone formation in man. *J. Clin. Invest.*, **47,** 1043
21. Adler, R. D., Bennion, L. J., Duane, W. C. and Grundy, S. M. (1975). Effects of low dose chenodeoxycholic acid feeding on biliary lipid metabolism. *Gastroenterology*, **68,** 326
22. LaRusso, N. F., Hoffman, N. E., Hofmann, A. F., Northfield, T. C. and Thistle, J. L. (1975). Effect of primary bile acid ingestion on bile acid metabolism and biliary lipid secretion in gallstone patients. *Gastroenterology*, **69,** 1301
23. Tangedahl, T. N., Hofmann, A. F. and Kottke, B. A. (1979). Biliary lipid secretion in hypercholesterolaemia. *J. Lipid Res.*, **20,** 125
24. Von Bergmann, K., Gutsfeld, M., Schulze-Hagen, K. and Von Unruh, G. (1979). Effects of ursodeoxycholic acid on biliary lipid secretion in patients with radiolucent gallstones. In Paumgartner, G., Stiehl, A. and Gerok, W. (eds.). *Biological Effects of Bile Acids*, p. 61. (Lancaster: MTP Press)
25. Schersten, T. and Lindblad, L. (1979). Biliary cholesterol output during ursodeoxycholic

acid secretion in man. In Paumgartner, G., Stiehl, A. and Gerok, W. (eds.). *Biological Effects of Bile Acids*, p. 53. (Lancaster: MTP Press)

26. Salen, G., Nicolan, G., Shefer, A. and Mosbach, E. H. (1975). Hepatic cholesterol metabolism in patients with gallstones. *Gastroenterology*, **69,** 676
27. Coyne, M. J., Bonorris, G. G., Goldstein, L. I. and Schoenfield, L. J. (1975). Effect of chenodeoxycholic acid and phenobarbital on the rate-limiting enzymes of hepatic cholesterol and bile acid synthesis in patients with gallstones. *J. Lab. Clin. Med.*, **87,** 281
28. Miettinen, T. A. (1970). Detection of changes in human cholesterol metabolism. *Ann. Clin. Res.*, **2,** 300
29. Thistle, J. L., Ott, B. J. and Ellefson, R. D. (1978). Serum lipoprotein cholesterol changes during bile acid ingestion for gallstone dissolution. *Gastroenterology*, **75,** 990 (abstr.)
30. Kannel, W. B., Castelli, W. P. and Gordon, T. (1979). Cholesterol in the prediction of atherosclerotic disease: new perspectives based on the Framingham study. *Ann. Inter. Med.*, **90,** 85
31. Albers, J. J., Cheung, M. C. and Hazzard, W. R. (1978). High-density lipoproteins in myocardial infarction survivors. *Metabolism*, **27,** 479
32. Williams, P., Robinson, D. and Bailey, A. (1979). High-density lipoprotein and coronary risk factors in normal men. *Lancet*, **1,** 72
33. Miller, G. J. and Miller, N. E. (1975). Plasma-high-density-lipoprotein and development of ischaemic heart disease. *Lancet*, **1,** 16
34. Small, D. M. (1971). Prestone gallstone disease — is therapy safe? *N. Engl. J. Med.*, **284,** 214

36
Effects of bile acid feeding and depletion on plasma and biliary squalene, methyl sterols and lathosterol

T. A. MIETTINEN

A decrease in cholesterol biotransformation to bile acids during bile acid therapy for cholesterol gallstones may result in cholesterol accumulation unless cholesterol production (synthesis and/or absorption) were decreased. Some studies have suggested that cholesterol absorption is reduced by oral chenodesoxycholate (CDCA)[1,2]; others, however, have not revealed any change[3,4]. Total body pools of cholesterol appear to be unaltered after prolonged bile acid therapy[5,6]. The hepatic activity of the rate-limiting enzyme for cholesterol synthesis, hydroxymethylglutaryl coenzyme-A reductase, has been reported to be decreased by CDCA[7] but no exact information is available as far as the overall cholesterol synthesis is concerned. Some of the cholesterol precursors in plasma and bile appear to reflect changes in cholesterol synthesis in many, albeit not all, clinical and experimental conditions[8]. Therefore, plasma and biliary squalene, lanosterol and other methyl sterols, and lathosterol were studied before and after chenotherapy in gallstone patients and ileal bypass in patients with familial hypercholesterolaemia. These treatments evidently should decrease and increase cholesterol synthesis, respectively. In an earlier series CDCA actually reduced the precursor levels in the plasma and bile[9].

EFFECTS OF CDCA

Five non-obese patients (two males and three women) with a functioning gallbladder and radiolucent gallstones were treated with 1 g/day of CDCA for up to 18 months. A sixth patient with gallstones and obesity discontinued the treatment after 14 days. From one to three fasting serum and duodenal bile samples were collected before and after the treatment from each patient. Serum was analysed for free methyl sterols and total and free cholesterol. In the bile squalene, methyl sterols, lathosterol, cholesterol, bile acids and phospholipids were quantitated. Gas–liquid chromatographic methods were used for the determination of squalene, sterols and bile acids[9,10]. The precursor values are presented per free or total cholesterol in serum or bile'

Table 1 Serum and biliary free methyl sterols and lathosterol and squalene before and after chenodeoxycholic acid (CDCA) therapy or ileal bypass (IB-P). Mean ± SE

Source	*Treatment*	*Free methyl sterols** *I*	*II*	*III*	*IV*	*V*	*Sum*	*Lathostetol**	*Squalene**
PATIENTS WITH GALLSTONES									
Serum	none	45 ± 10	37 ± 7	40 ± 15	41 ± 5	26 ± 8	189 ± 40	—	—
	CDCA	36 ± 6†	30 ± 5†	38 ± 7	28 ± 5†	20 ± 4†	151 ± 24†	—	—
Bile	none	682 ± 198	330 ± 95	355 ± 147	969 ± 270	492 ± 149	2829 ± 806	992 ± 300	98 ± 40
	CDCA	439 ± 105	249 ± 68	339 ± 111	600 ± 170†	286 ± 82†	1913 ± 473†	537 ± 225†	71 ± 11
PATIENTS WITH FAMILIAL HYPERCHOLESTEROLAEMIA									
Serum	none	24 ± 5	20 ± 4	14 ± 3	35 ± 5	19 ± 3	113 ± 17	15 ± 1	57 ± 40
	IB-P	145 ± 37†	120 ± 34†	33 ± 7†	110 ± 20†	88 ± 20†	495 ± 111†	397 ± 133†	45 ± 22
Bile	none	367 ± 138	212 ± 97	162 ± 47	906 ± 254	332 ± 132	1979 ± 656	271 ± 120	24 ± 6
	IB-P	1168 ± 306†	628 ± 173†	202 ± 30	2079 ± 417†	806 ± 201†	4879 ± 1094†	3647 ± 919†	83 ± 19†

* The values are given in 10^2 μg/mg of free cholesterol; in bile virtually all sterols were in unesterified form

† Statistically significant change ($p < 0.05$ or less). Tentative identification of methyl sterol fractions are as follows: I Δ^8-methostenol and some dihydrolanosterol, II Δ^8-(4α,β) dimethyl sterol, III methostenol, IV lanosterol and V $\Delta^{8,24}$(4α,β) dimethyl sterol

respectively, so as to eliminate the marked interindividual fluctuations in the cholesterol concentrations especially in the bile samples.

During the treatment the CDCA content increased from 27–55% to 72–94% (ranges) of biliary bile acids and the molar percentage of biliary cholesterol decreased from 5.0–15.6% to 3.5–7.9%. The molar percentage decreased by CDCA in all but one hypertriglyceridaemic patient. The dissolution of gallstones occurred in two cases only during the long-term CDCA treatment.

Table 2 Relative distribution of serum free and biliary methyl sterols before and after chenodeoxycholate (CDCA) treatment or ileal bypass (IB-P)

Source	*Treatment*	*Methyl sterol, percentage of total*				
		I	*II*	*III*	*IV*	*V*
PATIENTS WITH GALLSTONES						
Serum	none	22±3	21±3	18±4	26±5	13±2
	CDCA	24±1	20±1	24±1	19±1	13±1
Bile	none	24±1	12±1*	12±1	36±3	16±1
	CDCA	24±1	12±1*	16±3*	34±5	14±1
PATIENTS WITH FAMILIAL HYPERCHOLESTEROLAEMIA						
Serum	none	21±2	18±1	13±2	31±1	17±1
	IB-P	28±2†	21±3	8±2*	26±4†	17±1*
Bile	none	17±1*	10±1	9±1	49±3*	15±1
	IB-P	23±2†	12±1†	4±1*†	45±3†	16±1

* Statistically different ($p < 0.05$ or less) from the respective value in the patients with gallstones

† Statistically significant change

The serum free total methyl sterol level was significantly decreased mainly due to a reduction in lanosterol (Tables 1 and 2). A similar decrease was found also in the bile where, in addition, the lathosterol level was lowered by CDCA while squalene was unaffected. Highly significant positive correlations were found between the serum and biliary methyl sterol values (Figure 1), and between the biliary lathosterol and serum methyl sterol levels. Biliary squalene, however, tended to correlate negatively with serum methyl sterols. Since, in addition, biliary and serum lathosterol, but not squalene, were correlated with each other in our earlier series[9] it can be inferred that the post-mevalonate cholesterol precursors of the two sources have a site of origin in common and that the decrease of these precursors in serum and bile may signify reduced cholesterol synthesis during CDCA therapy. The pretreatment serum triglyceride level tended to correlate with serum lanosterol ($r = 0.687$), biliary lathosterol ($r = 0.697$) and biliary lanosterol ($r = 0.52$) but poorly with squalene ($r = 0.037$).

EFFECTS OF ILEAL BYPASS OPERATION

Cholesterol precursors were studied in serum and bile in six patients with familial hypercholesterolaemia before, and for up to 6 years after, an ileal

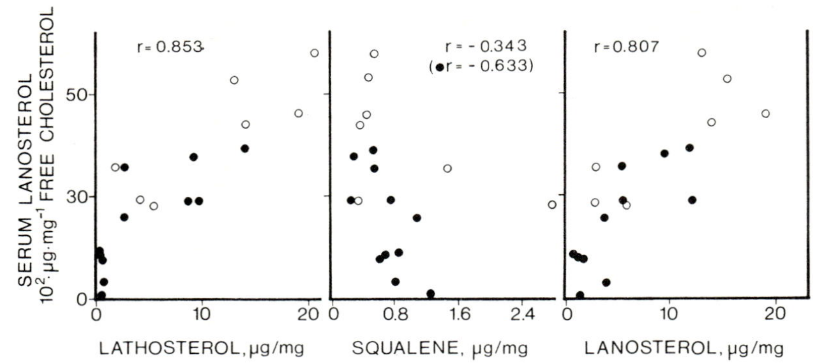

Figure 1 Correlation of serum-free lanosterol with biliary lathosterol, squalene and lanosterol. Open symbols before; closed symbols during CDCA therapy. Biliary values are expressed per mg of cholesterol

bypass operation performed to decrease serum cholesterol. The mean cholesterol synthesis measured with the sterol balance technique[10] increased about 3.5-fold (from 1129 to 3911 mg/day). This was associated with up to 6-fold and 3-fold increases in the serum and biliary methyl sterol levels, respectively. The respective increases in serum lathosterol were even higher (Table 1). Serum squalene was not affected consistently but biliary squalene appeared to increase by a factor of 3.5. The relative increase in methyl sterols was highest for subfractions I and II both in the serum and the bile, resulting in significant changes in the methyl sterol patterns (Table 2). A significant correlation was found between the serum and biliary methyl sterols (shown in Figure 2 for lanosterol) and lathosterol (r = 0.900) but not for squalene (−0.038). The correlations of biliary lathosterol (r = 0.522, $p < 0.05$) and

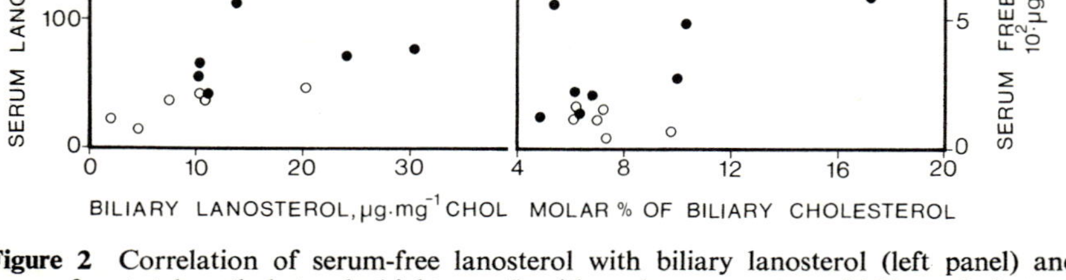

Figure 2 Correlation of serum-free lanosterol with biliary lanosterol (left panel) and serum-free total methyl sterols (right panel) with molar percentage of biliary cholesterol before (○) and after (●) ileal bypass operation. FCH = free cholesterol

squalene ($r = 0.466$) with serum lanosterol were less constant than in the CDCA study. Serum methyl sterols were weakly correlated with the molar percentage of biliary cholesterol (Figure 2).

DIURNAL VARIATION

Since the serum squalene and methyl sterol levels show normally a marked diurnal variation with a nocturnal or early morning peak[11] and since the molar percentage of biliary cholesterol correlated with the serum methyl sterols, the precursors and lipids were measured serially over a period of 24 h in the bile samples and in the serum lipoproteins. Figure 3 shows the typical nocturnal rise[12] in the molar percentage of biliary cholesterol. The diurnal fluctuation in the lipoprotein precursor levels is seen to be associated to some

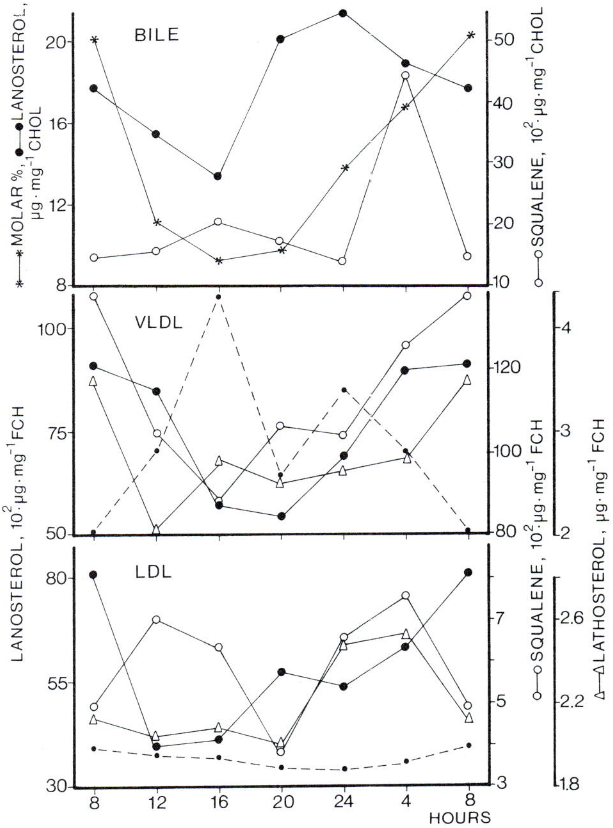

Figure 3 Diurnal variation of cholesterol molar percentage in bile, and of cholesterol precursors in bile, plasma very-low density lipoprotein (VLDL) and low-density lipoprotein (LDL) in a patient with closed T-tube in common bile duct after cholecystectomy for cholesterol gallstones. Meals were consumed at 0800, 1200 and 1600 hours and snack at 2000 hours, after plasma and bile samples were obtained. Concentration curves for free cholesterol (FCH) shown by dashed lines for VLDL (mean 10 mg%) and LDL (mean 36 mg%) cholesterol

extent with those in the bile, the molar percentage partially follows the time-course of biliary methyl sterols and almost perfectly follows that in VLDL precursors and LDL methyl sterols.

DISCUSSION

The major purposes of the present study were to investigate whether the serum and biliary cholesterol precursors are interrelated and whether an increase in cholesterol synthesis caused by ileal bypass, and especially a decrease in that supposedly caused by CDCA therapy, would affect the precursor levels in the two sources. The methyl sterol pattern of the bile differed from that of the serum lipoproteins mainly in that lanosterol (fraction V) was markedly higher in the bile especially in familial hypercholesterolaemia. This suggests, provided the biliary methyl sterols are of hepatic (newly synthesized) origin, that some other organ(s) than the liver also contributes to methyl sterols of the serum lipoproteins. Despite this possible difference in the site of origin, and despite some differences in the methyl sterol patterns of the patients with hypercholesterolaemia from those with gallstones, the serum and biliary methyl sterol levels were significantly correlated with each other during both low and high cholesterol synthesis. This indicates that a site of origin in common, most likely the liver, contributed strongly to methyl sterols both in the serum and the bile. The same seems to apply to lathosterol while squalene behaves differently. The methyl sterol values fall rapidly early in the morning due to diurnal variation apparently in hepatic production of cholesterol[11]. This may dissociate transiently the release of the precursors into the morning samples of the bile and serum lipoproteins especially in ileal bypass, impairing the correlation between the bile and serum.

A decrease in serum methyl sterols was first demonstrated during a total fast in obese human subjects and was interpreted to indicate reduced cholesterol synthesis[3]. The decrease in plasma and biliary methyl sterols and lathosterol (Table 1) during the CDCA treatment provides a new kind of evidence, in that in patients with gallstones oral bile acid therapy actually reduces cholesterol synthesis. In patients with cerebrotendinous xanthomatosis, biliary lathosterol and lanosterol has been mentioned to disappear 1 day after CDCA was started[13]. This was interpreted to indicate depression of elevated cholesterol synthesis. In none of the patients of the present and previous series lanosterol or lathosterol were disappearing totally, even though in several subjects the values became very low. In general the relative decrease in biliary methyl sterols tended to be higher than that in serum, as if the hepatic cholesterol synthesis had been effectively inhibited.

Serum methyl sterols and biliary lathosterol appear to increase parallel with the increase in cholesterol synthesis when enterohepatic circulation of bile acids is interrupted[8,10]. The present results confirm this observation. They also indicate that enhanced cholesterol synthesis increased biliary output of cholesterol precursors between squalene and lathosterol at least, while in serum the increase is detectable between lanosterol and lathosterol only. Serum total squalene is not consistently related to overall cholesterol synthesis[8] because other factors, such as dietary squalene[14] (possibly intestinal squalene synthesis, too), hypertriglyceridaemia[15] and adaptation of squalene cyclization, can affect its serum level.

The present results indicate that the biliary and serum free methyl sterols and lathosterol levels are closely associated with each other, that methyl sterols and lathosterol increase both in the bile and serum when cholesterol synthesis is stimulated by interrupted enterohepatic circulation of bile acids, that their levels are decreased during CDCA therapy – most likely secondary to reduced cholesterol synthesis, and that serum and biliary squalenes are less consistently correlated with each other or with changes in cholesterol synthesis.

Acknowledgments

This work was supported by grants from the Finnish National Council for Medical Sciences.

References

1. Adler, R. D., Bennion, L. J., Duane, W. C. and Grundy, S. M. (1975). Effects of low dose chenodesoxycholic acid feeding on biliary lipid metabolism. *Gastroenterology*, **68**, 326
2. Ponz de Leon, M., Carulli, N., Loria, P., Iori, R. and Zironi, F. (1979). The effect of chenodeoxycholic acid (CDCA) on cholesterol absorption. *Gastroenterology*, **77**, 223
3. Tangedahl, T. N., Matseshe, J. W., Thistle, J. L. and Hofmann, A. F. (1977). Plant sterols increase effectiveness of chenodeoxycholic acid therapy in lowering cholesterol saturation of fasting-state bile in patients with radiolucent gallstones (abstr.). *Gastroenterology*, **72**, 1138
4. Mok, H. Y. J. and Grundy, S. M. (1980). Cholesterol and bile acid absorption during bile acid therapy in obese subjects undergoing weight reduction. *Gastroenterology*, **78**, 62.
5. Hoffman, N. E., Hofmann, A. F. and Thistle, J. L. (1974). Effect of bile acid feeding on cholesterol metabolism in gallstone patients. *Mayo Clin. Proc.*, **49**, 236
6. Pedersen, L., Arnfred, T. and HessThaysen, E. (1974). Cholesterol kinetics in patients with cholesterol gallstones before and during chenodeoxycholic acid treatment. *Scand. J. Gastroenterol.*, **9**, 787
7. Coyne, M. J., Bonorris, G. G., Goldstein, L. I. and Schoenfield, L. J. (1976). Effect of chenodeoxycholic acid and phenobarbital on the rate-limiting enzymes of hepatic cholesterol and bile acid synthesis in patients with gallstones. *J. Lab. Clin. Med.*, **87**, 281
8. Miettinen, T. A. (1970). Detection of changes in human cholesterol metabolism. *Ann. Clin. Res.*, **2**, 300
9. Tarpila, S. and Miettinen, T. A. (1978). Effects of chenodesoxycholic acid on biliary and plasma squalene, methylsterols and lathosterol in patients with gallstones. Presented at the *XIIth Scandinavian Conference on Gastroenterology*, 24–26 August, Lund, Sweden. Abstract Book, p. 49
10. Miettinen, T. A. (1976). Methods for evaluation of hypolipidaemic drugs in man: mechanisms of their action. In Paoletti, R. and Glueck, C. J. (eds.). *Lipid Pharmacology*, Vol. II, pp. 83–125. (New York: Academic Press)
11. Miettinen, T. A. (1980). Diurnal variation of serum methyl sterols and squalene in controls, ileal dysfunction and subjects on cholestyramine. Presented at *VII International Symposium on Drugs Affecting Lipid Metabolism*, May, Milan. Abstract Book, p. 10
12. Metzger, A. L., Adler, R., Heymsfield, S. and Grundy, S. M. (1973). Diurnal variation in biliary lipid composition. *N. Engl. J. Med.*, **288**, 333
13. Salen, G., Meriwether, T. W. and Nicolau, G. (1975). Chenodeoxycholic acid inhibits

increased cholesterol and cholestanol synthesis in patients with cerebrotendinous xanthomatosis. *Biochem. Med.*, **14,** 57

14. Liu, G. C. K., Ahrens, E. H. Jr., Schreibman, P. H. and Crouse, J. R. (1976). Measurement of squalene in human tissues and plasma: validation and application. *J. Lipid Res.*, **17,** 38
15. Saudek, C. D., Frier, B. M. and Liu, G. C. K. (1978). Plasma squalene: lipoprotein distribution and kinetic analysis. *J. Lipid Res.*, **19,** 827

37
Effect of chenodeoxycholic acid on interrelations between serum squalene, biliary cholesterol saturation and endogenous triglyceride synthesis

F. BEGEMANN, M. PAPENHAGEN AND S. NIELSEN

INTRODUCTION

The cholelitholytic effect of ursodeoxycholic acid (UDCA) or chenodeoxycholic acid (CDCA) relies on reduced biliary cholesterol secretion, which in turn appears to be related to a decreased hepatic cholesterol synthesis, as evidenced by lower activities of the rate-limiting enzyme, HMG-CoA reductase.

However, recent observations cast some doubts on this concept. Thus, HMG-CoA reductase is an interconvertible enzyme, the total activity of which, as measured *in vitro*, need not reflect cholesterol synthesis *in vivo*[1]. Accordingly, enzyme activity has not been found to correlate with biliary cholesterol secretion during cholelitholytic treatment[2,3]. Furthermore, the major part of biliary cholesterol seems to originate from circulating liproprotein cholesterol and not from hepatic *de novo* synthesis[4].

In view of these findings, more information is needed on cholesterol biosynthesis during cholelitholytic treatment.

Currently some obligate bioprecursors of cholesterol, such as squalene, are thought to parallel newly synthesized proportions of cholesterol in serum or other compartments, thus reflecting under many conditions the state of endogenous cholesterol synthesis[5-7]. The present study therefore compares serum squalene to other relevant parameters in gallstone patients, in order:

(a) to obtain additional information on the role of newly synthesized cholesterol for biliary cholesterol saturation;
(b) to examine whether such mechanisms are predominantly responsible for the desaturating effect of CDCA on bile.

METHODS

Examinations

In 19 patients, presented with radiolucent gallstones for cholelitholytic therapy, a sample of serum and of cholecystokinine-stimulated intraduodenal bile was obtained at the same time under fasting conditions, for determination of biliary cholesterol saturation and of serum squalene. Similar studies were repeated in 14 of them after treatment with CDCA (13–16 mg kg^{-1} day^{-1}) for 6–10 weeks. In 10 of these subjects endogenous triglyceride synthesis was determined simultaneously, both before and after treatment[8].

Analyses

Biliary cholesterol saturation: as 'lithogenic index', with saturation lines including a physiological zone of metastability for cholesterol solubility[9,10].

Serum squalene: by gas–chromatography, according to the methods of Liu *et al.*[6].

Endogenous triglyceride synthesis: by a precursor labelling method, using [^{14}C]palmitic acid, as reported elsewhere[8].

RESULTS

When serum squalene concentrations were compared to lithogenic index of bile before treatment, a significant curvilinear correlation appeared (r_{tot} = 0.52, $p < 0.05$; Figure 1). Following CDCA treatment, there was no longer a significant association (Figure 2). Expressed as mean value before and after

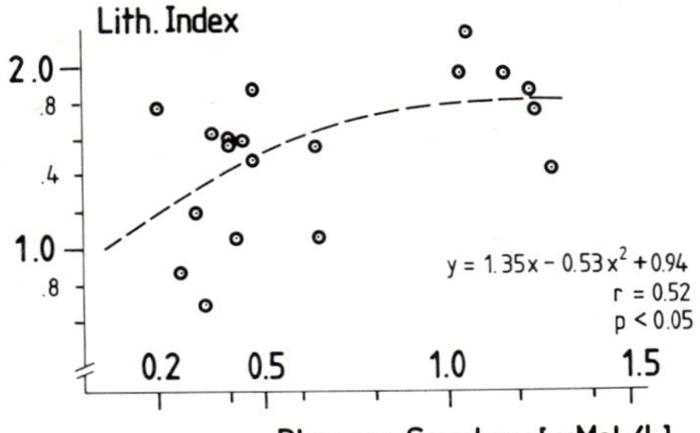

Figure 1 Correlation between plasma squalene and biliary cholesterol saturation in gallstone patients before CDCA treatment

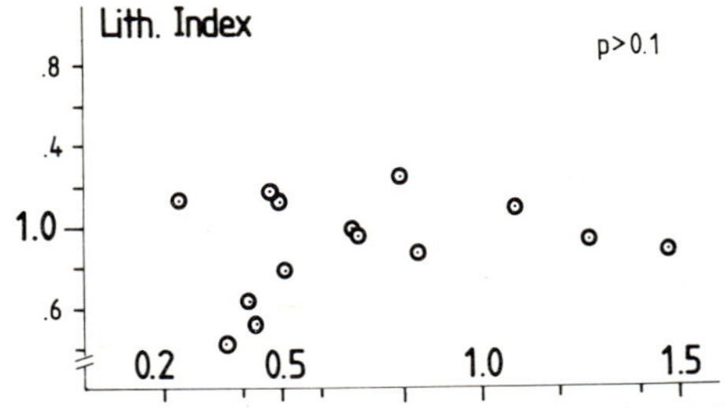

Figure 2 Lack of correlation ($p > 0.1$) between plasma squalene and lithogenic index after CDCA

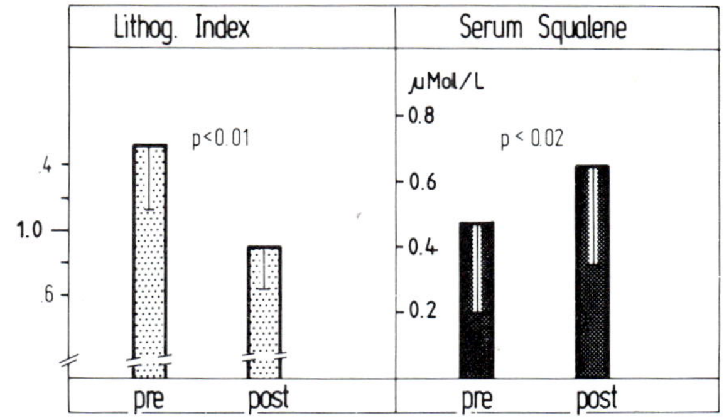

Figure 3 Mean values before and after CDCA (see Figures 1 and 2)

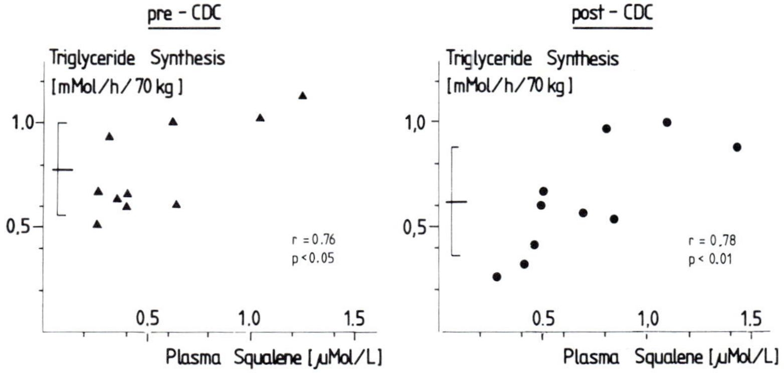

Figure 4 Correlation between plasma squalene concentration and triglyceride synthesis before and after CDCA

treatment, lithogenic index had decreased from 1.45 to 0.85, as expected. However, serum squalene concentration had unexpectedly risen from 0.55 to 0.70 μmol/l on average ($p<0.02$; Figure 3). To further clarify the origin of increasing serum squalene concentrations, these were compared to available results of endogenous triglyceride synthesis[8] in 10 patients.

Both before and after CDCA, a significant correlation was noted (Figure 4), though triglyceride synthesis, in contrast to serum squalene, fell from 0.78 to 0.62 mmol h^{-1} per 70 kg on average with CDCA ($p<0.01$).

DISCUSSION

Any conclusions from squalene analysis, relating to cholesterol metabolism, must meet two prerequisites:

(a) Actual concentrations of serum squalene should originate essentially from endogenous sources. In fact, this may be assumed for samples collected after an overnight fast, since trace amounts from ordinary foodstuff disappear within a few hours[11].

(b) Endogenous serum squalene should reliably reflect influx of newly synthesized cholesterol; thus possibly, though not necessarily, paralleling the state of cholesterol synthesis. Recent reports support this view, although still on preliminary evidence[5–7].

Under these criteria the significant association of serum squalene to lithogenic index, shown here, indicates that cholesterol synthesis significantly influences biliary cholesterol saturation.

These mechanisms are also involved in the desaturating effect of CDCA, since relative biliary squalene values have been found to decrease in these patients upon treatment with CDCA, as reported earlier[12]. However, hepatic cholesterol synthesis may not be the most important determinant of biliary cholesterol saturation during CDCA treatment, since lithogenic indices are no longer correlated to serum squalene. Moreover, serum squalene unexpectedly increases on average.

This elevation is difficult to explain, if hepatic cholesterol synthesis is reduced by CDCA, and if serum squalene mainly originates from the liver[13]. Increased extrahepatic release of squalene into serum after treatment with CDCA cannot be excluded. However, a significant correlation to endogenous triglyceride synthesis indicates that serum squalene is associated with VLDL secretion both before and after treatment, suggesting its hepatic origin.

Taken together, these findings are consistent with the following hypothesis: besides suppressing hepatic cholesterol synthesis, CDCA withholds newly synthesized cholesterol from biliary secretion and diverts it into plasma, thus contributing additionally to decreased biliary secretion.

This mode of action would simultaneously explain why CDCA should leave plasma cholesterol unaffected, although it diminishes endogenous cholesterol synthesis and perhaps even intestinal cholesterol absorption[14].

It is clear, however, that this tentative hypothesis needs to be substantiated or refuted by additional work.

References

1. Nordstrom, J. L., Rodwell, V. W. and Mitschelen, J. J. (1977). Interconversion of active and inactive forms of rat liver hydroxymethylglutaryl-CoA reductase. *J. Biol. Chem.*, **252,** 8924
2. Key, P. H., Bonnorris, G. G., Marks, J. W. and Schoenfield, L. J. (1978). Mechanism of cholesterol desaturation of bile by chenodeoxycholic acid in gallstone patients. *Gastroenterology*, **74,** 1161
3. Maton, P. N., Reuben, A., Ellis, H. J. and Doowling, R. H. (1979). Hepatic cholesterol synthesis in cholelithiasis: role of HMG CoA reductase in determining biliary cholesterol secretion. *Clin. Sci.* **56** (Suppl. Medical Research Society, Report No. 46), pp. 15–16
4. Schwartz, C. C., Berman, M., Vlahcevic, Z. R., Halloran, L. G., Gregory, H. and Swell, L. (1978). Multicompartmental analysis of cholesterol metabolism in man. *J. Clin. Invest.*, **61,** 408
5. Nestel, P. I. and Kudchodkar, B. (1975). Plasma squalene as an index of cholesterol synthesis. *Clin. Sci.*, **49,** 621
6. Liu, G. C. K., Ahrens, E. H. Jr., Schreibman, P. H. and Crouse, J. R. (1976). Measurement of squalene in human tissues and plasma: validation and application. *J. Lipid Res.*, **17,** 38

7. Miettinen, T. A. (1969). Serum squalene and methyl sterols as indicators of cholesterol synthesis *in vivo*. *Life Sci.*, **8,** 713
8. Begemann, F. (1978). Influence of chenodeoxycholic acid on the kinetics of endogenous triglyceride transport in man. *Eur. J. Clin. Invest.*, **8,** 283
9. Admirand, W. and Small, D. M. (1968). The physico-chemical basis of gallstone formation in man. *J. Clin. Invest.*, **47,** 1043
10. Carey, M. and Small, D. M. (1975). Solubility of cholesterol in bile. In Matern, S., Hackenschmidt, J., Back, P. and Gerok, W. (eds.). *Advances in Bile Acid Research*, pp. 277–283. (Stuttgart: Schattauer)
11. Lewis, R. W. (1976). Effect of alimentation on human serum squalene levels. *Lipids*, **11,** 430
12. Begemann, F., Papenhagen, M. and Nielsen, S. (1979). Effect of chenodeoxycholic acid on endogenous cholesterol precursor: variations in biliary and plasma squalene. Presented at the 14th Meeting of the European Association of the Study of the Liver, 13–15 September, Düsseldorf
13. Goodman, D. W. (1964). Squalene in human and rat blood plasma. *J. Clin. Invest.*, **43,** 1480
14. Ponz de Leon, M., Carulli, N., Loria, P., Iori, R. and Zironi, F. (1979). The effect of chenodeoxycholic acid (CDCA) on cholesterol absorption. *Gastroenterology*, **77,** 223

38
Cholesterol and bile acid metabolism in diabetes mellitus

E. ANDERSEN AND K. HELLSTRÖM

Diabetes mellitus (DM) of the adult-onset type is in general characterized by insulin resistance and often also by overweight and/or hypertriglyceridaemia. Hyperinsulinism and glucose intolerance are commonly encountered in obese subjects and in patients with hyperlipoproteinaemia (HLP) of the type IV pattern. Excessive obesity and HLP type IV are to a variable extent associated with enhanced cholesterogenesis and increased elimination of cholesterol as bile acids[1–4]. The overall regulation of these processes is incompletely known. In order to study the possible influence of overt DM this chapter deals with bile acid kinetics and steroid balance in patients with this disease.

MATERIAL AND METHODS

The patients

The study comprised 14 insulin-independent and seven insulin-dependent middle-aged patients who have had DM for 0.5–7 years. There was no evidence of neuropathy, diseases in the thyroid, liver, kidneys or intestine. None of the patients showed addiction to alcohol or narcotics. Eight of the insulin-independent, but none of the insulin-dependent, patients were

Table 1 Basal data

	Insulin-independent	*Insulin-dependent*
n	8 F, 6 M	2 F, 5 M
Age (years)	59 ± 2	53 ± 6
RBW (%)	118 ± 5.0	92 ± 4.4
Glucose (mmol/l)	12.1 ± 1.1	9.6 ± 4.4
Tg (mmol/l)	2.4 ± 0.2	1.1 ± 0.2
Cholesterol (mmol/l)	5.9 ± 0.2	4.7 ± 0.3
CGD (*n*)	8	0

CGD = cholesterol gallstone disease

cholecystectomized or suffered from cholesterol gallstone disease. Five of the insulin-independent patients were slightly obese (relative body weight >120%). Insulin-independent and insulin-dependent patients differed with regard to the plasma triglyceride (Tg) level being higher among the former. The fasting blood glucose was elevated in both groups (Table 1).

Experimental protocol

The patients were hospitalized for some days before and during the studies. They were fed a diet in which 44%, 33%, and 23% of the energy was supplied as carbohydrate, fat, and protein, respectively. The caloric intake, calculated from standard foodstuff tables, was adjusted to keep the body weight constant. The daily intake of cholesterol was less than 1 mmol. A total of seven patients with DM of adult-onset type were examined twice. In some cases the first study was performed before the institution of therapy. When reinvestigated these patients had been treated with sulphonylurea (glibenclamide, Daonil®) for 1–3 months. Three patients had been taking the drug for about 2 years before the first study. In these cases the second investigation was undertaken when therapy had been withdrawn for 1–3 months. These seven patients were also studied with regard to plasma very low density lipoprotein (VLDL)–Tg kinetics with the [^{3}H]glycerol technique.

[^{14}C]cholic acid and [^{14}C]chenodeoxycholic acid as sodium salts were dissolved in water and administered orally to the subjects, who had fasted overnight. Four samples of duodenal bile were collected from each patient at 2–4-days intervals. Cholecystokinin was administered intravenously and 5–10 ml of concentrated bile were drawn into ice-chilled tubes. The bile samples were analysed for lipid composition and the specific radioactivities of cholic acid (CA) and chenodeoxycholic acid (CDCA) were determined. Blood glucose, serum Tg and cholesterol were measured repeatedly. Faeces collected for 7–10 days were pooled and analysed for neutral steroids.

VLDL–Tg kinetics were studied immediately following the procedure for bile acid turnover. After an overnight fast the patients received an intravenous injection of [^{3}H]glycerol (40 μCi), dissolved in 10 ml saline. Venous blood samples were obtained from an indwelling catheter in the opposite arm at intervals of 30 min from 2 to 6 h and then at 7, 8 and 10 h after the administration of label. The VLDL fraction was isolated in all blood samples and analysed for radioactivity. The first meal was served 8 h after the isotope injection.

Methods

Blood glucose, serum cholesterol and triglycerides were measured using a discrete multichannel analyser (Autochemist, LKB Clinicon, Bromma, Sweden). The techniques used for determination of biliary bile lipids[5], and bile acid kinetics[3], steroid balance[4] and plasma VLDL–Tg kinetics[6] have been reported in earlier publications. In the studies of bile acid kinetics the correlation coefficient for CA and CDCA averaged 0.994±0.003 and 0.996±0.002 respectively.

Table 2 Steroid balance

	Bile acid formation		Neutral steroid excretion		Steroid balance	
	mmol/day	μmol kg⁻¹ day⁻¹	mmol/day	μmol kg⁻¹ day⁻¹	mmol/day	μmol kg⁻¹ day⁻¹
Insulin-independent	1.63 ± 0.19**	21.7 ± 3.0*	2.83 ± 0.19***	37.1 ± 2.4***	3.61 ± 0.21***	47.7 ± 4.3***
Insulin-dependent	1.29 ± 0.25	18.6 ± 3.0	1.39 ± 0.12*	20.5 ± 1.4**	1.83 ± 0.29	26.4 ± 3.3
Normolipidaemic controls	1.00 ± 0.12	14.1 ± 1.7	1.07 ± 0.13	15.1 ± 1.8	1.83 ± 0.22	25.8 ± 3.1

* Significently different from controls ($p < 0.05$)
** Significantly different from controls ($p < 0.01$)
*** Significantly different from controls ($p < 0.001$)

Table 3 Steroid balance in patients with insulin-independent diabetes

	Bile acid formation		Neutral steroid excretion		Steroid balance	
	mmol/day	μmol kg⁻¹ day⁻¹	mmol/day	μmol kg⁻¹ day⁻¹	mmol/day	μmol kg⁻¹ day⁻¹
Normolipidaemic RBW <120% ($n = 4$)	1.7 ± 0.08**	22.3 ± 1.7*	3.2 ± 0.26**	41.1 ± 3.0**	4.0 ± 0.26**	51.7 ± 3.9**
Hyperlipidaemic RBW <120% ($n = 5$)	1.9 ± 0.46	28.2 ± 7.3	3.0 ± 0.43*	42.9 ± 4.0**	4.0 ± 0.68*	58.4 ± 8.6*
Normolipidaemic RBW >120% ($n = 4$)	1.4 ± 0.26	15.6 ± 2.7	2.5 ± 0.19**	28.3 ± 2.1**	3.0 ± 0.13*	35.2 ± 1.7*
Hyperlipidaemic RBW >120% ($n = 1$)	0.9	10.6	2.3	27.8	2.3	27.9

* Significantly different from controls ($p < 0.05$)
** Significantly different from controls ($p < 0.01$)

Statistical analyses

Data are presented as mean ± SEM. Student's *t*-test and paired *t*-test were used for evaluating the significance of differences. Linear regressions were calculated by the method of least squares and their significance was tested by estimating the correlation coefficient, '*r*'[7].

RESULTS

Bile acid formation

Bile acid synthesis in insulin-independent patients averaged 1.63 mmol/day or 21.7 μmol kg^{-1} day^{-1}, i.e. values significantly higher than those previously observed in normolipidaemic controls (Table 2). Values within the normal range among the insulin-independent patients were only encountered in the normolipidaemic, overweight subgroup (Table 3). Bile acid production in the insulin-dependent patients did not differ from that of the controls (Table 2).

Steroid balance

Due to the highly significant rise in the excretion of neutral steroids in faeces, the steroid balance (calculated as bile acid formation + faecal excretion of cholesterol and cholesterol neutral metabolites minus cholesterol intake) in the insulin-independent patients exceeded corresponding data in the normolipidaemic controls (Table 2). The highest values were found in the normo- and hyperlipidaemic non-obese subgroups, but the steroid balance was slightly elevated also in the four normolipidaemic, obese patients (Table 3).

Although the faecal excretion of neutral steroids was somewhat supranormal in the insulin-dependent patients the net steroid balance remained normal (Table 3).

Sulphonylurea treatment

Under basal conditions the pool size and synthesis of cholic acid (CA) ranged from 0.5 to 3.5 mmol and 0.5 to 2.0 mmol/day, respectively, in the seven insulin-independent patients also studied when treated with glibenclamide. During treatment, the CA pool size decreased in three, and the CA synthesis in all but one patient (patient T.P.). The mean pool size and formation of CDCA remained unchanged. Upon re-examination during

Table 4 Net steroid balance in seven insulin-independent patients when treated or untreated with sulphonylurea

	Neutral steroid excretion (mmol/day)	*Bile acid formation* (mmol/day)	*Net steroid balance* (mmol/day)
Untreated	3.1 ± 0.33	1.8 ± 0.33	4.0 ± 0.50
Treated	3.5 ± 0.25	1.6 ± 0.3	4.2 ± 0.42

therapy the neutral faecal excretion had increased in five of the seven patients. As these losses were partly compensated for by a reduced biosynthesis of bile acids the mean net steroid balance was the same during both studies (Table 4). When the patients were examined without treatment the serum level and apparent formation of VLDL–Tg averaged 2.1 mmol/l and 6.5 μmol kg^{-1} h^{-1}, respectively. During treatment with glibenclamide the VLDL–Tg concentration and apparent production decreased in all subjects except patient T.P.; i.e. the one who differed from the others also with regard to the response in bile acid production.

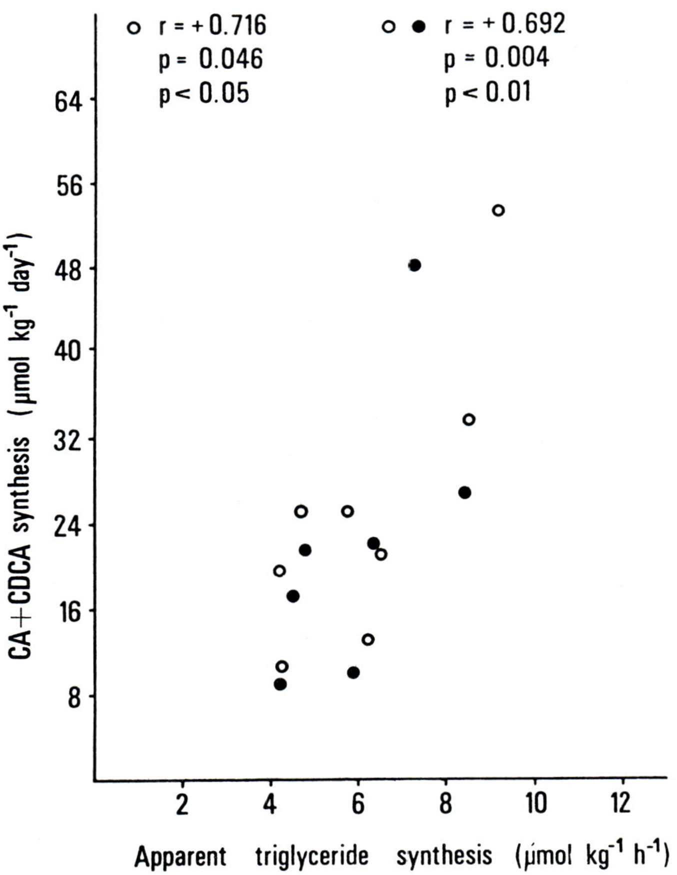

Figure 1 Relation between total bile acid formation (μmol kg^{-1} day^{-1}) and apparent triglyceride synthesis (μmol kg^{-1} h^{-1}) when the patients were untreated (open rings) and treated (closed rings) with sulphonylurea. Equation of the regression line: $y = 5.11\times -6.89$ (open rings), $y = 5.30\times -8.49$ (open and closed rings)

Relationship between VLDL–Tg formation and bile acid synthesis

The relationship between the apparent production of VLDL–Tg and bile acids is demonstrated in Figure 1. On the basis of without-treatment data the synthesis of VLDL–Tg correlated significantly with the total bile acid formation ($p<0.05$). Using all results for VLDL–Tg production before and during therapy, this parameter correlated with corresponding data for CA, CDCA, and CA + CDCA ($p<0.01$). No significant correlation was found between the apparent synthesis of VLDL–Tg and the net steroid balance.

DISCUSSION

The plasma level of VLDL–Tg is influenced by the blood concentration of free fatty acids, glucose and insulin, factors that may stimulate VLDL–Tg synthesis both independently and by interfering with the action of the other. Plasma Tg is also controlled by mechanisms regulating extrahepatic utilization of Tg. Accordingly, HLP type IV in non-diabetic patients[6] as well as hypertriglyceridaemia in diabetics[9] have been found to be associated with overproduction and/or decreased clearance of VLDL. Irrespective of the rate of VLDL–Tg formation it correlated closely with that of the bile acids in non-diabetics, suggesting a parallel regulation and possibly an integrated metabolism[6].

In keeping with current knowledge insulin-independent and insulin-dependent diabetic patients differed in several respects. Whereas the former tended to be obese and hypertriglyceridaemic the latter were almost underweight and normolipidaemic. Furthermore, more than half of the insulin-independent patients but none of the insulin-dependent patients had or have had cholesterol gallstone disease. As evidenced by the current study the two types of DM also differed with regard to cholesterol metabolism. While the insulin-dependent patients synthesized cholesterol and bile acids at the same rate as normolipidaemic non-diabetic controls these variables were significantly enhanced in the insulin-independent patients.

The abnormalities in cholesterol metabolism in the insulin-independent patients might be related to DM itself, to overweight, hypertriglyceridaemia and/or unknown factors. The blood glucose level appears to be of minor importance, being about the same in insulin-independent and insulin-dependent patients. Although excessive obesity is reported to be associated with enhanced cholesterogenesis[1,2] the overweight patients in the current study had a steroid balance below the average of the group. These findings are in line with a recent report demonstrating normal values for steroid balance when calculated per kg body weight in normolipidaemic overweight subjects[10].

During treatment with glibenclamide the blood glucose dropped towards normal levels in all patients but the means for bile acid formation and steroid balance remained essentially unchanged. However, all six patients who responded to therapy with a reduced formation of VLDL–Tg also showed a decrease in the amount of bile acids produced. In analogy patient

T.P., who for unknown reasons had increased VLDL–Tg synthesis during therapy, also accelerated the formation of bile acids. The parallel changes in VLDL–Tg and bile acid biosynthesis observed in this study are in keeping with previous findings in non-diabetics, as discussed above. A decrease in bile acid excretion following treatment with sulphonylurea or insulin has been observed by others[11–13]. However, therapy primarily aimed to normalize the blood glucose level may be without effect on total cholesterol synthesis which in the current study remained supranormal. The possible consequence of such a defect in terms of being a risk factor for atherosclerosis remains to be established.

References

1. Miettinen, T. A. (1971). Cholesterol production in obesity. *Circulation*, **44,** 842
2. Nestel, P. J., Schreibman, P. H. and Ahrens, E. A. Jr (1973). Cholesterol metabolism in human obesity. *J. Clin. Invest.*, **48,** 982
3. Einarsson, K., Hellström, K. and Kallner, M. (1974). Bile acid kinetics in relation to sex, serum lipids, body weights and gallbladder disease in patients with various types of hyperlipoproteinaemia. *J. Clin. Invest.*, **54,** 1301
4. Angelin, B., Einarsson, K., Hellström, K. and Kallner, M. (1976). Elimination of cholesterol in hyperlipoproteinaemia. *Clin. Sci. Mol. Med.*, **51,** 393
5. Andersén, E. and Hellström, K. (1979). The effect of cholesterol feeding on bile acid kinetics and biliary lipids in normolipidemic and hypertriglyceridemic subjects. *J. Lipid Res.*, **20,** 1020
6. Angelin, B., Einarsson, K., Hellström, K. and Leijd, B. (1978). Bile acid kinetics in relation to endogenous triglyceride metabolism in various types of hyperlipoproteinaemia. *J. Lipid Res.*, **19,** 1004
7. Snedecor, G. W. and Cochran, W. G. (1974). *Statistical Methods*, 6th Edn. (Ames, IA: Iowa State University Press)
8. Bagdade, J. D., Porte, D. Jr and Bierman, E. L. (1967). Diabetic lipemia. A form of acquired fat-induced lipemia. *N. Engl. J. Med.*, **276,** 427
9. Nikkilä, E. and Kekki, M. (1973). Plasma triglyceride transport kinetics in diabetes mellitus. *Metabolism*, **22,** 1
10. Leijd, B. (1980). Cholesterol metabolism in obesity and type IV hyperlipoproteinaemia. *Clin. Sci. Mol. Med.* (In press)
11. Bennion, L. G. and Grundy, S. M. (1977). Effects of diabetes mellitus on cholesterol metabolism in man. *N. Engl. J. Med.*, **296,** 1365
12. Saudek, C. D. and Brach, E. L. (1978). Cholesterol metabolism in diabetes. I. The effect of diabetic control on sterol balance. *Diabetes*, **27,** 1059
13. Nestel, P. J. (1979). *Cholesterol Metabolism in Diabetes Mellitus*. International Congress Series No. 500. Diabetes 1979

Workshop on Dissolution of Gallstones

WORKSHOP ON DISSOLUTION OF GALLSTONES

PART I
Staging of Cholesterol Gallstone Disease

Staging gallstone and gallbladder disease and its relevance to medical treatment: speculations and scenarios

A. F. HOFMANN AND C. WOLPERS

INTRODUCTION

Cholesterol gallstone disease can be successfully treated by chenodeoxycholic acid (CDCA) or ursodeoxycholic acid (UDCA) only at an early stage[1]. Thus, staging of gallstone disease by the physician is essential for a judicious decision about treatment. In this chapter we wish to consider the staging of gallstone and gallbladder disease and how staging categories bear on medical treatment. The overall pathology of gallstone and gallbladder disease is summarized in Figure 1.

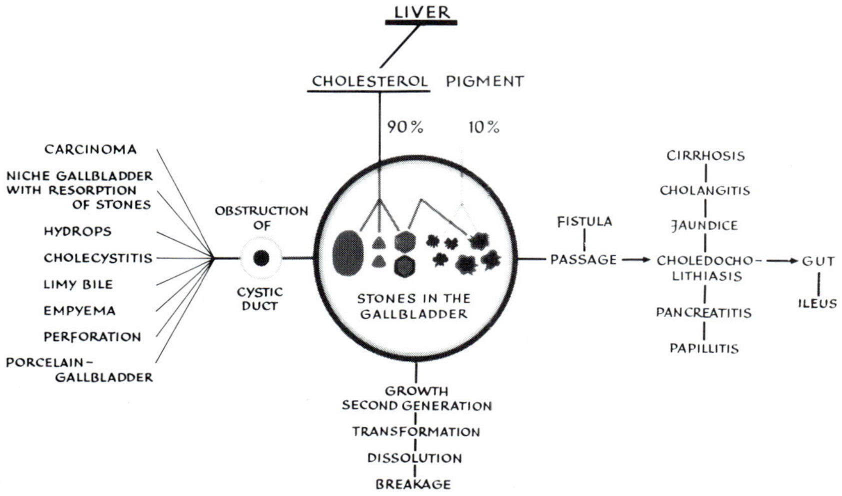

Figure 1 The pathology of gallstone and gallbladder disease. The gallbladder is shown schematically in the centre with cholesterol stones on the left, combination stones in the centre, and pigment stones on the right. The consequences of cystic duct obstruction are shown on the left; those of stone passage are shown on the right

STAGING GALLSTONE DISEASE

The staging of gallstone disease was impossible until the development of oral cholecystography permitted the detection of asymptomatic gallstones. It became clear that there was a stage in the history of at least some gallstones when they were completely asymptomatic[2,3]. This stage had been predicted from autopsy studies, but obviously accurate posthumous assessment of symptomatology was impossible.

Donald Small, after brilliantly defining the physical chemistry of model systems simulating bile[4], applied these concepts to gallbladder bile from patients. Together with Admirand[5], he showed that the bile in a majority of gallstone patients is supersaturated with cholesterol, whereas bile from patients without gallstones is usually unsaturated with cholesterol.

Table 1 Staging of gallstone and gallbladder disease

Stage	*Event*	*Diagnosis*	*Recommended treatment*
I Supersaturated bile	secretion of hepatic bile containing an excess of cholesterol	duodenal drainage; biochemical analysis; calculation of percentage saturation	none
II Crystallization	nucleation and crystallization of cholesterol; retention of cholesterol crystals	duodenal drainage; microscopy	none; if patient symptomatic, medical
III Uncomplicated gallstone disease with unimpaired gallbladder function	aggregation of crystals to form stone; stone growth	imaging: ultrasonography or cholecystography	medical
IV Gallstone disease with impaired gallbladder function	inflammation of gallbladder; fibrosis; perhaps cystic duct obstruction	imaging: cholecystography or scintigraphy	surgical
V Acute cholecystitis	acute obstruction of cystic duct by gallstone	clinical; confirmation by scintigraphy	surgical; possibly medical, if patient recovers and returns to Stage III

With this information, plus the accepted medical knowledge about cholelithiasis, Small proposed five stages of gallstone disease[6]. There was first a genetic–metabolic stage, undetectable by current techniques. This was followed by a chemical stage, detected chemically by the finding of supersaturated gallbladder bile. This was followed by a physical stage, when crystallization had occurred; diagnosis was by a physical technique – microscopy which indicated the presence of cholesterol crystals in bile. The fourth stage was that of gallstone growth, when the patient was symptomatic and cholecystography revealed gallstones or a non-visualizing gallbladder. The final stage was a clinical stage in which the gallbladder became obstructed (acute cholecystitis) or bile flux was obstructed by a stone in the common duct.

A NEW STAGING CLASSIFICATION (TABLE 1)

Supersaturated bile: the chemical stage

Bile is readily obtained by duodenal drainage and its degree of cholesterol saturation calculated from the molar proportions of bile acids, lecithin and cholesterol. All of these three major biliary lipids may now be determined enzymatically[7–9], so that the measurement of bile saturation of any bile sample can be carried out in any clinical laboratory.

Bile which is supersaturated with cholesterol is termed 'supersaturated'. Small proposed that this stage be termed the 'chemical stage of gallstone disease' and this proposal seems useful.

The natural history of the patient who has supersaturated bile in his gallbladder is not known. There are at least three possibilities. First, the patient may stop forming supersaturated bile and bile may revert to its unsaturated state, if the metabolic disturbance causing supersaturation is self-limited. The patient may continue to form supersaturated bile for his entire life without nucleation ever occurring. Third, nucleation may occur and cholesterol monohydrate crystals may form. These may be passed or may be retained. If they aggregate, and the aggregate continues to grow, gallstones will occur.

Formation of cholesterol crystals: the physical stage

Crystal formation is not synonymous with gallstone formation. Individuals have been observed using ultrasonography with 'sludge' in the gallbladder; at subsequent examination the sludge was no longer present, suggesting it had dissolved or had been emptied[10]. In some instances sludge is composed of cholesterol crystals[11].

With the demonstration by Holzbach and his co-workers[12] that gallstone patients nucleate rapidly, and the finding by both Sedaghat and Grundy[13] and the Holzbach group[12] that patients without gallstones may have supersaturated bile yet nucleate extremely slowly, it seems that gallstone patients may well lack an anti-nucleating factor.

It seems useful to define a stage characterized by the presence of crystals without gallstones. In some patients with acalculous cholecystitis, there are crystals without stones and symptomatic improvement after cholecystectomy[14].

Gallstones without gallbladder disease

Gallstones may be detected by ultrasonography and radiology; it is claimed that the two techniques now have similar accuracy[15], although we believe that for the detection of very small stones cholecystography is more sensitive. The current view is that, when gallstones are of sufficient size to be detected by imaging techniques, spontaneous passage or dissolution is extremely rare[16]. If this is true, the natural history of gallstones is to grow and either cause no mucosal response, to grow and induce chronic mucosal inflammation, or to grow and obstruct the cystic duct, causing cholecystitis.

That gallstones may be present without mucosal inflammation is well documented in the autopsy studies of Schein *et al.*[17] and Lindstrom[18], although it can only be assumed that many of the gallstones present in healthy gallbladders at autopsy could have been visualized by conventional imaging techniques in life. In the study of Schein *et al.*[17], it was shown that the prevalence of chronic cholecystitis was much greater in patients with larger stones.

Thus, the key question is whether gallstones can be detected by imaging techniques before irreversible gallbladder disease has occurred. If so, and if as noted previously autopsy studies strongly support this hypothesis, then gallstone dissolution will result in unsaturated bile in a healthy gallbladder. How often gallstones which are detected by cholecystography or ultrasound occur in a healthy bladder can be answered easily by retrospective studies from institutions which carry out elective cholecystectomy for the completely silent stone, provided care is taken to examine the gallbladder carefully and immediately after its removal.

Gallstones with impaired gallbladder function

If the majority of gallstones can be detected only after gallbladder disease has occurred, i.e. if most stones do not reach a detectable size until they have induced chronic cholecystitis, then the question is what degree of cholecystitis causes irreversible impairment of function, i.e. defective filling and emptying. Thus, it seems that gallstone disease should be staged by its effect on gallbladder structure and function, i.e. that Small's stage of gallstone growth should be subdivided according to the amount of induced gallbladder inflammation (Table 2).

Gallstones with total cystic duct occlusion

The end stage of gallstone disease may be occlusion of the cystic duct by the stone. When this occurs symptoms may subside. Surgery is unnecessary unless acute cholecystitis occurs, but is often recommended because of the possibility of cancer.

Hypotheses

These considerations lead to two mutually exclusive hypotheses:

(a) Cholesterol gallstone disease should be treated only when there is little or no gallbladder inflammation or impairment of gallbladder function. The aim here is to produce healthy bile in a healthy gallbladder.

(b) Gallstone disease can be treated irrespective of the degree of gallbladder inflammation provided the functional activity of the gallbladder, i.e. filling and emptying, is sufficiently maintained that unsaturated bile reaches the gallstones and can dissolve them. The goal is to eliminate stones because they cause pain or because they can obstruct the ducts and cause acute or chronic cholecystitis or jaundice; the goal of therapy is thus to prevent symptoms or surgical complications. The magnitude of the inflammatory process is irrelevant, provided it is asymptomatic and stable. Many patients are found to have severe chronic cholecystitis at autopsy, yet were symptom-free in life.

It may also be that in some patients the inflammatory process is minimal and will disappear when stones are dissolved. Thus, stone dissolution will result in unsaturated bile in a healthy gallbladder.

Table 2 Ultrasound screening to detect gallstone disease at a stage qualifying for medical treatment

Screening requirement[1]	*Application to medical treatment of gallstones*
1. Leads to an improvement in end-results	replacement of surgical therapy by medical therapy eliminates surgical mortality and morbidity
2. Medical therapy favourably alters natural history	medical therapy prevents occurrence of acute cholecystitis or complications from gallbladder or duct obstruction
3. Available health services must be sufficient to confirm diagnosis and provide care	confirmation of gallstone disease by cholecystography considered sensitive and specific; medical therapy should be widely available
4. Claims for effectiveness must have been shown in clinical trials	effectiveness of medical therapy documented in numerous clinical trials; increased survival must occur if surgical mortality is eliminated and drug is shown to be fully safe
5. Compliance among asymptomatic patients in whom diagnosis has been achieved must be sufficient	adequate compliance for stone dissolution observed in most clinical trials
6. Beneficial results must outweigh side-effects of treatment	efficacy of medical therapy is high; risk (hepatotoxicity) is extremely low
7. Mechanism for formal periodic weighing of costs and benefits must be developed	(not yet proposed): to date no detailed benefit/cost analysis comparing medical versus surgical therapy has been constructed
8. Burden of disability must warrant action	cholecystectomy is fifth leading cause of hospitalization and an important cause of surgical death

[1] Modified from Sackett[22].

IMPLICATIONS FOR MEDICAL PRACTICE

As has been discussed elsewhere, medical therapy for gallstones is best considered a preventive approach to gallbladder disease[19].

It is clearly impossible at present to stage gallbladder disease non-invasively. At present, one can only infer from the cholecystodynamic behaviour of the gallbladder during ultrasonography or cholecystography that gallbladder filling and emptying are unimpaired, and that fibrosis is minimal. As noted, with smaller, younger stones which are often spherical, chronic cholecystitis is less advanced than with larger, older stones which are often elliptical or faceted. Criteria for cholecystometrics have not been proposed, but newer imaging techniques with gamma-emitting isotopes[20] or real-time ultrasonography[21] appear to be useful for this purpose.

With the development of grey-scale ultrasonography, and the claim that its accuracy is equal or superior to that of conventional cholecystography[15], the possibility of regular screening of the gallbladder for the presence of early stone disease has become a reality.

The criteria for screening techniques have been discussed at length[22] and, as indicated in Table 2, ultrasonography screening for treatable gallstone disease would appear to meet the required criteria. It is assumed that routine screening would be applied only to patients at increased risk for gallstones in the world. This would apply to women over 20, men over 50, and all individuals with American Indian ancestry. There seems little point in screening Black patients.

If it is elected to screen and treat all patients with stones irrespective of symptoms, some patients will be treated unnecessarily. However, if the transfer coefficients shown in Figure 2 can be estimated accurately, then it should be possible to calculate for society the relative costs of screening and medical therapy versus surgery for symptomatic cases or acute cholecystitis.

Our prediction is that it will be marginally cheaper to 'screen and treat' than to 'wait and cut'. However, this conclusion applies only to the United States and Western Europe and does not apply to developing countries where surgery will probably be cheaper than screening and medical treatment.

If it became conventional medical practice to screen and treat rather than to wait and cut, there would be some major effects on health. First, surgical deaths associated with cholecystectomy would be decreased by the fraction of individuals whose stones dissolved, perhaps 50% of all patients undergoing biliary tract surgery. Second, gallbladder disease would cease being a major cause for hospitalization; it is now the fifth leading cause[22] of hospitalization and among the five most common surgical procedures[23]. Third, many gallstone patients would no longer have to suffer the pain, inconvenience, and cost of surgery. From an economic standpoint, in countries with national medical insurance, the flow of the tax dollar would be diverted away from the surgeon and hospital costs, and move toward the physician, the radiologist, and the pharmaceutical industry.

FUTUROLOGY

There are at least three scenarios.

The first scenario is a continuation of the present. Some physicians will screen and treat; others will recommend waiting for symptoms followed by eventual surgery.

A second scenario in these days of increasing government regulation is the calling of a 'technical consensus' conference by the appropriate government agency[24]. Here epidemiologists, decision analysis experts, or medical-care cost experts would meet with physicians and surgeons; a consensus would be hammered out which might decide, for example, that the policy of screen and treat was cost-effective.

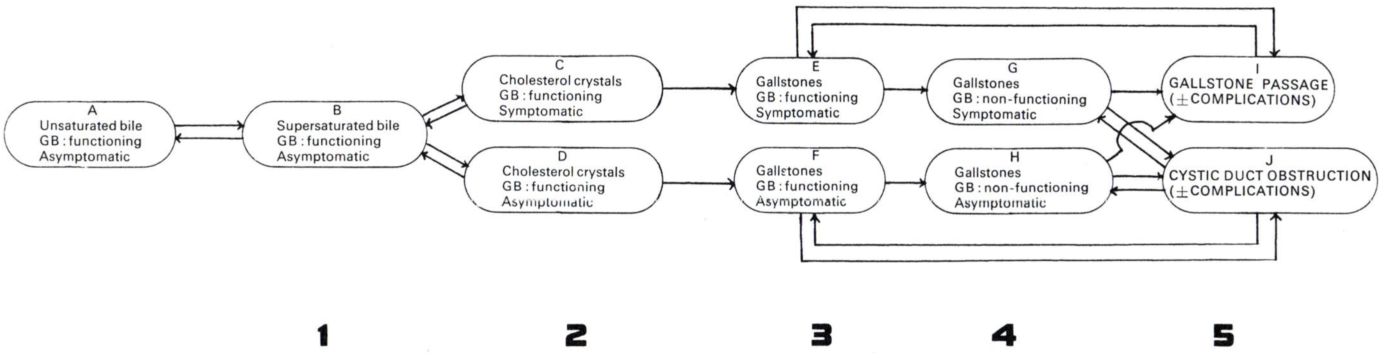

Figure 2 The five stages of gallstone disease shown in a compartment model. Compartment C denotes 'acalculous cholecystitis'. Compartments C, E, and F are eligible for medical therapy. If the fraction of the population in the various compartments can be estimated and transfer coefficients defined, it will indicate the natural history of gallstone disease

Were this recommendation to be made, and were it to be propagated to the community of practising gastroenterologists, the policy of screening by ultrasonography followed by cholecystography and medical treatment of eligible patients would become conventional medical practice. Were this to occur, the patient who was not screened and who developed acute cholecystitis followed by a complex cholecystectomy could argue, aided by a malpractice lawyer, that his care was sub-optimal and that redress was in order. Were this to occur and were the courts to sympathize, the policy of 'screen and treat' would become routine, not because of cost-effectiveness but because of medicolegal reasons, i.e. fear of a malpractice suit if it were not done. This scenario has perhaps already occurred with the practice of screening for cardiac disease using electrocardiography.

It is also possible that a technical consensus conference would come to the conclusion that the policy of screening and treatment was not cost-effective. Were this to be the case, any move towards screening and medical treatment in the future would depend on physician attitudes, as well as policies of third-party reimbursement.

A final scenario, unlikely to be seen in our lifetime, is the development of a new drug, effective in microgram amounts, which can be added to toothpaste or salt and which will prevent supersaturated bile and subsequent gallstone disease in the population.

EPILOGUE

In the long history of biliary tract disease, the two most significant advances were the safe one-stage cholecystectomy and oral cholecystography. Now it appears that medical dissolution and ultrasonography are advances of comparable magnitude.

The latter two methods apply only to patients with cholesterol gallstones. Nonetheless, since cholesterol gallstones compose the majority of gallstones in the Western world, the majority of patients with gallstones are eligible for these exciting, even revolutionary, new diagnostic and therapeutic techniques. If these techniques were applied globally, then gallbladder disease would persist only in patients with non-cholesterol stones. Realization of the magnitude of this unsolved problem might highlight our ignorance of the neglected area of gallstone disease and might stimulate research on the cause and treatment of other types of cholelithiasis.

Acknowledgments

The work of A.F.H. is supported in part by NIH Grant AM 21506, as well as grants-in-aid from the Rorer Company, and from the Falk Foundation.

References

1. Wolpers, C. (1976). Auswahl der Gallensteinträger zur Litholyse. *Leber Magen Darm*, **6,** 43
2. Comfort, M. W., Gray, H. K , and Wilson, J M. (1948). The silent gallstone: a ten to twenty year follow-up study of 112 cases. *Ann. Surg.*, **128,** 931

3. Peskin, G. W. (1973). The treatment of silent gallstones. *Surg. Clin. N. Amer.*, **53,** 1063
4. Small, D. M. (1967). Physicochemical studies of cholesterol gallstone formation. *Gastroenterology*, **52,** 607
5. Admirand, W. H. and Small, D. M. (1968). The physicochemical basis of cholesterol gallstone formation in man. *J. Clin. Invest.*, **47,** 1043
6. Small, D. M. (1975). The formation and treatment of gallstones. In Schiff, L. (ed.). *Diseases of the Liver*, pp. 146–162. (Philadelphia: J. B. Lippincott)
7. Iwata, T. and Yamasaki, K. (1964). Enzymatic determination and thin layer chromatography of bile acids in blood. *J. Biochem.* (*Japan*), **56,** 424
8. Gurantz, D., Laker, M. F. and Hofmann, A. F. (1981). Enzymatic measurement of choline-containing phospholipids in bile. *J. Lipid Res.* (In press)
9. Fromm, H., Amin, P., Klein, H. and Kupke, I. (1980). Use of a simple enzymatic assay for cholesterol analysis in human bile. *J. Lipid Res.*, **21,** 259
10. Gosink, B. B. and Leopold, G. R. (1976). Ultrasound and the gallbladder. *Semin. Roentgenol.*, **11,** 185
11. Filly, R. A., Allen, B., Minton, M. J., Bernhoft, R. and Way, L. W. (1980). *In vitro* investigation of the origin of echoes within biliary sludge. *J. Clin. Ultrasound*, **8,** 193
12. Holan, K. R., Holzbach, R. T., Hermann, R. E., Cooperman, A. M. and Claffey, W. J. (1979). Nucleation time: a key factor in the pathogenesis of cholesterol gallstone disease. *Gastroenterology*, **77,** 611
13. Sedaghat, A. and Grundy, S. M. (1980). Cholesterol crystals, a prerequisite for cholesterol gallstone formation. *N. Engl. J. Med.*, **302,** 1274
14. Porterfield, G., Cheung, L. Y. and Berenson, M. (1977). Detection of occult gallbladder disease by duodenal drainage. *Am. J. Surg.*, **134,** 702
15. Cooperberg, P. L. and Burhenne, H. J. (1980). Real-time ultrasonography. *N. Engl. J. Med.*, **302,** 1277
16. Wolpers, C. (1968). Spontanauflösung von Gallenblasensteinen. *Dtsch. med. Wschr.*, **93,** 2525
17. Schein, C. J., Hurwitt, E. S. and Rosenblatt, M. A. (1955). The significance of calculus size in determining the indication for elective cholecystectomy. *Gastroenterology*, **29,** 377
18. Lindstrom, C. G. (1977). Frequency of gallstone disease in a well-defined Swedish population. A prospective necropsy study in Malmo. *Scand. J. Gastroenterol.*, **12,** 341
19. Hofmann, A. F. (1980). The medical treatment of cholesterol gallstones: a major advance in preventive gastroenterology. *Am. J. Med.*, **69,** 4
20. Shaffer, E. A., McOrmond, P. and Duggan, H. (1980). Quantitative cholescintigraphy: assessment of gallbladder filling and emptying and duodenogastric reflux. *Gastroenterology*, **79,** 899
21. Everson, G. T., Braverman, D. Z., Johnson, M. L. and Kern, F. Jr. (1980). A critical evaluation of real-time ultrasonography for the study of gallbladder volume and contraction. *Gastroenterology*, **79,** 40
22. Sackett, D. L. (1975). Laboratory screening: a critique. *Fed. Proc.*, **34,** 2157
23. Luft, H. S., Bunker, J. P. and Enthoven, A. C. (1979). Should operations be regionalized? *N. Engl. J. Med.*, **301,** 1364
24. Perry, S. and Kalberer, J. T. Jr. (1980). The NIH consensus-development program and the assessment of health-care technologies. *N. Engl. J. Med.*, **303,** 169

The staging of cholesterol gallstones with respect to nucleation and growth

D. M. SMALL

Crystalline cholesterol monohydrate[1] is a major constituent of gallstones and stones formed from cholesterol dissolved in bile[2], therefore cholesterol monohydrate crystallization is a prerequisite to cholesterol gallstone formation. Five stages leading to the formation of symptomatic cholesterol gallstone disease have been proposed[3,4], and each stage is a prerequisite for the next (see Figure 1). The first is a genetic–metabolic stage, in which the genetic propensity or metabolic abnormality which can lead to production of supersaturated bile is present, but not yet manifest. The second stage is a *chemical* stage in which gallbladder bile becomes supersaturated with cholesterol. This stage is diagnosed by measuring the chemical composition of bile and calculating cholesterol saturation[5]. The third stage is a *physical* stage in which the supersaturated bile is nucleated and growth of cholesterol monohydrate crystals is initiated. This stage is diagnosed by observing

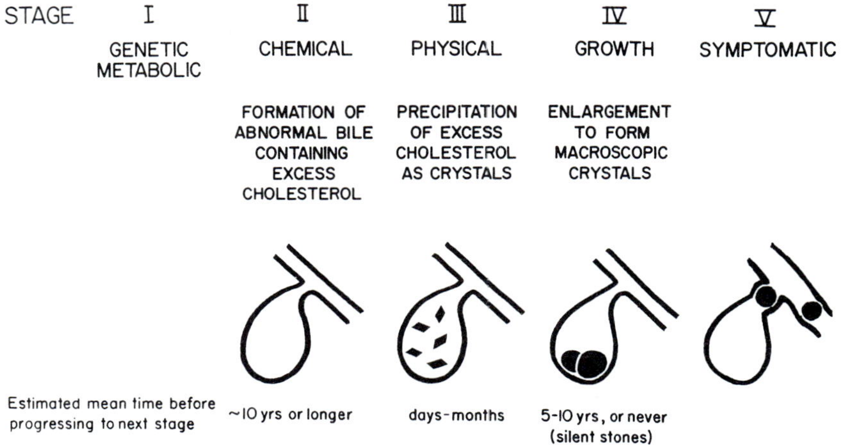

Figure 1 The stages of cholesterol gallstone formation[3,4]. The mean estimations of the times during which each stage exists before progressing to the next stage are given below. Thus, on the average about 10 years are required for the formation of stones from supersaturated bile (i.e. between stages 2 and 4), and approximately 10 years between stages 4 and 5. About half the people probably never develop stage 5. Stage 3 is the shortest of all stages, and probably only exists for days or weeks

Figure 2 Cholesterol monohydrate crystal under crossed polars. The crystal is a flat rhomboid structure much greater in breadth and width than in thickness. The edge angles are 79.2 and 100.8°[15].

microscopic crystals of cholesterol monohydrate in fresh bile on subjects who do not yet have stones (see Figure 2). In stage four, microscopic crystals grow or agglomerate into macroscopic stones, and in the fifth stage, macroscopic stones cause symptoms by initiating cholecystitis and/or blocking of the cystic or common duct.

An illustration of these stages comes from studies of American Indians, in particular the Pima Indians. About 70% of Pima women will ultimately develop gallstones, thus a large proportion of them have a predisposition to gallstones[6]. The chemical stage appears at around the time of puberty or by age 15, and by age 18 many young Indian women have supersaturated duodenal bile[7,8], but do not yet have stones[6]. However, by age 25, more than half of these women will have developed gallstones large enough to be found by cholecystography[4]. This suggests the mean time between the development of stage 2 and 4 is about 10 years. Finally, about half of such patients will ultimately develop symptoms, on average some 10 years after the initial appearance of stones[2,4]. Thus, the chemical stage can apparently exist for several years before stones are found. Since cholesterol crystals are rarely reported without stones, the duration of the physical stage (nucleation and precipitation of cholesterol crystals) must be a rather short stage leading quickly to the formation of macroscopic stones. The specific details of each of these sequential events are not known, but answers will be obtained by following these events in patients who have undergone stone dissolution with bile acid therapy and are followed by duodenal drainage and ultrasonography, for recurrence of stages 2, 3 and 4.

Certain people without gallstones have supersaturated bile without crystals. In fact, some populations (e.g. American Indians, Scandinavians), have a high prevalence of supersaturated bile in subjects without stones. However, it appears that populations with highly supersaturated bile are at risk for gallstone formation, since the overall prevalence of gallstone disease is related to the supersaturation of bile in subjects without gallstones[9]. The greater the supersaturation of bile, the greater the prevalence of gallstones[9] (see Figure 3). Many years ago we noted that hepatic bile from monkeys with interrupted enterohepatic circulation could be quite supersaturated[10], yet not precipitate its cholesterol readily. Recently it has been noted that highly supersaturated bile from gallstone patients did not precipitate crystals even after 48 h[11]. This raises the question of how cholesterol precipitates from bile to form crystals and stones. That is, what really happens during the physical stage of gallstone formation (nucleation and growth)?

Crystallization is similar whether it is from an undercooled melt, or a supersaturated solution; *nucleation comes first and crystal growth follows*[12,13].

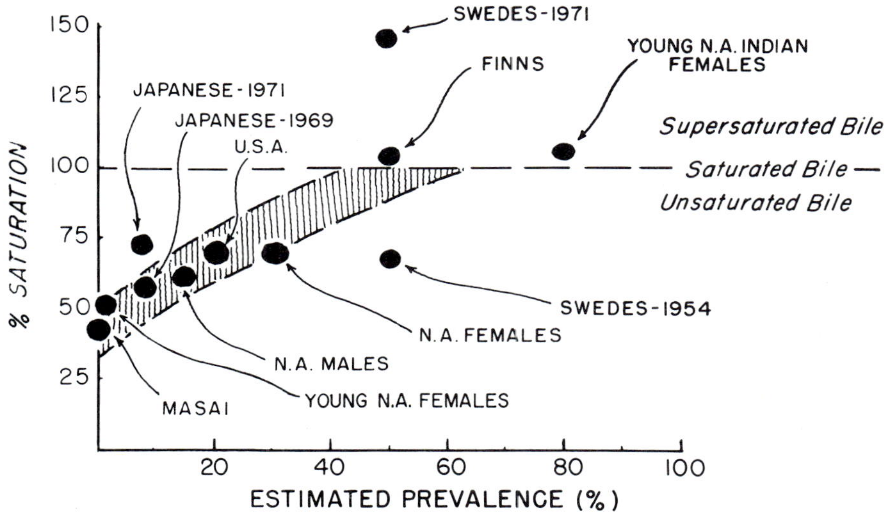

Figure 3 Percentage saturation of control gallbladder bile (according to Admirand and Small)[2] *vs.* estimated prevalence of gallstones in different populations. Control biles having lowest percentage cholesterol saturation appear to come from populations with lowest prevalence of cholesterol gallstones, while populations with supersaturated control biles have very high prevalences of cholesterol gallstones. Several populations with intermediate saturation (i.e. 65–75%) have intermediate prevalences of cholesterol stones as estimated from post mortem, hospital admission and cholecystogram evidence of gallstones (from Small, ref. 9). N.A. = North America.

HOMOGENEOUS NUCLEATION

In either an undercooled or supersaturated liquid, small clusters of molecules are continuously forming and breaking up (see Figure 4, top, from ref. 14). A critical cluster size must be reached so that the rate of breaking up is less than the rate of formation. The critical size depends on the system, but is of the order of a few tens to a few hundred molecules. The probability of forming such an aggregate is greater the greater the supersaturation, or the greater the undercooling. Marked supersaturation and undercooling occur in many systems before spontaneous or *homogeneous nucleation* occur. In fact, the ratio between the true freezing point and the temperature of homogeneous nucleation in °K is equal to about 0.8 for many substances[12]. Thus, pure water may be undercooled some 50 °C below its true melting point before it crystallizes. The process of crystallization from supersaturated solutions is similar. Very high degrees of supersaturation are reached (in some cases

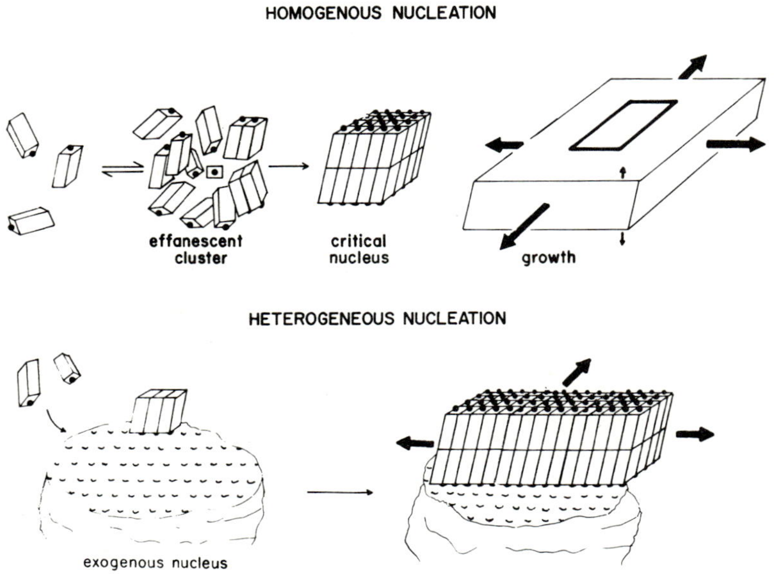

Figure 4 Diagrammatic illustrations of the processes of nucleation and crystal growth. Above, homogeneous nucleation; below, heterogeneous nucleation. On the left, cholesterol molecules in solution above their true saturation point are in constant rapid equilibrium with small clusters whose rate of formation is equal to their rate of disintegration. Proceeding towards the right, as supersaturation becomes higher a level is reached at which a critical aggregate size is formed and the molecules align in a minute crystal. This critical size contains tens to hundreds of molecules; once formed, spontaneous growth of all such nuclei occurs, rapidly producing a large number of small crystals. Growth of cholesterol monohydrate, shown on the right, is most rapid along the two faces in which molecules come together side by side, rather than end to end, thus producing the flat parallelogram-shaped crystals seen in Figure 2. Below illustrates heterogeneous nucleation. A relatively large particle (exogenous nucleus) having a surface which has a similar lattice allows the cholesterol molecules to adsorb, align and crystallize at a concentration lower than the maximum supersaturation level found with homogeneous nucleation shown above. Anti-nucleating agents can disturb the formation of critical-sized nuclei, adsorb to exogenous nuclei, and anti-growth agents can adsorb to small crystals to prevent or retard further growth (from ref. 15, with permission)

many times greater than true saturation) before homogeneous nucleation takes place[13]. The characteristics of homogeneous nucleation are: the absence of contaminating foreign nuclei which permit a very high supersaturation, the spontaneous formation of many critical-sized clusters at the maximum supersaturation, and the rapid precipitation of massive numbers of small crystals ($>10^6$/ml).

HETEROGENEOUS NUCLEATION

Nucleation of a less supersaturated solution can be brought about by adding particular nucleating agents such as a small amount of the same crystalline material or certain foreign substances; this process is called *heterogeneous nucleation* (see Figure 4, bottom). It is easy to understand nucleation if the nuclei added are only small crystals of the same material. These crystals act as centres of growth. In fact, the number of larger crystals formed is essentially equal to the number of small crystal nuclei added. They are effective nuclei which permit crystallization at very low levels of supersaturation. However, many foreign substances will also act as nuclei. For instance, small amounts of crystalline platinum are very effective nucleating agents for crystallization of tin, virtually preventing undercooling[12]. It is well known that dust can nucleate supersaturated salt solutions. However, the situation in which a

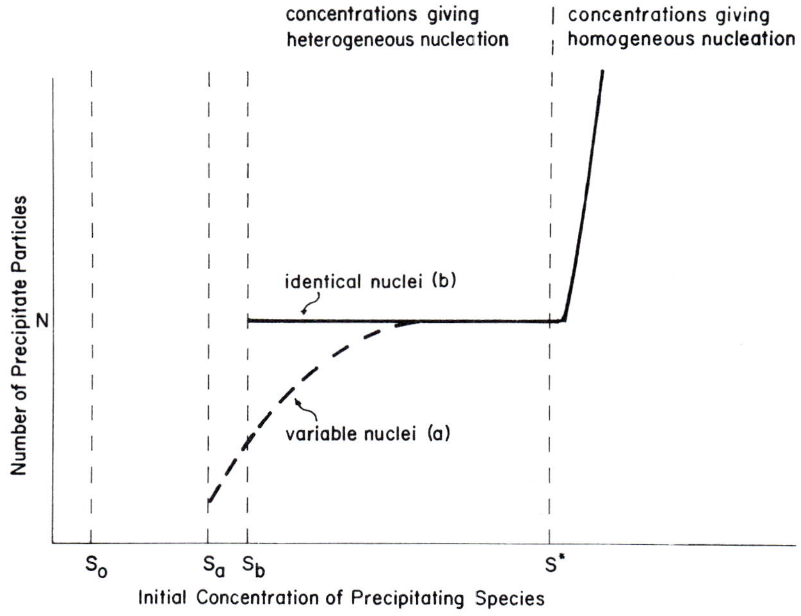

Figure 5 Heterogeneous nucleation from identical nuclei and variable nuclei. A number of precipitate particles are represented on the vertical axis, and the initial concentration of the precipitating species on the horizontal axis. S_o represents the true absolute solubility of the precipitating species, and S^* represents the concentration at which homogeneous nucleation occurs. Heterogeneous nucleation may occur between these two concentrations. If *n* identical nuclei are introduced into the solution, then provided the supersaturation reaches the critical level S_b, *n* particles of precipitate will form around each nuclei. The number of particles is constant over the nucleating range (b). The nucleation depends upon the degree of supersaturation, but not on the number of particles. If variable nuclei, each with different capacity to nucleate, are added (curve a), then those with the greatest capacity to nucleate will do so at very low supersaturations, i.e. at point S_a, and those which are less efficient at nucleation will nucleate at higher levels of supersaturation; thus the number of particles will vary with the concentration at which the precipitating species is introduced (along curve a). (Adapted from ref. 13, with permission)

single species of identical nuclei is used and that in which variable nuclei (such as dust) are used produce different results (see Figure 5).

The effectiveness of nucleation of foreign substances varies. Some will nucleate nearly as effectively as native crystals, that is, at low supersaturation; while others nucleate only at higher levels of supersaturation. In part, the effectiveness depends on the 'lattice match'. That is, if the molecular surface of the foreign material is highly matched to the crystal of the material to be precipitated, molecules will adsorb at low levels of supersaturation, align along the similar lattice and crystallize at the surface. *The greater the lattice mismatch, the higher the level of supersaturation necessary to indicate nucleation.* The characteristics of heterogeneous nucleation are: requires particles of considerable size (100–1000 Å dia.), always occurs at supersaturation levels less than that causing homogeneous nucleation, the number of crystals formed is about equal to the number of nuclei (but see Figure 3), and the effectiveness of foreign nuclei is related to their molecular structure.

To complicate the problem there are also molecules which may act as anti-nucleating agents even in small concentrations. In the absence of heterogeneous nucleation these molecules in some way prevent critical-sized nuclei from forming, and thus extend maximum supersaturation. They may also interact with potential nucleating agents binding to the active surface and thus prevent or retard heterogeneous nucleation. Small peptides and proteins are putative anti-nucleating agents for certain inorganic crystallization.

CRYSTAL GROWTH

Once nucleation occurs crystal growth follows. The rate at which crystals grow depends on a number of factors within a given system; the following promote growth:

(a) a large area of surface available for growth;
(b) a rapid movement or diffusion of molecules to the surface;
(c) a facile re-orientation at the surface;
(d) a large driving energy for crystallization, that is, a large difference in free energy between the molecule in the dissolved state and in the crystal;
(e) and a high degree of supersaturation.

The cholesterol monohydrate crystal structure as defined by Craven[15] is a crystal in which tilted bilayers of cholesterol molecules are hydrogen bonded to a layer of water (see Figure 6). The molecules pack side to side along their long axes with their hydroxyl groups and in a plane and their isopentyl tails in a parallel plane displaced about one molecular length. The surfaces on which rapid growth occurs are those surfaces in which the molecules come together side by side rather than end to end, such as the face shown in Figure 6. Roughly equally rapid rates of growth occur along the two faces intersecting at angles of 79.2 and 100.8°[16] while growth along the face roughly perpendicular to the molecular axis is many times slower (see Figure 4, above). This gives rise to the flat plate-like parallelogram, cholesterol monohydrate crystals (shown in Figure 2).

As there are nucleating and anti-nucleating agents, there are also agents

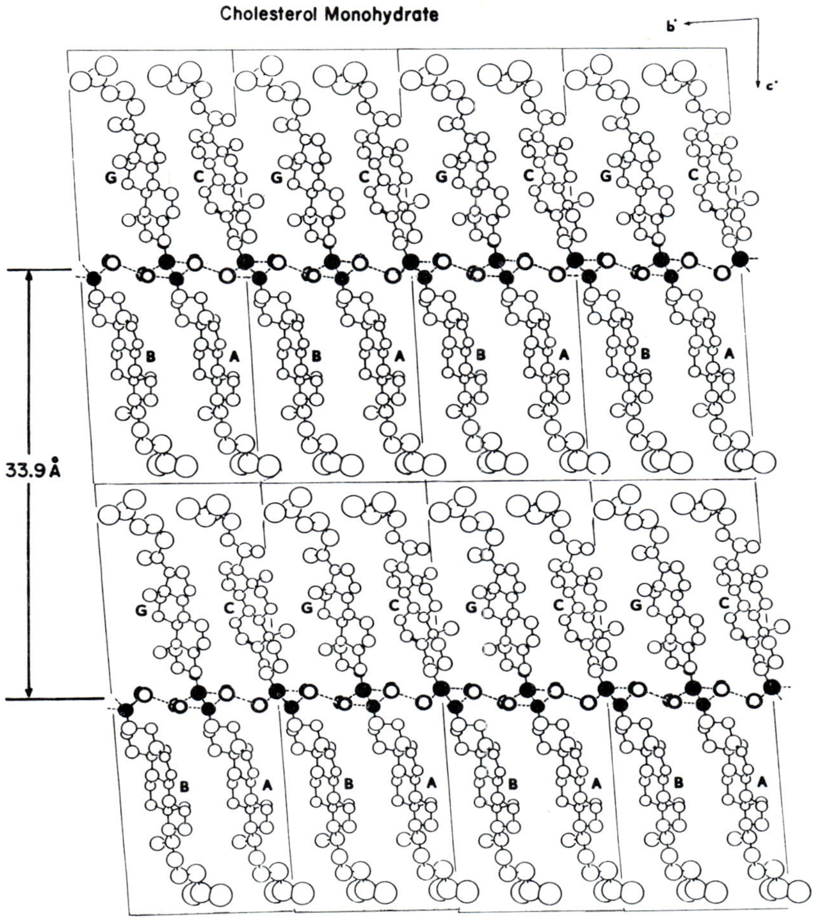

Figure 6 One of the faces of the cholesterol monohydrate crystal showing the bilayered packing of the molecules in the crystalline lattice. The black dots show the oxygens of the cholesterol molecules and the heavier circles show the oxygens of the water molecules hydrogen-bonded to the oxygen to the cholesterol. The repeat spacing along this plane is 33.9 Å (redrawn from ref. 15, with permission)

which can potentiate or slow growth. Potentiating materials cause defects in the crystal which allow new surface to form. Anti-crystallizing materials interfere with the growing surface and thus slow or prevent growth. Certain substances may adsorb only to one face of a crystal, allowing other more slowly growing faces to grow relatively more rapidly. This gives the crystal a different morphology; for instance, needles instead of plates.

BILE AND NUCLEATION

In the context of human bile and cholesterol gallstones, there is no doubt that bile can be highly supersaturated, but not contain microscopically visible crystals. Much has been made of the metastable (very slow crystallization) and labile (rapid crystallization) zones of crystallization as determined by Carey and me[5], as illustrated in Figure 7. However, some cautions must be expressed. Our studies were carried out in bile salt–lecithin–cholesterol model systems and not in native bile. It is certain that these systems were not entirely dust-free and that exogenous nucleating agents were undoubtedly present. It is known that the common source of nuclei is the solvent. In fact, the number of nuclei is roughly proportional to the volume of solvent[13]. However, the solutes, glassware, adjacent glass, stirrers, etc, may all provide nucleating agents. Thus, nucleation must have occurred at much lower levels of supersaturation than would be expected for homogeneous nucleation. Therefore the metastable and labile zones only apply to our model system[5] and not necessarily to native bile.

Thus, according to Walton[13] homogeneous nucleation of cholesterol from ethanol–H_2O occurs at a supersaturation ratio of about 13; that is, 13 times greater than true solubility. Thus, I suspect that homogeneous nucleation of

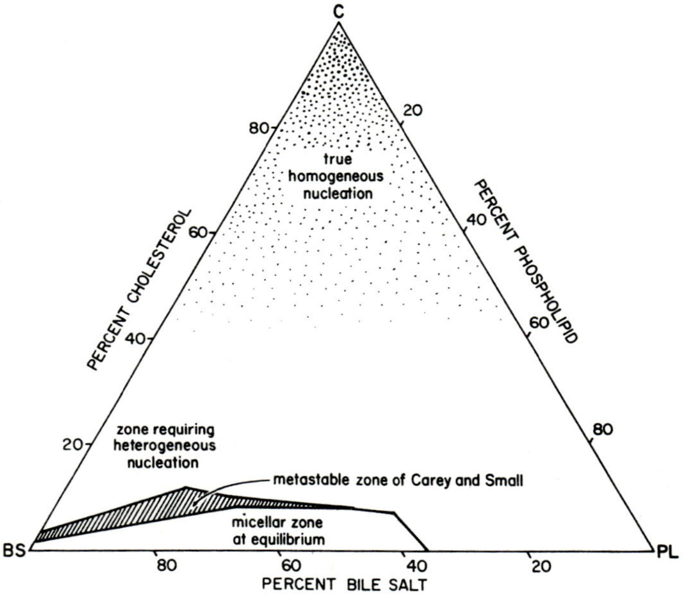

Figure 7 The sodium taurocholate–phospholipid–cholesterol system at 10% solids according to Carey and Small[5]. The micellar zone at equilibrium is shown at the bottom. Just above the metastable zone, which did not nucleate readily after several hours, is shown. Carey and Small implied that homogeneous nucleation occurred above this zone[5] but, as discussed in the text, it is probable that the zone requiring heterogeneous nucleation extends well above the metastable zone, and that true homogeneous nucleation only occurs at very high levels of supersaturation. While the exact level at which homogeneous nucleation occurs is not known, it is probably higher than the saturation ratio, S* (concentration at homogeneous nucleation ÷ concentration at true saturation) of 3 (i.e. 300% saturated), and could be as high as 13, as appears to be the case for cholesterol crystallization from supersaturated solutions in ethanol–water systems[13]

(Small (1981))

cholesterol from bile occurs only at very high supersaturation, for example above a saturation ratio of 3 (> 300% saturation). Thus, given the measured levels of supersaturation (< 300%), heterogeneous nucleation and conditions favourable for growth must be necessary for cholesterol crystal formation in bile (see Figure 7). Heterogeneous nucleation requires relatively large particles as nuclei. The liver may secrete some protein and glycoproteins which are probably not large enough to act as nuclei. Therefore, such *nuclei must form in, or be introduced into, bile.* Under certain circumstances particulate material may form in bile as a result of abnormal secretion or precursors and physicochemical changes occurring subsequently in bile. For example, pigments precipitate with calcium as a result of excessive secretion of unconjugated pigments. In the gallbladder, mucus may coagulate to form a lattice for nucleation[17], or calcium and fatty acid may precipitate to form nuclei of calcium soaps. External particles including bacteria may be introduced from the duodenum, especially after surgical intervention. In fact, many cholesterol monohydrate stones contain potential nucleating agents such as bile acids[18], bile pigments and bacteria[19], mucoid material[20], calcium soaps[21], and carbonates[22].

In addition to the concept that normal bile can be highly supersaturated and requires heterogeneous nuclei to initiate the physical stage, other possible explanations for the high supersaturation without microscopically visible crystals in subjects without stones include:

(a) the presence of an anti-nucleating agent(s) in supersaturated bile which prevent nucleation;
(b) the presence of anti-growth agent(s) (i.e. submicroscopic crystals have been nucleated but do not grow because of an anti-growth factor(s)), and
(c) the absence of anti-nucleating or anti-growth agents in the bile of gallstone patients.

In the future nucleating and growth factors must be understood.

Acknowledgments

This work was supported by Research Grants HL18623, HL12362, and Training Grant HL07291 from the National Institutes of Health, United States Public Health Service.

References

1. Bogren, H. and Larsson, K. (1963). An x-ray diffraction study of crystalline cholesterol in some pathological deposits in man. *Biochim. Biophys. Acta*, **75**, 65
2. Admirand, W. H. and Small, D. M. (1968). The physico-chemical basis of cholesterol gallstone formation in man. *J. Clin. Invest.*, **47**, 1045
3. Small, D. M. (1974). Management of gallstones particularly the silent variety: advantages of a varied and individualized approach. In Ingelfinger, F. J., Ebert, R. B., Finland, M. and Relman, A. S. (eds.). *Controversy in Internal Medicine*, pp. 545–559. (Philadelphia: W. B. Saunders)
4. Shaffer, E. A. and Small, D. M. (1976). Gallstone disease: pathogenesis and management. In Ravitch, M. M.. Austen, W. G., Scott, H. W., Jnr., Fonakalsrud, E. W., Polk,

H. C., Jnr. and Steichen, F. M. (eds). *Current Problems in Surgery*, Vol. XIII, No. 7, pp. 1–72. (Chicago: Year Book Medical Publishers)

5. Carey, M. C. and Small, D. M. (1978). The physical chemistry of cholesterol solubility in bile: relationship to gallstone formation and dissolution in man. *J. Clin. Invest.*, **61,** 998
6. Sampliner, R. E., Bennett, P. H., Comess, L. J., *et al.* (1970). Gallbladder disease in Pima Indians. *N. Engl. J. Med.*, **283,** 1358
7. Bennion, L. J., Knowler, W. C., Mott, D. M., Spagnola, A. M. and Bennett, P. H. (1979). Development of lithogenic bile during puberty in Pima Indians. *N. Engl. J. Med.*, **300,** 873
8. Thistle, J. L. and Schoenfield, L. J. (1971). Lithogenic bile among young Indian women: lithogenic potential disease with chenodeoxycholic acid. *N. Engl. J. Med.*, **284,** 177
9. Small, D. M. (1972). Current concepts of the etiology of gallstones. Implications and therapy. *Postgrad. Med.*, **51,** 187
10. Small, D. M., Dowling, R. H. and Redinger, R. N. (1972). The enterohepatic circulation of bile salts. *Arch. Intern. Med.*, **130,** 552
11. Sedaghat, S. and Grundy, S. M. (1980). Cholesterol crystals and the formation of cholesterol gallstones. *N. Engl. J. Med.*, **302,** 1274
12. Ubbelohde, A. R. (1965). *Melting and Crystal Structure*. (Oxford: Clarendon Press)
13. Walton, A. G. (1967). In Elving, P. J. and Kolthoff, J. M. (eds). *The Formation and Properties of Precipitates*. Vol. 23. (New York: Interscience Publishers)
14. Small, D. M. (1980). Cholesterol nucleation and growth in gallstone formation. *N. Engl. J. Med.*, **302,** 1305
15. Craven, B. M. (1976). Crystal structure of cholesterol monohydrate. *Nature* (*London*), **260,** 727
16. Loomis, C. R., Shipley, G. G. and Small, D. M. (1978). The phase behaviour of hydrated cholesterol. *J. Lipid Res.*, **20,** 525
17. Lee, S. P., LaMont, J. T. and Carey, M. C. (1980). The prevention of cholesterol (CH) gallstones with aspirin (ASA). *Gastroenterology*, **78,** 1205 (abstr.)
18. Schoenfield, L. J., Sjövall, J. and Sjövall, K. (1966). Bile acid composition of gallstones from man. *J. Lab. Clin. Med.*, **68,** 1856
19. Rains, A. J. H. (1964). *Gallstones: Causes and Treatment*. (Springfield: Thomas)
20. Womack, N. A. (1971). The development of gallstones. *Surg. Gynaecol. Obstet*, **133,** 973
21. Cowie, A. G. A., Sutor, D. J., Wooley, S. E. *et al.* (1973). The calcium palmitate gallstone. *Br. J. Surg.*, **60,** 16
22. Sutor, D. J. and Wooley, S. E. (1971). A statistical survey of the composition of gallstones in eight countries. *Gut*, **12,** 55

Discussion

Dr Kern I correctly anticipated that Drs Hofmann and Small would not leave me much to say about staging of gallstone disease, and therefore I will not talk about staging in gallstone disease. I would like to concentrate a little bit on what I think are the key problems that we do not know much about in the pathogenesis of gallstones and gallstone disease, and the major directions for research in the future, some of which has already been covered.

I would like to emphasize and stress the importance of real time ultrasound as a major technological advance which will now, I believe, allow us to learn about the natural history of gallstone disease, that is to acquire information that was impossible to acquire by oral cholecystography or other means. This equipment is portable, the resolution that one gets is extremely good and the stones can be detected, as small as 1 mm. The patients can now be followed to determine the rate of growth of those stones, to determine whether they shrink in size, whether they disappear and in short to acquire information about the natural history of the so-called silent gallstones, information that was not available to us before.

We know very little about the factors that are responsible for the increasing incidence of gallstones with age. We are just beginning to learn something about the factors responsible for predominance in females or the males, we still do not know whether there are hereditary factors that are important, we know little about diet except that patients who eat a high calorie, high cholesterol diet are more prone to get gallstones, but again there may be other factors involved in such patients. We know, thanks to Scott Grundy and his colleagues, quite a bit about the pathogenesis of stones in obesity and we are trying to learn something about stones in pregnancy. But I stress the large areas of gaps of our knowledge.

On the subject of supersaturated bile, it is worth mentioning that in every study supersaturated bile is found in the gallbladder after an overnight fast in normal people. We believe that patients with gallstones have bile which is more supersaturated and which is supersaturated for a longer period of time. I think that it is probably true but I wonder if the data in support of that are really adequate.

The hepatic contribution to the pathogenesis of gallstones is the secretion of supersaturated bile, and the contribution of the gallbladder is the nucleation of bile, precipitation of crystals, and retention of crystals. Growth of crystals and growth of stones are brand new areas that we need to learn a great deal more about. I call your attention to the important work that is coming from Dr Carey's laboratory, which strongly suggests that at least in the prairie dog model the secretion of supersaturated bile itself has an effect on gallbladder function. Once again I have tried to emphasize areas for research in the future that I think we need for a thorough understanding of the pathogenesis and staging of gallstone disease.

Dr Schersten In the discussion of the change from the chemical to the physical stage of gallstone disease it is very important to take into account the diurnal variation of the bile composition. I think that most of us in the morning have a supersaturated bile (with the possible exception of those days when we are eating continuously) but in the rest of the day, there is high variation between individuals and many factors can influence the diurnal variation. The partition between the gallbladder and the intestine for instance, and the ability of the gallbladder to respond to different types of stimuli are examples. I think that diurnal variation may be of considerable importance to the interval between the chemical and the physical stage in the development of gallstones.

Dr Hofmann I think that the literature is not as clear as it might be, in my opinion. What we have in the morning emerging from the liver is bile which is close to supersaturated; what is in the gallbladder in the majority of the young population is unsaturated because it was stored there after the evening meal. One thing that Dr Kern did not discuss and I do not know how he feels about it, is whether the healthy gallbladder makes the bile better. Does the healthy gallbladder desaturate bile by absorbing cholesterol? My opinion is that it does, based on the study of Duane and Bennion. So my opinion is that actually one of the steps in developing gallbladder disease, or one of the advanced steps may be cholecystitis so that the gallbladder never improves bile composition.

Dr Begemann I would just like to say that I think that the study of Duane and Bennion showing cholesterol absorption from the gallbladder is terribly important, but as far as I know, it has not been confirmed and I think it is an area that needs to be investigated further.

Dr Hofmann What Duane and Bennion showed was that after a 5-days fast bile was less saturated in, I think, five out of seven individuals. Now whether those two people are going to be the people that get gallstones, and the other five are not, we do not know. We certainly need much more information on that kind of study.

Dr Paumgartner Is there direct evidence that cholesterol can be absorbed by the normal human gallbladder?

Dr Hofmann I am not aware of any such studies, maybe Dr Small will be.

Dr Small Neiderhiser and Roth looked years ago for that, but they really could not show it. They could show that lecithin was absorbed and some fatty acids, and way back people showed that an inflamed gallbladder absorbed bile salts. One thing I would like to point out though is the study by Carey on cholesterol solubility which he did when he was with me. He showed that if you have more concentrated bile, you can get more cholesterol in solution. We do not really know just how concentrated the early morning bile is. In some surgical patients it rises to 25% solids, whereas the bile that is coming out from the liver is much more dilute, The mixture of these two biles in the gallbladder and how they behave is still a mystery.

Dr Paumgartner We must now stop the discussion about absorption of cholesterol from the gallbladder. I take it from what was said here that we do not have hard evidence that the normal gallbladder can or does absorb cholesterol.

Dr Thistle I would like to ask a question of Dr Small. The subject of prophylaxis of gallstones I think will be a more important subject at future Falk meetings, because perhaps half of the patients who acquire dissolution may have a recurrence. With regard to nucleation and the rate of precipitation, is it likely that one may be able to accomplish prophylaxis by bringing the bile saturation just down close to the saturation line? And also, are patients who have a sufficient nidus to facilitate precipitation or who still have a little bit of debris after

SLCG RIA

**(Sulfolithocholylglycine Radioimmunoassay)
Diagnostic Kit**

This radioactive material may be received, acquired, possessed, and used only by physicians, clinical laboratories, blood banks or hospitals and only for *in vitro* clinical or laboratory tests not involving internal or external administration of the material, or the radiation therefrom, to human beings or animals. Its receipt, acquisition, possession, use, and transfer are subject to the regulations and a general license, or a specific license, of the regulatory authorities of the user's country.
ABBOTT Laboratories

Name and Intended Use
ABBOTT Laboratories' SLCG RIA Diagnostic Kit is a method for the quantitative measurement of total circulating serum sulfolithocholic acid conjugates.

Summary and Explanation of the Test
Sulfolithocholic acid conjugates (SLCG) are secondary bile acids which circulate in human serum bound to albumin. This test system (radioimmunoassay) is designed to measure the concentration of SLCG in human serum. The assay is standardized against sulfolithocholylglycine (SLCG) and results are reported as SLCG.

Radioimmunoassay has been applied in various forms to the measurement of bile acids including SLCG[1-5]. The major differences are in the methods of extraction of the bile acids from serum binding proteins (albumin) and in techniques of separating the free or unbound bile acid from the bile acid which is bound to antibody during an incubation period. This test system is stabilized to extract SLCG from its binding proteins. The SLCG antibody complex is precipitated by addition of polyethylene glycol (PEG) and separated from the free (unbound) SLCG by centrifugation.

The two primary bile acids in humans, cholic acid and chenodeoxycholic acid, are formed from cholesterol by the hepatic cells and are excreted into the bile as conjugates of taurine and glycine.[6] The bile acid (or salt) conjugates are stored in the gallbladder in the fasting state and then enter the duodenum upon stimulation from food in the stomach. The bile salts accelerate lipolysis and promote solubilization and absorption of fatty acids and monoglycerides. The secondary bile salts are formed from bacterial dehydroxylation in the intestines. The two secondary bile salts found in greatest amounts are deoxycholate (from cholate) and lithocholate (from chenodeoxycholate). Sulfated esters of the bile acids are also formed in the liver cells and all of the bile acids in their various chemical states participate in the enterohepatic circulation. Demers and Hepner[7] have reported that serum bile acid levels, particularly sulfolithocholylglycine, are a very sensitive index of hepatic cell dysfunction. In a series of 110 patients with liver disease (alcoholic cirrhosis, hepatitis, cholestasis, and hepatic malignancy), SLCG was elevated in all patients, even though bilirubin, SGOT and alkaline phosphatase levels were normal in 14.

Chemical and Biological Principles of the Procedure
The following competitive reactions describe the radioimmunoassay procedure:

$$\begin{array}{lcl} \text{SLCG} & & \rightleftharpoons \text{SLCG} \cdot \text{Antibody} \\ & + \text{Antibody} & \\ {}^{125}\text{I-SLCG} & & \rightleftharpoons {}^{125}\text{I-SLCG} \cdot \text{Antibody} \end{array}$$

SLCG, whether radiolabeled or not, will bind to specific antiserum. In a mixture of both types of SLCG (^{125}I-SLCG and SLCG), each will be bound to a limited amount of antiserum in proportion to its concentration in the mixture. When SLCG from blood, or a standard solution, is equilibrated with ^{125}I-SLCG and SLCG antiserum, the amount of ^{125}I-SLCG that is bound to the antiserum will be inversely proportional to the amount of nonradioactive SLCG present in the sample or standard solution. By separating the antiserum complex from unbound SLCG and measuring the radioactivity of ^{125}I-SLCG bound in the complex, concentrations of added SLCG can be plotted versus percent of ^{125}I-SLCG bound. The standard curve so prepared can then be used to determine the amount of SLCG in patient blood.

There are four requisites for radioimmunoassay:

1. A highly purified antigen.
2. A specific antibody (antiserum) produced by injection of that antigen into another animal species.
3. Radioactively labeled purified antigen (or antigen derivative) having appropriate specific activity.
4. A satisfactory method for the separation of the antigen-antibody complex from the free antigen.

Free antigen can be separated from antigen bound to antibody and, depending upon the method of separation, either *free* or *bound* antigen can be measured by counting the radioactivity.

SLCG RIA utilizes polyethylene glycol (PEG) to separate the bound labeled SLCG from the free SLCG. After incubation of the antigen and antibody, a standard amount of PEG is added and vigorously agitated with the mixture. Next the PEG precipitate is separated by centrifugation. The supernatant is discarded and the precipitate counted to determine the amount of ^{125}I-SLCG bound to antibody. This amount will vary *inversely* with the quantity of non-labeled antigen present in the original known or unknown mixture.

Reagents

1. ^{125}I-Sulfolithocholylglycylhistamine Reagent Solution, Phosphate Buffered Saline containing 0.75% Bovine Gamma Globulin and 0.02 *M* Sodium Salicylate. Activity: 0.50 μCi or less/ml. Preservative: 0.01% Thiomersal (mercury derivative).
2. Sulfolithocholylglycine Antiserum (Rabbit) in Phosphate Buffered Saline containing 0.75% Bovine Gamma Globulin and 0.02 *M* Sodium Salicylate. Preservative: 0.01% Thiomersal (mercury derivative).
3. Sulfolithocholylglycine Standards: 0, 10, 25, 50, 100 and 250 μg/100 ml Normal Saline containing 4% Human Serum Albumin and 1% Bovine Gamma Globulin. Preservative: 0.01% Thiomersal (mercury derivative).
4. PBS-BGG Buffer, Phosphate Buffered Saline containing 0.75% Bovine Gamma Globulin and 0.02 *M* Sodium Salicylate. Preservative: 0.01% Thiomersal (mercury derivative).
5. Polyethylene Glycol 6000, 18% Solution in 0.09 *M* Barbital Buffer.

Warnings or Precautions for Users

1. For *in vitro* Diagnostic Use.
2. Do not mix materials from different master lots.
3. Do not use kit components beyond the expiration date.
4. The general licensee shall store the by-product material until used in the original shipping container or in a container providing equivalent radiation protection.
5. The following precautions should be observed in handling radioactive material:
   a) Handling should preclude any pipetting by mouth.
   b) There should be no smoking or eating where radioactive materials are being handled.
   c) Hands should be covered with rubber gloves during and thoroughly washed after handling of radioactive materials.
   d) Spills should be wiped up quickly and thoroughly and the contaminated materials added to radioactive waste matter.
   e) Concerning the disposal of radioactive waste refer to the appropriate regulations applicable to your laboratory.

Storage Instructions

1. Store kit reagents in a refrigerator at 2° to 8°C. Do **not** freeze.
2. Protect reagents containing salicylate from direct light.

Physical, Biological or Chemical Indications of Instability or Deterioration

Precipitates in the reagent solutions and/or unusual control test results are generally considered indications of reagent instability or deterioration.

Instruments

Commercially available well scintillation counters are routinely employed to determine radioactivity. Reference to the operational manual for each counting system should be made for a description of:

1. Installation procedures and special requirements.
2. Principles of operation.
3. Performance characteristics and specifications.
4. Operating instructions.
5. Calibration procedures.
6. Operational precautions and limitations.
7. Hazards.
8. Service and maintenance information.

Specimen Collection and Preparation

At least eight hours after the patient has eaten, withdraw 2 ml of venous blood with a sterile syringe and needle, and transfer it to a regular glass test tube. Let the blood clot and separate the serum. No additives or preservatives are necessary to maintain the integrity of the specimen. All glassware or plastic material coming into contact with the specimen should be void of any residues from former specimens, reagents or cleaning compounds.

If the test is to be run within 24 hours, the serum may be stored in the refrigerator. If a longer time will elapse before performance of the test, the serum should be frozen. As in the case of most proteinaceous material, alternate freezing and thawing should be avoided. At the time the test is to be performed, the serum and all reagents should be brought to room temperature.

Procedure

Materials Provided
No. 5768, SLCG RIA Diagnostic Kit, 100 test units
Kit contains:

1 Vial (20 ml) ^{125}I-Sulfolithocholylglycylhistamine Reagent Solution. Phosphate Buffered Saline containing 0.75% Bovine Gamma Globulin and 0.02 *M* Sodium Salicylate, Activity: 0.50 μCi or less/ml. Preservative: 0.01% Thiomersal (mercury derivative).

1 Vial (20 ml) SLCG Antiserum (Rabbit) in Phosphate Buffered Saline containing 0.75% Bovine Gamma Globulin and 0.02 *M* Sodium Salicylate. Preservative: 0.01% Thiomersal (mercury derivative).

1 Vial (2.5 ml) SLCG Standard, 0 μg/100 ml Normal Saline containing 4% Human Serum Albumin and 1% Bovine Gamma Globulin. Preservative: 0.01% Thiomersal (mercury derivative).

5 Vials (0.5 ml each) SLCG Standards: 10, 25, 50, 100 and 250 μg/100 ml Normal Saline containing 4% Human Serum Albumin and 1% Bovine Gamma Globulin. Preservative: 0.01% Thiomersal (mercury derivative).

1 Vial (2.5 ml) PBS-BGG Buffer, Phosphate Buffered Saline containing 0.75% Bovine Gamma Globulin and 0.02 *M* Sodium Salicylate. Preservative: 0.01% Thiomersal (mercury derivative).

1 Bottle (200 ml) Polyethylene Glycol 6000, 18% Solution in 0.09 *M* Barbital Buffer.

No. 5768, SLCG RIA Diagnostic Kit, 300 test units
Kit contains:

3 Vials (20 ml each) ^{125}I-Sulfolithocholylglycylhistamine Reagent Solution. Phosphate Buffered Saline containing 0.75% Bovine Gamma Globulin and 0.02 *M* Sodium Salicylate, Activity: 0.50 μCi or less/ml. Preservative: 0.01% Thiomersal (mercury derivative).

3 Vials (20 ml each) SLCG Antiserum (Rabbit) in Phosphate Buffered Saline containing 0.75% Bovine Gamma Globulin and 0.02 *M* Sodium Salicylate. Preservative: 0.01% Thiomersal (mercury derivative).

2 Vials (2.5 ml each) SLCG Standard, 0 μg/100 ml Normal Saline containing 4% Human Serum Albumin and 1% Bovine Gamma Globulin. Preservative: 0.01% Thiomersal (mercury derivative).

5 Vials (0.5 ml each) SLCG Standards: 10, 25, 50, 100 and 250 μg/100 ml Normal Saline containing 4% Human Serum Albumin and 1% Bovine Gamma Globulin. Preservative: 0.01% Thiomersal (mercury derivative).

3 Vials (2.5 ml each) PBS-BGG Buffer, Phosphate Buffered Saline containing 0.75% Bovine Gamma Globulin and 0.02 *M* Sodium Salicylate. Preservative: 0.01% Thiomersal (mercury derivative).

2 Bottles (335 ml each) Polyethylene Glycol 6000, 18% Solution in 0.09 *M* Barbital Buffer.

Materials Required But Not Provided
The following generally available laboratory equipment is also required for performance of the SLCG RIA Diagnostic Test:

Test tubes – 12 x 75 mm roundbottom tubes capable of withstanding a force of 1000 x g during centrifugation
Test tube rack
Ordinary glass test tubes for collection of blood specimen
Refrigerator and freezer
Calibrated pipettes or automatic syringe to deliver 2 ml
Micropipetting device to deliver 25 μl and 200 μl
Scintillation well counter capable of counting ^{125}I
Sample mixer (Vortex, or equivalent)
Centrifuge capable of 1000 x g, swinging bucket head
Timer
Paper towels for blotting lips of test tubes after decantation
Parafilm® or equivalent for covering test tubes during incubation
Waterbath capable of maintaining 37° ± 2°C

SLCG RIA Test Procedure

A Standard Curve *must* be prepared each time that a group of unknown samples is assayed.

Caution:

Precision pipetting can be achieved only when all reagents and unknowns are at the same temperature (room temperature). Time intervals between steps are critical. When samples are processed in groups, best results are obtained when the first and last samples in the group are separated by no more than 10 minutes.

1. Bring all test kit reagents to room temperature including the polyethylene glycol reagent and the serum samples.
2. Label tubes for performance of the test as follows:
   a) Tubes 1 and 2, labeled TCT (Total Count Tubes), will contain aliquots of the ^{125}I-Sulfolithocholylglycylhistamine Reagent Solution. These are to be used in determination of total radioactivity.
   b) Tubes 3 and 4 are to be used to detect Nonspecific Binding (NSB) if this determination is to be made.
   c) Tubes 5 through 16 are standards from which the standard curve is prepared.
   Tubes 5 and 6, 0 μg/100 ml SLCG
   Tubes 7 and 8, 10 μg/100 ml SLCG
   Tubes 9 and 10, 25 μg/100 ml SLCG
   Tubes 11 and 12, 50 μg/100 ml SLCG
   Tubes 13 and 14, 100 μg/100 ml SLCG
   Tubes 15 and 16, 250 μg/100 ml SLCG
   d) Tubes 17, etc. are for unknown samples in duplicate.
3. a) Pipette 25 μl of SLCG Standards into appropriately labeled tubes 5 through 16.
   b) Pipette 25 μl of unknown samples into properly identified tubes beginning with 17.
   c) Pipette 25 μl SLCG Standard, 0 μg/100 ml, and 200 μl PBS-BGG Buffer into tubes 3 and 4 (NSB).
4. Pipette 200 μl ^{125}I-Sulfolithocholylglycylhistamine Reagent Solution into all tubes. Mix on sample mixer 3 to 5 seconds, or shake the test tube rack manually.
5. Carefully and without delay, pipette 200 μl SLCG Antiserum (Rabbit) into all tubes except 1 through 4. Mix on sample mixer 3 to 5 seconds, or shake the test tube rack manually.
6. Cover all tubes with Parafilm or equivalent and incubate at 37° ± 2°C for one hour.
7. After incubation, pipette 2 ml Polyethylene Glycol Solution into all tubes except 1 and 2 (Total Count Tubes). Total elapsed time for PEG addition should not exceed 10 minutes. Mix vigorously on sample mixer for 5 seconds.
8. Immediately (within 15 minutes after PEG addition) centrifuge tubes containing PEG for 10 minutes at room temperature at 1000 x g.
9. Remove tubes carefully from centrifuge (not disturbing the precipitate). Decant the supernatant solution and blot the lip of the tube on absorbent paper.
10. Count the radioactivity remaining in each tube including TCT (1 and 2) for a minimum of one minute each. If necessary, subtract background and record as net cpm.
11. For calculations, see **Results** section.

The final reaction material in the SLCG RIA test is the PEG precipitate which contains both radioactive and nonradioactive antibodybound SLCG. After incubation, centrifugation and decantation, the tubes should be counted as soon as practicable.

Satisfactory results will depend on many factors, including accuracy of pipetting, equilibration of reagents, temperature control, careful timing, proper storage and control of reagents. Any foreign substances on the glassware or plastic materials may affect protein binding when in contact with the specimens. The efficiency of the counting instruments should be reconfirmed in case of unsatisfactory results in testing.

Duplicate determinations should be performed with each patient's specimen until experience proves it no longer necessary.

Dilution Factor

Values greater than 250 μg/100 ml require repeat testing. Start with a dilution of at least 1:4 of the unknown serum in the 0 μg/100 ml standard solution. Multiply the results found for the diluted specimen by the dilution factor when reporting the results.

Results

Rectilinear Method

1. Calculate mean value for the duplicates of TCT.
2. Calculate the percentage of ^{125}I-SLCG bound to antiserum in the PEG precipitate as follows:

$$\frac{\text{cpm precipitate (Standard)}}{\text{cpm TCT}} \times 100$$
= % Bound (Standard)

$$\frac{\text{cpm precipitate (Unknown)}}{\text{cpm TCT}} \times 100$$
= % Bound (Unknown)

3. On rectilinear graph paper, plot the % Bound for each SLCG Standard on the vertical (Y) axis vs. the corresponding SLCG concentration on the horizontal (X) axis. Using these points, draw the best fit smooth curve.
4. To determine the concentration of serum SLCG in unknown samples, extend a horizontal line from the calculated % Bound found on the Y axis to the curve. At the point of intersection, extend a vertical line to the X axis and read the corresponding SLCG value for the unknown.

Log-Logit Method

1. The average cpm for the SLCG Standard, 0 μg/100 ml, is designated B_0. Calculate the Logit percentage (B/B_0) of ^{125}I-SLCG bound to antiserum in the PEG precipitate as follows:

$$\frac{\text{cpm precipitate (Standard)}}{\text{cpm } B_0} \times 100$$
= % B/B_0 for Standard

$$\frac{\text{cpm precipitate (Unknown)}}{\text{cpm } B_0} \times 100$$
= % B/B_0 for Unknown

2. On Log-Logit paper, construct a standard curve by plotting % B/B_0 for each of the standards on the vertical (Y) axis vs. the corresponding SLCG concentration on the horizontal (X) axis. Note that on log-logit paper, the first standard value is 10 μg/100 ml, **not zero**. The 0 μg/100 ml standard is provided for determination of % B/B_0, NSB and dilution of patient specimens. Construct the best single straight line through the points.
3. To determine the concentration of SLCG in unknown samples, find the calculated % B/B_0 on the Y axis and extend a horizontal line to the curve. At the point of intersection, extend a vertical line to the X axis and read the corresponding SLCG value for the unknown. Specimens with SLCG levels less than 10 μg/100 ml should be reported as normal.

Example: Assume the following values for standards and unknowns "A" and "B".

SLCG RIA Worksheet

Tube Number	Sample Identity	cpm	% Bound	Average % Bound	% B/B_0	Average % B/B_0	SLCG (μg/100 ml)
1	TCT	35714	–				
2		35338	–				
	Average	35526					
3	NSB	4185	11.8	11.6	19.4	19.0	
4		4035	11.4		18.7		
5	0 μg/100 ml	21713	61.1	60.6	100	100	
6		21343	60.1		100		
7	10 μg/100 ml	16803	47.3	47.9	78.0	79.0	
8		17211	48.5		79.9		
9	25 μg/100 ml	14452	40.7	40.2	67.1	66.3	
10		14093	39.7		65.5		
11	50 μg/100 ml	11448	32.2	31.4	53.2	51.9	
12		10900	30.7		50.6		
13	100 μg/100 ml	8660	24.4	24.5	40.2	40.4	
14		8740	24.6		40.6		
15	250 μg/100 ml	6284	17.7	17.0	29.2	27.9	
16		5789	16.3		26.6		
17	"A"	9347	26.3	26.2	43.4	43.3	78.8
18		9248	26.1		43.2		
19	"B"	7501	21.1	21.1	34.8	34.8	155.0
20		7480	21.0		34.7		

See examples of Standard Curves, pages 7 and 8.

Limitations of the Procedure

For diagnostic purposes, the SLCG concentration should be used merely as an adjunct to other data (e.g., symptoms, results of other tests, clinical impressions, etc.) available to the physician.

Post-prandial studies carried out at ABBOTT Laboratories on 20 normal subjects indicate that SLCG values may be elevated for at least four hours after eating. Values rose to a maximum within one hour and declined to their original values by eight hours. Therefore, it is necessary to draw the blood specimen from fasting patients (at least eight hours after eating).

Serum SLCG values from patients with various non-liver illnesses were obtained in several clinical studies. The results indicated that 95% of these SLCG values were within the normal range.

It was determined in a study at ABBOTT Laboratories that certain anticoagulants might interfere with the SLCG RIA test by lowering the SLCG level in serum. These anticoagulants are: sodium citrate, sodium oxalate, acid citrate dextrose, EDTA and possibly heparin. In these studies heparin did not lower SLCG levels in plasma, but since it is an anticoagulant, caution is advised.

Expected Values

Based upon data derived from several investigations, the normal range (mean ± 2 standard deviations) is 0.0 to 80.0 μ g/100 ml.

Note:

The above normal range is merely a suggested normal range. Each laboratory should ascertain the range of normal values appropriate to the population it serves.

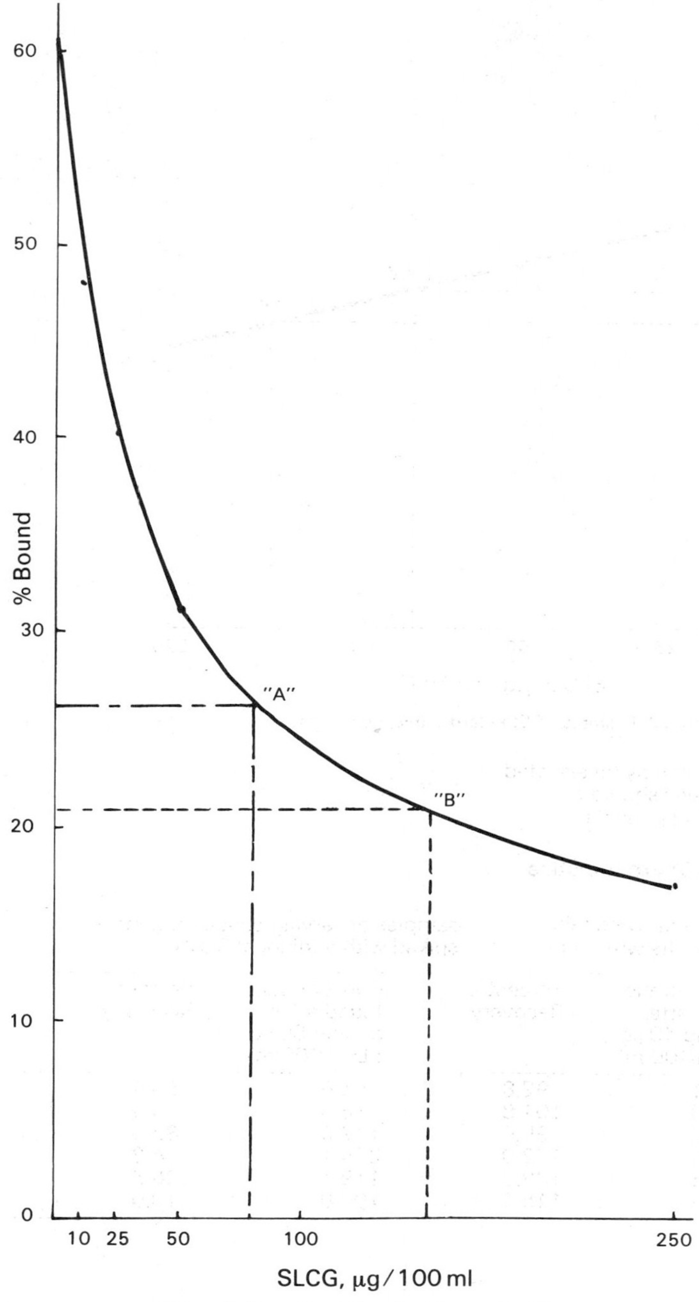

Figure 1. Example of Standard Curve, Rectilinear

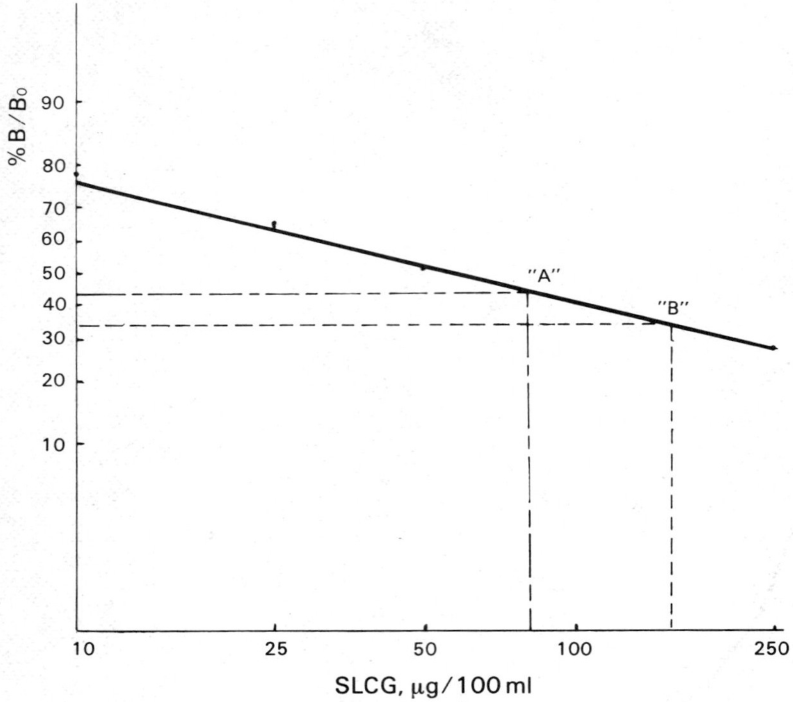

Figure 2. Example of Standard Curve, Log-Logit

Since SLCG concentration may be elevated after eating, the specimens should be obtained only from fasting patients.

Specific Performance Characteristics

Accuracy:
Recovery Studies – The following table summarizes recovery results when six samples of varying concentrations were spiked with additional SLCG.

Initial SLCG Concentration (μg/100 ml)	Concentration found after adding 40 μg SLCG/100 ml	Percent Recovery	Concentration found after adding 80 μg SLCG/100 ml	Percent Recovery
10.0	47.1	92.8	81.6	89.5
39.1	79.8	101.8	116.3	96.5
81.2	119.2	95.0	147.6	83.0
157.7	198.5	102.0	225.1	84.2
33.8	77.5	109.2	119.1	106.6
19.1	65.3	115.0	107.0	110.0

Precision:
The precision of the SLCG RIA test was evaluated by assaying a panel of four serum pools in replicates of ten on three consecutive occasions using one lot of material. Three estimates of the variability of the assay were computed: Inter-assay (between), Intra-assay (within) and Total variability. $\bar{\bar{x}}$ is defined as the grand mean over the three occasions of testing.

Precision Studies

SLCG Concentration (μg/100 ml)

Sample Identification	$\bar{\bar{x}}$	Inter-assay* S. D.	Inter-assay* % C.V.	Intra-assay** S. D.	Intra-assay** % C.V.	Total Assay*** S. D.	Total Assay*** % C.V.
SA-2	10.8	1.5	13.9	0.9	8.3	1.6	14.8
SB-2	43.3	1.8	4.2	2.2	5.0	2.5	5.8
SC-2	81.4	1.2	1.5	2.7	3.3	2.9	3.6
SD-2	147.1	0.1	0.1	6.4	4.3	6.2	4.2

* Measure of the variation of the means of the assays.
** Based on the pooled variances of the 10 replicates for each of the 3 assays.
*** Variation of the 30 independent observations about the grand mean ($\bar{\bar{x}}$).

Specificity:
The steroidal compounds listed below were assayed using the SLCG RIA kit. The % Cross Reactivity listed in the table is the mean of the values found for the concentrations indicated.

Cross Reactivity

Compound	Concentration (μg/ml)	Mean % Cross Reactivity
Cholic acid (CA)	1, 10, 100, 1000	0
Glycocholic acid (GCA)	1, 10, 100, 1000	0
Taurocholic acid (TCA)	1, 10, 100, 1000	0
Deoxycholic acid (DCA)	1, 10, 100, 1000	0
Glycodeoxycholic acid (GDCA)	1, 10, 100, 1000	0.02
Taurodeoxycholic acid (TDCA)	1, 10, 100, 1000	0.01
Chenodeoxycholic acid (CDCA)	1, 10, 100, 1000	0.05
Glycochenodeoxycholic acid (GCDCA)	1, 10, 100, 1000	0.05
Taurochenodeoxycholic acid (TCDCA)	1, 10, 100, 1000	0.01
Lithocholic acid (LCA)	1, 10, 100, 1000	0.05
Glycolithocholic acid (GLCA)	1, 10, 100, 1000	0.40
Taurolithocholic acid (TLCA)	1, 10, 100, 1000	0.10
Sulfodeoxycholic acid (SDCA)	1, 5, 10, 20	0
Cholesterol	500, 1000, 1500, 3000	0
Testosterone	0.25, 0.5, 1.0, 2.0	0
Dehydroepiandosterone	0.25, 0.5, 1.0, 2.0	0
Progesterone	0.25, 0.5, 1.0, 2.0	0
Estradiol	0.25, 0.5, 1.0, 2.0	0
Prednisone	2.5, 5, 10, 20	0
Digoxin	0.5, 1.0, 2.0, 10	0
Digitoxin	0.5, 1.0, 2.0, 10	0
Sulfochenodeoxycholic acid (SCDCA)	1, 5, 10, 20	4.30
Sulfolithocholic acid (SLCA) (unconjugated)	0.1, 0.5, 1.0, 5.0	13.90*
Sulfolithocholyltaurine (SLCT)	10, 25, 50, 100	71.00*

* Since the SLCG RIA test measures SLCA conjugates, cross reactivity with SLCA and other conjugates is acceptable.

Drug interference was studied by performing the SLCG RIA test on normal human serum before and after the addition of various substances. The results are shown in the following table:

Substance added to Pooled Human Serum	SLCG Value (μg/100 ml) found in the presence of varying amounts of substance	
	10 μg/ml added	100 μg/ml added
Water blank	47	46
Methanol blank	44	45
Aminophylline	43	46
Amobarbital	47	47
Caffeine	46	46
Cephalothin Sodium	47	47
Chloramphenicol	45	48
Chlorpromazine	45	47
Chlorpheniramine Maleate	45	47
Codeine	47	46
Cyclamate Sodium	46	49
Diphenhydramine	51	49
Diazepam	44	47
Digitoxin	47	52
Diphenylhydantoin	47	49
Erythromycin	46	46
Furosemide	48	49
Hydrochlorthiazide	45	48
Imipramine	46	48
Indomethacin	45	47
Isoproterenol	43	47
Meprobamate	46	45
Methimazole	48	49
Methyldopa	46	47
Nicotine	46	49
Penicillin	47	48
Phenacetin	46	47
Phenobarbital	45	47
Phenylbutazone	44	49
Phenylephrine · HCl	47	49
Propylthiouracil	42	36
Ouabain	53	43
Quinine Sulfate	59	44
Saccharin Sodium	52	52
Streptomycin	50	50
Sulfadiazine	55	39
Tetracycline	53	50
Tolbutamide	55	49
Ascorbic Acid (50 μg/ml)	51	

Sensitivity:
Using the methods described by Rodbard and Lewald,[8] the sensitivity of the SLCG RIA test was found to be 2.2 μg/100 ml and the affinity constant was found to be 8.3 x 10^7 liters/mole.

Bibliography

1. Van den Berg, J. W. O., et al., Solid Phase Radioimmunoassay for Determination of Conjugated Cholic Acid in Serum, Clin. Chim. Acta 73:277-283, 1976.
2. Matern, S., Krieger, R., and Gerok, W., Radioimmunoassay of Serum Conjugated Cholic Acid, Clin. Chim. Acta 72:39-48, 1976.
3. Murphy, G. M., et al., The Preparation and Properties of an Antiserum for the Radioimmunoassay of Serum Conjugated Cholic Acid, Clin. Chim. Acta 54:81-89, 1974.
4. Schalm, S. W., et al., Diurnal Variation of Serum Bile Acids Determined by Multiple Specific Bile Acid Radioimmunoassays, Clin. Res. 23:396A, 1975.
5. Demers, L. M., and Hepner, G., Radioimmunoassay of Bile Acids in Serum, Clin. Chem. 22:602-606, 1976.
6. Javitt, N. B., Bile Acids and Hepatobiliary Disease, (in) Schiff, L., ed. "Diseases of the Liver", 4th ed. J. P. Lippincott Co., 1975, pp. 111-145.
7. Demers, L. M., and Hepner, G. W., Levels of Immunoreactive Glycine-conjugated Bile Acids in Health and Hepatobiliary Disease, Am. J. Clin. Path. 66:831-839, 1976.
8. Rodbard, S. D., and Lewald, J. E., Computer Analysis of Radioligand Assays and Radioimmunoassay Data, Karolinska Symposia, Research Methods in Reproductive Endocrinology, Geneva, March, 1970, Acta Endocr. 64: Suppl. 147, 79-103, 1970.

ABBOTT GmbH
Diagnostics Division
Postfach 1760
D-6070 Langen
West Germany

Bile Acids SLCG May 78 / 3.0 e
US-C. 05/693-5233/R1–3–REV. DEC., 1977

Printed in West Germany

gallstone dissolution more likely to get recurrences and should they be selected out as patients who should continue on prophylactic treatment?

Dr Small The closer to saturation level that you get the better. That is for certain. I think Dr Mazer and Dr Carey may have some interesting information on what urso may do to mucus, which could be a nucleating agent. But I do not have an answer to your other questions.

Dr Carey All that I can say about the cholesterol saturation of bile in relation to gallbladder mucus production is that the mucus production parallels the relative cholesterol content of the bile. When you desaturate bile, I would presume, you would decrease the gallbladder mucin production. We have shown in the prairie dog that the gallbladder mucin production is increased tenfold when bile reaches supersaturation. I would assume that with urso or with cheno, if you get desaturation, you would probably reduce the amount of mucus produced by the gallbladder.

Dr Ostrow I hate to toss in another type of gallstone but I still think that one of the biggest problems we face is, how to tell, what kind of a gallstone a patient has. I wonder whether anybody has any comment on better ways of excluding pigment gallstones and cholesterol stones with enough calcium that do not dissolve.

Dr Paumgartner In relation to this question I wondered whether the improved methods of measuring radio density by computer tomography would help. I was talking to the X-ray people in our hospital about this problem but they were not very optimistic about this approach.

Unidentified discussant We have conducted a study using CT scanning to detect calcifications or calcium contents which cannot be detected by ordinary X-ray, and we have found about 30% increase in the sensitivity by using CT scanning.

Dr Schoenfield I would like to raise what I think are two difficult questions relating to the staging of gallstone disease. To my knowledge, patients with cholesterol crystals without gallstones have not been identified. I am not aware of any patients who had cholesterol crystals without the presence of gallstones. I wonder if perhaps you might explain this for us.

The second question relates to a comment Dr Hofmann made regarding the finding of sludge in ultrasonography and the possible interpretation of sludge as cholesterol crystals. I think that there is some controversy about this interpretation. I wonder what the evidence is, that sludge does represent cholesterol crystals.

Dr Carey Could I comment that in the surgical literature you will find at least two papers in which they have looked at crystals in bile and they have equated that with biliary symptoms and there have been no stones in the gallbladder. As you know there are some people who maintain that bile crystals are an indication for cholecystectomy in the absence of stones.

Dr Schoenfield I think the papers referred to in the surgical literature are actually poorly controlled anecdotal observations. I am absolutely certain that there will be in the next year excellent data documenting crystals on duodenal drainage without gallstones as determined by cholecystectomy. The person who did it is Dr Richard Strong at the Naval Hospital in San Diego.

Dr Hofmann I think Dr Schoenfield has raised a very important point. First of all, I cannot quote accurately, but from my memory of Juniper's paper in *Gastroenterology* in 1965 the presence of microcrystals was a non-specific finding with a certain number of false positives and false negatives. Microcrystals could be present in the absence of gallstones. But I am open to correction on that.

Secondly, if we are talking about staging of disease in its relevance to prophylaxis the only way at present that we can demonstrate this is by duodenal intubation and aspiration, or perhaps by ERCP. We are surely not suggesting that this is a practical way of screening a population, so that we can decide who ought to be treated. I think we have got to attain some clinical perspective from this.

Thirdly, about a question of acalculus cholecystitis, I think Dr Noel Williams from Halifax is probably in the audience. He and his colleagues have done an extensive study on bile analysis and the phenomenon of acalculus cholecystitis. Perhaps they might offer a comment, with the chairman's permission.

I wonder if you would kindly comment on your experience of acalculus cholecystitis in the presence of microcrystals in bile or supersaturated bile as a clinical entity warranting treatment.

Dr Williams You are probably referring to the paper we did some years ago. We were looking at patients who presented with typical biliary colic and had negative cholecystograms. A lot of these patients in fact were given cholecystokinin to see whether the pain was reproduced and we had a nasal duodenal tube there at the same time. And of these patients there were a whole group of them who had cholecystitis (evidenced by, at least, fibrosis plus the usual parameters of inflammation) with subsequent cholecystectomy. Most of the ones who had cholesterolosis had supersaturated bile but no stones.

Dr Paumgartner And crystals in the bile?

Dr Williams Crystals in some but not in all.

Dr Kern To my knowledge, there is no extensive literature on the chemical composition of sludge which is seen by real-time ultrasound. There is a recent paper in the radiological literature (one of the authors is Larry Way). In the majority this sludge was calcium bilirubinate, in the minority cholesterol monohydrate. The number of patients was small and what I meant to say in my talk was that in some instances this sludge will be cholesterol monohydrate.

Dr Heaton I hope you will forgive me if I come back to this question of the effect of fasting, and particularly of absorption of cholesterol by the gallbladder. I am rather worried by the implication by Alan Hofmann that the demonstration of a fall in saturation of bile with a fast implies absorption of cholesterol. It is true that the only published evidence of this is the 5-day fast of Duane, but we have in press a paper showing that between 15 and 20 hours of fasting there is a significant drop in the cholesterol saturation of gallbladder bile. This, I think, is much too early and quick to be explained by absorption of cholesterol by the gallbladder. Our suggestion is that the gallbladder is in fact contracting and refilling during a fast and is refilling with less saturated bile because during a fast the liver gradually slows down its synthesis and secretion of cholesterol. In animal work HMG-CoA reductase activity does in fact drop at around 15 to 16 hours after fasting, and I would have thought that this was a very reasonable alternative explanation to the absorption of cholesterol.

Dr Hofmann I have not read your paper in press, but all that I really meant to say is that we need to know the effect of fasting on hepatic bile and on gallbladder bile, and that these are not necessarily the same thing. We need to define these because we have the idea that initially acute interruption of the enterohepatic circulation causes hepatic bile to become more saturated as shown by Dr Small in the monkey, by Dr Javitt and McSherry in the monkey and by Dr Grundy and his colleagues in man. But then we may have a subsequent situation in time, indeed as you say, where synthesis goes down and the hepatic bile, despite interruption becomes less saturated.

Dr Paumgartner We have to proceed to the next section of this workshop. The most important point that has emerged from this discussion in my opinion is that so far we have paid a lot of attention to cholesterol saturation of bile but did not pay enough attention to nucleation factors. Dr Small has pointed out the difference between homogeneous and heterogeneous nucleation and I learnt from his discussion that we probably have to pay attention to a number of substances which are present in bile and will influence nucleation because we are probably dealing with heterogeneous nucleation. I think we must pay more attention to crystals than to supersaturated bile. When we see crystals we must accept this as an abnormal situation, whereas when we find supersaturated bile this is not always abnormal but occurs under certain conditions such as an overnight fast also in normals.

WORKSHOP ON DISSOLUTION OF GALLSTONES

PART II
Effects of Chenodeoxycholic Acid and Ursodeoxycholic Acid on Bile Acid and Biliary Lipid Metabolism

Effects of chenodeoxycholic acid and ursodeoxycholic acid on bile acid and biliary lipid metabolism in patients with radiolucent gallstones. Correlation with efficacy and toxicity

A. STIEHL

During chenodeoxycholic acid (CDCA) treatment of patients with cholesterol gallstones several authors have observed an increase of ursodeoxycholic acid (UDCA) in bile[1,2]. In some patients, although the amount of UDCA in bile exceeded the amount of CDCA, nevertheless cholesterol gallstones dissolved[3]. Subsequently UDCA was tested for its cholesterol gallstone dissolving capacity and was found to be effective; even more important, in contrast to CDCA treatment, side-effects were not observed[4–17].

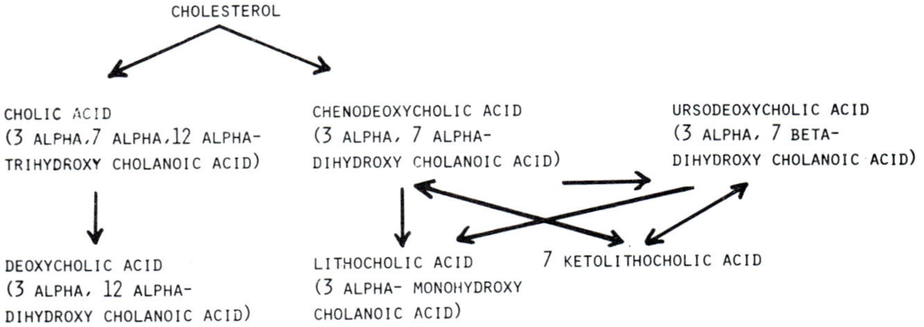

Figure 1 Metabolism of bile acids. Cholic acid and chenodeoxycholic acid are primary bile acids. Deoxycholic acid and lithocholic acid are secondary bile acids

CDCA and UDCA differ in structure only in the orientation of the hydroxyl group at the C-7 position, but administration of the two bile acids to man induces different alterations of bile acid and bile lipid metabolism[1–4,9,10,13–16,18–26].

After oral administration of a bile acid it is reabsorbed in the intestine, reaches the liver via the portal blood, is conjugated in the liver with the amino acids taurine or glycine, and is excreted into the bile. In the intestine the bile acid is subjected to bacterial degradation. The bile acids formed in the liver from cholesterol – cholic acid (CA) and chenodeoxycholic acid – thus are degradated in the intestine to the secondary bile acids deoxycholic acid (DCA) and lithocholic acid (LCA). Recent studies indicate that CDCA can not only be dehydroxylated to LCA but also to 7-ketolithocholic acid (7KLCA) (Figure 1). Most of CDCA is degraded by bacteria to LCA which in man is a biological end product; relatively little CDCA is transformed to 7KLCA which if reabsorbed, can be transformed in the liver mainly to CDCA but also to UDCA[27–30].

UDCA is degradated by bacteria in the intestine to LCA and 7KLCA acid[27,28]. Degradation of UDCA to LCA is less and formation of 7KLCA is greater than that of CDCA. 7KLCA can be transformed in the liver to CDCA and UDCA. According to Salen *et al.*[29] there is considerable evidence that CDCA can be transformed to UDCA directly. In Fromm's opinion the transformation of CDCA to UDCA requires 7KLCA as an intermediary product[30].

In a previous study[14] we investigated the effects of CDCA and UDCA in a prospective study in ten patients in which every patient served as his own control. During treatment with CDCA there were increases of LCA, LCA sulphate, CDCA and UDCA and decreases of CA and DCA. During treatment with UDCA, only this bile acid increased in bile while all other bile acids decreased. The data indicate that the amounts of UDCA in bile during UDCA treatment are considerably lower than the amounts of CDCA during CDCA treatment. The increases of UDCA and CDCA during the treatment periods, however, were comparable. Apparently both bile acids are efficiently reabsorbed in the intestine.

LCA and LCA sulphate were significantly lower during UDCA treatment than during CDCA treatment[14,15,31]. These data are in agreement with the observation that bacterial degradation of UDCA to LCA is not as effective as the degradation of CDCA to LCA[28]. Of especial interest are the amounts of unsulphated LCA, since it has hepatotoxic properties. The very small amounts of LCA formed during UDCA treatment would favour the use of this drug. The amounts of unsulphated LCA during CDCA treatment were increased[14], but were much smaller than in animals with LCA associated liver toxicity. No correlation between LCA in bile and plasma transaminases was detected. It seems unlikely therefore that the measured amounts of unsulphated LCA have liver toxic properties[32–34].

Bile acids which are reabsorbed in the intestine are transported to the liver by the portal blood. Bile acids which are not taken up by the liver appear in the peripheral blood. Therefore plasma bile acids reflect the spillover of the enterohepatic circulation. During treatment with CDCA[14] this bile acid increased in plasma from 0.9 ± 0.2 μg/ml to 1.7 ± 0.4 μg/ml. The spillover therefore was little. During treatment with UDCA this bile acid increased in plasma from less than 0.1 μg/ml to 2.5 ± 0.3 μg/ml. The greater increase of UDCA in plasma in comparison to CDCA could reflect a more slowly hepatic uptake. The measured plasma concentrations of bile acids in patients on tréatment indicate that the spillover of CDCA and UDCA into the peripheral blood is little.

Cholesterol formation in the liver is thought to be regulated by HMG-CoA reductase. All authors who studied the effect of CDCA on this enzyme agree that CDCA decreases the activity of HMG-CoA reductase[7,21,35–37]. A similar effect of UDCA was observed by some but not by all authors (Figure 2).

	CDCA	*UDCA*
HMG-CoA reductase	↓ Coyne *et al.* 1976[35]	↓ Maton *et al.* 1977[10]
	↓ Maton *et al.* 1980[21]	↓ Salen *et al.* 1980[13]
		→ Einarsson *et al.* 1980[36]
Cholesterol absorption	↓ Adler *et al.* 1975[38]	
	↓ Ponz de Leon *et al.* 1979[39]	↓ Ponz de Leon *et al.* 1980[45]
	→ Mok *et al.* 1978[40]	
	→ Tangedahl *et al.* 1979[41]	
	→ La Russo *et al.* 1980[42]	→ La Russo *et al.* 1980[42]
	→ Roda *et al.* 1980[43,44]	→ Roda *et al.* 1980[43,44]

Figure 2 Mechanism of action of CDCA and UDCA in man

CDCA and UDCA treatment decrease biliary cholesterol excretion. Besides cholesterol formation in the liver, cholesterol absorption in the intestine could also affect biliary excretion of cholesterol[38,39], but most authors agree that there is no such effect of UDCA on cholesterol absorption[40,42,43,46] (Figure 2).

During treatment with UDCA biliary cholesterol was significantly lower than during treatment with CDCA (Figure 3). Apparently, relatively low doses of UDCA effectively decrease biliary cholesterol excretion[24,47].

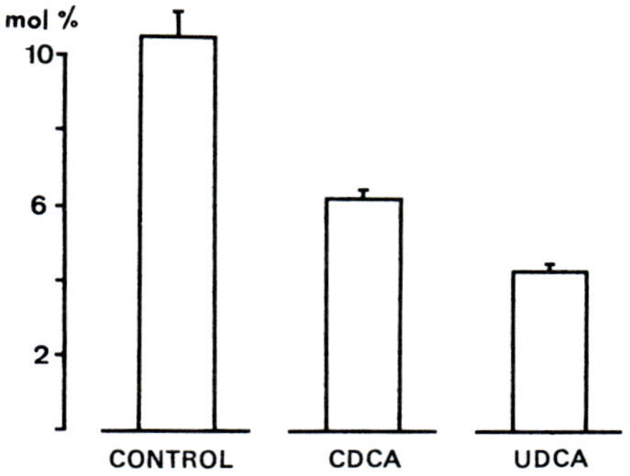

Figure 3 Effect of treatment on biliary cholesterol. (From Stiehl *et al. Gastroenterology*, **75**, 1016–1020, 1978.)

Plasma transaminases increased in four out of ten patients during treatment with CDCA but not during treatment with UDCA (Figure 4). No correlation was observed between plasma transaminases and plasma LCA concentrations (Figure 5). In contrast patients with elevated serum transaminases also had elevated plasma concentrations of CDCA (Figure 6).

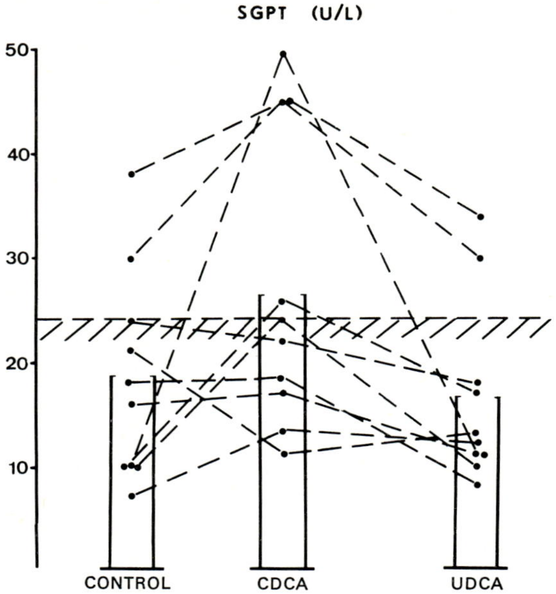

Figure 4 Serum transaminases during treatment with UDCA and CDCA

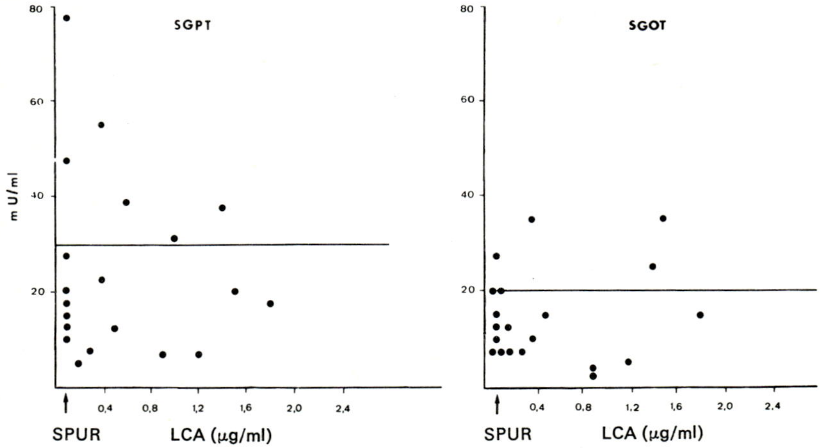

Figure 5 Correlation between LCA in plasma and SGOT and SGPT in gallstone patients on CDCA treatment. (From Stiehl *et al.*, *Inn. Med.*, **3**, 75–80, 1975.)

Recent physiocochemical studies suggest that increases of UDCA conjugates in bile may diminish the micellar capacity to dissolve cholesterol[48–50]. Especially glycine conjugated UDCA, but also taurine conjugated UDCA, forms micelles which dissolve less cholesterol than the CDCA conjugates[48,51]. Therefore glycine and taurine conjugation of UDCA was studied during UDCA treatment[15]. During treatment with UDCA the amounts of glyco-UDCA in bile were positively correlated to the dose of

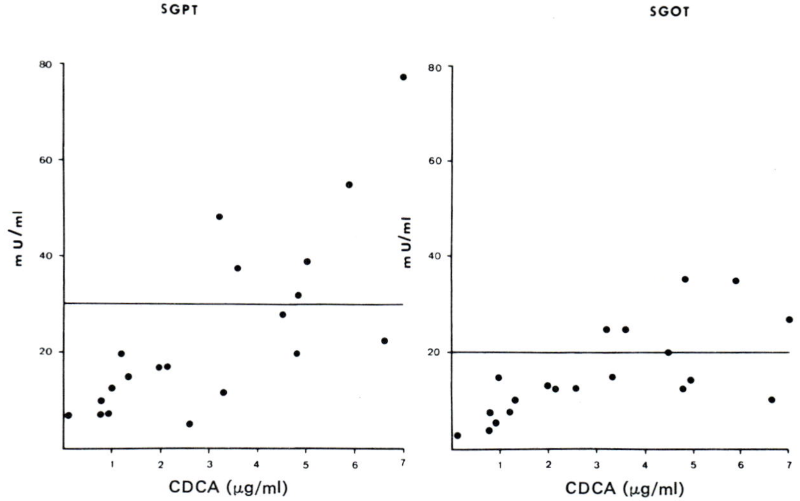

Figure 6 Correlation between CDCA in plasma and SGOT and SGPT in gallstone patients on CDCA treatment. (From Stiehl *et al.*, *Inn. Med.*, **3**, 75–80, 1975.)

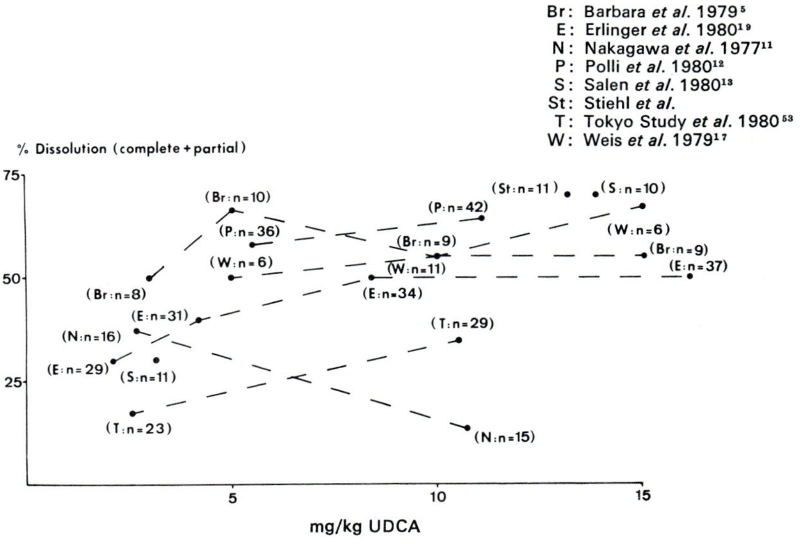

Figure 7 UDCA efficacy. Data from the literature. At doses of greater than 10 mg/kg no increase in the dissolution rates was observed

UDCA administered[15]. No correlation existed between the UDCA dose and the amounts of tauro-UDCA in bile. Biliary cholesterol was markedly decreased during UDCA treatment, but due to the increase of glyco-UDCA in bile at doses greater than 13 mg/kg in six out of seven patients, bile became supersaturated[15].

Studies on the efficacy of UDCA treatment in fact indicate that UDCA doses greater than 10 mg/kg do not increase the dissolution rates (Figure 7). For example, in the study by Erlinger *et al.*[19] with a dose of 8 mg/kg, dissolution was the same as with 16 mg/kg. These clinical efficacy studies are in good agreement with the observation that at doses of UDCA greater than 13 mg/kg, cholesterol saturation may increase[15]. In contrast, CDCA at high doses leads to greater reduction of biliary cholesterol saturation and better dissolution rates (Figure 8).

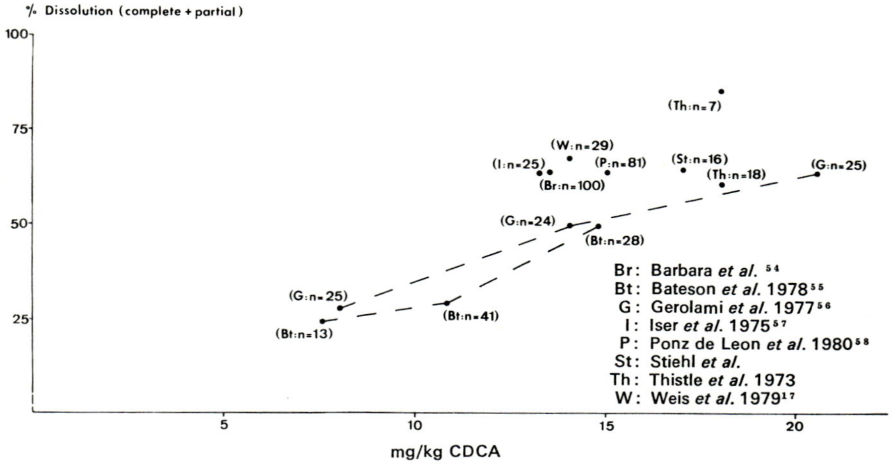

Figure 8 CDCA efficacy. Data from the literature. Dissolution rates increase with the dose

Apparently, cholesterol can be dissolved in micelles[60] but recent studies indicate that it also can be dissolved in liquid crystals. It seems possible that UDCA conjugates in particular can dissolve cholesterol out of relatively soft stones by formation of liquid crystals. It is not known how many cholesterol stones have a soft surface to allow mesophase formation. The importance of liquid crystals formation in gallstone dissolution is not completely clear at present. It seems possible, however, that both UDCA, by forming liquid crystals with cholesterol, and CDCA, by forming micelles with good cholesterol dissolving capacity, cooperate in gallstone dissolution.

Since the efficacy of UDCA is very high at relatively low doses and does not increase with doses greater than 10 mg/kg, while the efficacy of CDCA is better at higher doses, it seems possible that the combination of both drugs is the treatment of choice; CDCA–UDCA treatment effectively decreases biliary cholesterol, dissolves cholesterol gallstones, is free from side-effects, and saves approximately 25 % of treatment costs[15].

References

1. Salen, G., Tint, G. S., Eliav, B. *et al.* (1974). Increased formation of ursodeoxycholic acid in patients treated with chenodeoxycholic acid. *J. Clin. Invest*, **5?**, 612

2. Stiehl, A., Raedsch, R., Regula, M. *et al.* (1975). Treatment of patients with cholesterol gallstones with chenodeoxycholic acid: Alterations in the bile salt metabolism. *Inn. Med.*, **2,** 13
3. Fromm, H., Erbler, H. C. and Eschler, A. (1976). Veränderungen des Gallensäurenstoffwechsels unter der Behandlung mit Chenodeoxycholsäure. *Klin. Wochenschr.*, **54,** 1125
4. Attili, A. F., Angelico, M., Cantafora, A. *et al.* (1978). Effect of low doses of ursodeoxycholic acid on biliary lipid composition in nonobese gallstone patients. *Ital. J. Gastroenterol.*, **10,** 119
5. Barbara, L., Roda, E., Bazzoli, F. *et al.* (1978). Efficacy of ursodeoxycholic acid in dissolving cholesterol gallstones. A blind controlled trial. Europ. Soc. Study of The Liver, Padova. Abstract No. 74, 1978.
6. Bell, C. D., Whitney, B. and Dowling, R. H. (1972). Gallstone dissolution in man using chenodeoxycholic acid. *Lancet*, **2,** 1213
7. Danzinger, R. G., Hofmann, A. F., Schoenfield, L. S. *et al.* (1972). Dissolution of cholesterol gallstones by chenodeoxycholic acid. *N. Engl. J. Med.*, **289,** 1
8. Makino, I., Shinozaki, K., Yoshino, K. *et al.* (1975). Dissolution of cholesterol gallstones by ursodeoxycholic acid. *Jpn. J. Gastroenterol.*, **72,** 690
9. Makino, I. and Nakagawa, S. Changes in biliary lipid and biliary bile acid composition in patients after administration of ursodeoxycholic acid. *J. Lipid Res.*, **19,** 723
10. Maton, P. N., Murphy, G. M. and Dowling, R. H. (1977). Ursodeoxycholic acid treatment of gallstones. Dose–response study and possible mechanism of action. *Lancet*, **2,** 1297
11. Nakagawa, S., Makino, I. and Ishizaki, T. (1977). Dissolution of cholesterol gallstones by ursodeoxycholic acid. *Lancet*, **2,** 367
12. Polli, E. E., Bianchi, P. A., Conte, D. *et al.* (1981). Treatment of radiolucent gallstones with CDCA or UDCA: a multicenter trial. *Digestion* (In press)
13. Salen, G., Colallilo, A., Verga, D. *et al.* (1980). Effect of high and low doses of ursodeoxycholic acid on gallstone dissolution in humans. *Gastroenterology*, **78,** 1412
14. Stiehl, A., Czygan, P., Kommerell, B., *et al.* (1978). Ursodeoxycholic acid versus chenodeoxycholic acid. Comparison of their effects on bile acids and bile lipid composition in patients with cholesterol gallstones. *Gastroenterology*, **75,** 1016
15. Stiehl, A., Raedsch, R., Czygan, P. *et al.* (1980). Effects of biliary bile acid composition on biliary cholesterol saturation in gallstone patients treated with chenodeoxycholic acid and/or ursodeoxycholic acid. *Gastroenterology*, **79,** 1192
16. Thistle, J. L., Carlson, G. L., LaRusso, N. F. *et al.* (1979). Comparison of the effects of 5 and 10 mg/kg/day of ursodeoxycholic acid and chenodeoxycholic acid on cholesterol saturation of bile in patients with gallstones. In Paumgartner, G., Stiehl, A. and Gerok, W. (eds.) *Biological Effects of Bile Acids*, p. 67 (Lancaster: MTP Press)
17. Weis, H. J., Holtermüller, K. H., Stiehl, A. *et al.* (1979). Clinical experience and bile composition in patients taking ursodeoxycholic acid for gallstone dissolution. In Paumgartner, G., Stiehl, A. and Gerok, W. (eds.) *Biological Effects of Bile Acids* pp. 99–102 (Lancaster: MTP Press)
18. Allan, R. N., Thistle, J. L., Hofmann, A. F. *et al.* (1976). Lithocholate metabolism during chenotherapy for gallstone dissolution. I. Serum levels of sulphated and unsulphated lithocholates. *Gut*, **17,** 405
19. Erlinger, S. (1980). Discussion remark. VI. Int. Bile Acid Meeting, Freiburg i. Br., F.R.G.
20. Fedorowski, T., Salen, G., Colallilo, A. *et al.* (1977). Metabolism of ursodeoxycholic acid in man. *Gastroenterology*, **73,** 1131
21. Maton, P. N., Ellis, H. J., Higgins, J. P. *et al.* (1980). Hepatic HMG-CoA reductase in human cholelithiasis: effects of chenodeoxycholic and ursodeoxycholic acids. *Eur. J. Clin. Invest.*, **10,** 325
22. Mok, H. Y. I., Bell, G. D. and Dowling, R. H. (1974). Effect of different doses of chenodeoxycholic acid on bile-lipid composition and on frequency of side effects in patients with gallstones. *Lancet*, **2,** 253
23. Salvioli, G. and Salati, R. (1979). Faecal bile acid loss and bile acid pool size during short-term treatment with ursodeoxycholic and chenodeoxycholic acid in patients with radiolucent gallstones. *Gut*, **20,** 698

24. Scherstén, T. and Lindblad, L. (1979). Biliary cholesterol output during ursodeoxycholic acid secretion in man. In Paumgartner, G., Stiehl, A. and Gerok, W. (eds.) *Biological Effects of Bile Acids*, pp. 53–60 (Lancaster: MTP Press)
25. Stiehl, A., Ast, E., Czygan, P. *et al.* (1976). Elevated serum transaminases following treatment of patients with cholesterol gallstones with chenodeoxycholic acid. *Inn. Med.* **3,** 75
26. Thistle, J. L., Hofmann, A. F., Yu, P. Y. S. *et al.* (1977). Effect of varying doses of chenodeoxycholic acid on bile lipid and bile acid composition in gallstone patients: a dose response study. *Dig. Dis.*, **22,** 1
27. Fedorowski, T., Salen, G. and Mosbach, E. H. (1977). Formation of lithocholic acid from chenodeoxycholic acid and ursodeoxycholic acid by intestinal bacteria. Abstract. *Gastroenterology*, **73,** 1220
28. Fedorowski, T., Salen, G. S. and Tint, G. S. (1979). Transformation of chenodeoxycholic acid and ursodeoxycholic acid by human intestinal bacteria. *Gastroenterology*, **77,** 1068
29. Salen, G., Shefer, S., Tint, G. S. *et al.* (1980). The metabolism of 7 ketolithocholic acid in man. Abstract. VI. Int. Bile Acid Meeting, Freiburg i. Br., F.R.G.
30. Sarva, R. P., Fromm, H., Carlson, G. L. *et al.* (1980). Intracolonic conversion in man of chenodeoxycholic acid to ursodeoxycholic acid and the role of 7 ketolithocholic acid as an intermediate. Abstract. VI. Int. Bile Acid Meeting, Freiburg i. Br., F.R.G.
31. Stiehl, A., Czygan, P. and Raedsch, R. (1975). Sulfation of lithocholate in patients during chenodeoxycholate treatment. A protective mechanism. In Matern, S., Hackenschmidt, J. and Back, P. (eds.) *Advances in Bile Acid Research*, pp. 347–350. (Stuttgart-New York: F. K. Schattauer)
32. Bell, G. D., Mok, H. Y., Thwe, M. *et al.* (1974). Liver structure and function in cholelithiasis: effects of chenodeoxycholic acid. *Gut*, **15,** 165
33. Fromm, H., Holz-Slomezyk, M., Zobl, M. *et al.* (1975). Studies of liver function and structure in patients with gallstones before and during treatment with chenodeoxycholic acid. *Acta Hepatogastroenterol.*, **22,** 359
34. Pederson, L. and Bremmelgaard, A. (1976). Hepatic morphology and bile acid composition of bile and urine during chenodeoxycholic acid therapy for radiolucent gallstones. *Scand. J. Gastroenterol.*, **11,** 385
35. Coyne, M. J., Bonorris, G. G., Goldstein, L. I. *et al.* (1976). Effect of chenodeoxycholic acid and phenobarbital on the rate-limiting enzymes of hepatic cholesterol and bile acid synthesis in patients with gallstones. *J. Lab. Clin. Med.*, **87,** 281
36. Einarsson, K. and Ewerth, St. (1980). Bile acids and hepatic HMG-CoA reductase in man. Abstract. VI. Int. Bile Acid Meeting, Freiburg i. Br., F.R.G.
37. Salen, G., Nicolau, G., Shefer, S. *et al.* (1975). Hepatic cholesterol metabolism in patients with gallstones. *Gastroenterology*, **69,** 676
38. Adler, R. D., Bennion, L. J., Duane, W. C. *et al.* (1975). Effects of low dose chenodeoxycholic acid feeding on biliary lipid metabolism. *Gastroenterology*, **68,** 326
39. Ponz de Leon, M., Carulli, N., Loria, P. *et al.* (1979). The effect of chenodeoxycholic acid (CDCA) on cholesterol absorption in man. *Gastroenterology*, **77,** 223
40. Mok, H. Y. I. and Grundy, S. M. (1978). Bile acid and cholesterol absorption during BA therapy in obese subjects undergoing weight reduction. *Clin. Res.*, **26,** 151 A
41. Tangedahl, T. N., Thistle, J. L., Hofmann, A. F. *et al.* (1979). Effect of beta-sitosterol alone or in combination with chenic acid on cholesterol saturation of bile and cholesterol absorption in gallstone patients. *Gastroenterology*, **76,** 1341
42. LaRusso, N. F. and Thistle, J. L. (1980). Effect of urso and chenotherapy on cholesterol absorption in patients with cholelithiasis. Abstract. VI. Int. Bile Acid Meeting, Freiburg i. Br., F.R.G.
43. Roda, A., Bazzoli, F., Petronelli, A. *et al.* (1980). Intestinal cholesterol absorption during CDCA and UDCA administration in man. Abstract. VI. Int. Bile Acid Meeting, Freiburg i. Br., F.R.G.
44. Roda, E., Mazzella, G., Roda, A. *et al.* (1980). Effects of chenodeoxycholic acid and ursodeoxycholic acid administration on biliary lipid secretion in normal weight and obese gallstone patients. Abstract. VI. Int. Bile Acid Meeting, Freiburg i. Br., F.R.G.
45. Ponz de Leon, M., Carulli, N., Iori, R. *et al.* (1980). Medical treatment of radio-

lucent gallstones with chenodeoxycholic acid (CDCA): follow up report at four years. *Ital. J. Gastroenterol.*, **12,** 17
46. Sama, C. and LaRusso, F. (1980). Effect of primary bile acid administration on intestinal absorption of cholesterol in man. Abstract. VI. Int. Bile Acid Meeting, Freiburg i. Br., F.R.G.
47. von Bergmann, K., Gutsfeld, M., Schulze-Hagen, K. *et al.* (1979). Effects of ursodeoxycholic acid on biliary lipid secretion in patients with radiolucent gallstones. In Paumgartner, G., Stiehl, A. and Gerok, W. (eds.) *Biological Effects of Bile Acids*, pp.61–66. (Lancaster: MTP Press)
48. Carey, M. C. and Grace, K. O. (1979). The importance of total lipid concentration in determining cholesterol solubity in bile and the development of critical table for calculating percent cholesterol saturation with a correction factor for ursodeoxycholate-rich bile. In Paumgartner, G., Stiehl, A. and Gerok, W. (eds.) *Biological Effects of Bile Acids*, pp. 299–308. (Lancaster: MTP Press)
49. Corrigan, O. J., Su, C. C., Alkan, M. H. *et al.* (1980). Cholesterol dissolution in ursodeoxycholate-lecithin containing media: Involvement of mesophase formation *in vitro*. Abstract. VI. Int. Bile Acid Meeting, Freiburg i. Br., F.R.G.
50. Igimi, H. and Carey, M. C. (1980). pH-solubility relations of chenodeoxycholic and ursodeoxycholic acids: Physical-chemical basis for dissimilar solution and membrane phenomena. *J. Lipid Res.*, **21,** 72
51. Carey, M. C., Mazer, N. A., Benedek, G. B. *et al.* (1977). Novel physical-chemical properties of ursodeoxycholic acid and its conjugates: relevance to gallstone formation in man. Abstract. *Gastroenterology*, **72,** 1036
52. Tokyo Cooperative Gallstone Study Group (1980). Efficacy and indications of ursodeoxycholic acid treatment for dissolving gallstones. *Gastroenterology*, **78**, 542
53. Barbara, L., Roda, E., Roda, A. *et al.* (1977), Il trattamento medico della calcolosi biliare colesterolica nell' uomo con acido chenodesoxicolico. *Minerva Med.*, **68,** 3355
54. Bateson, M. C., Ross, P. E., Murison, J. *et al.* (1978). Comparison of fixed doses of chenodeoxycholic acid for gallstone dissolution. *Lancet*, **1,** 1111
55. Gerolami, A., Sarles, H., Brette, R. *et al.* (1977). Controlled trial of chenodeoxycholic acid therapy for radiolucent gallstones. *Digestion*, **16,** 299
56. Iser, J. H., Dowling, R. H., Mok, H. Y. I. *et al.* (1975). Chenodeoxycholic acid treatment of gallstones: a follow up report and analysis of factors influencing response to therapy. *N. Engl. J. Med.*, **293,** 378
57. Thistle, J. L. and Hofmann, A. F. (1973). Efficacy and specificity of chenodeoxycholic acid therapy for dissolving gallstones. *N. Engl. J. Med.*, **289,** 655
58. Admirand, W. H. and Small, D. M. (1968). The physical-chemical basis of cholesterol gallstone formation in man. *J. Clin. Invest.*, **47,** 1043.

Discussion

Dr Salen I want to congratulate Dr Stiehl for giving such a lucid and comprehensive presentation of the urso (UDCA) and cheno (CDCA) stories. Indeed, it is quite difficult for me to follow him, since he has said almost everything that I would like to discuss. However, I would like to review what I believe are the fundamental reasons why UDCA is less toxic than CDCA. This includes the bacterial metabolism of both bile acids and, of course, our studies in the Rhesus monkey, where we compared the effects of CDCA and UDCA on hepatic morphology and related these changes to biliary lithocholic acid concentrations (Figure 1).

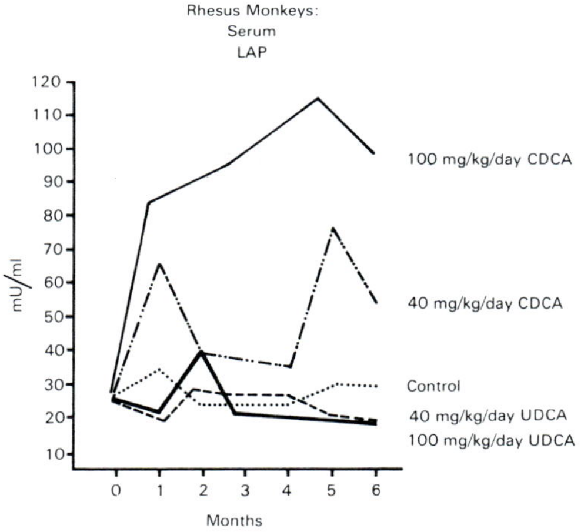

Figure 1 The effect of CDCA and UDCA on serum leucine aminopeptidase

This illustration shows the effect of CDCA and UDCA on serum leucine aminopeptidase levels (LAP) in Rhesus monkeys over a 6 month period. Two different doses of CDCA and UDCA were administered. Although the doses of CDCA and UDCA were higher than the dose given to humans, they are equivalent to the human dose because, in calculating animal doses, one must consider not only the weight of the animal and surface area, but also its metabolic rate. As you can see, levels of SLAP, an enzyme that reflects patency of the bile ducts, are quite abnormal in the CDCA-treated animals. The degree of abnormality appears to be dose-related, whereas in the UDCA-treated animals at the end of 6 months, there was little difference from control values.

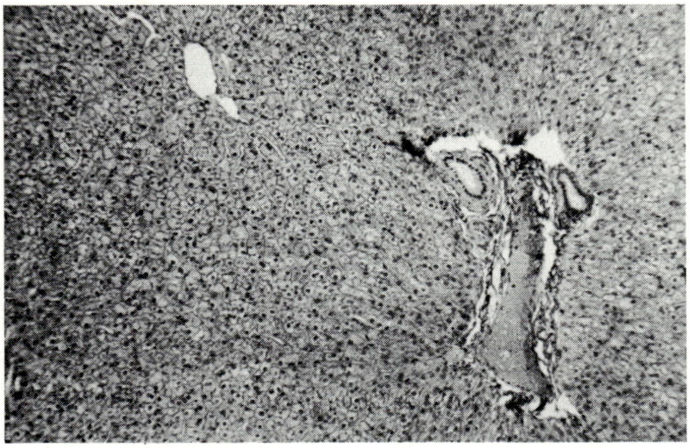

Figure 2 Hepatic histology of CDCA-treated monkey (40 mg/kg/day)

Figure 2 shows the histology of the liver of a CDCA-treated animal. Focus on the portal area which shows the characteristic lesions that includes periportal inflammation and bile duct hyperplasia. These findings are considered an early indication of cholestasis.

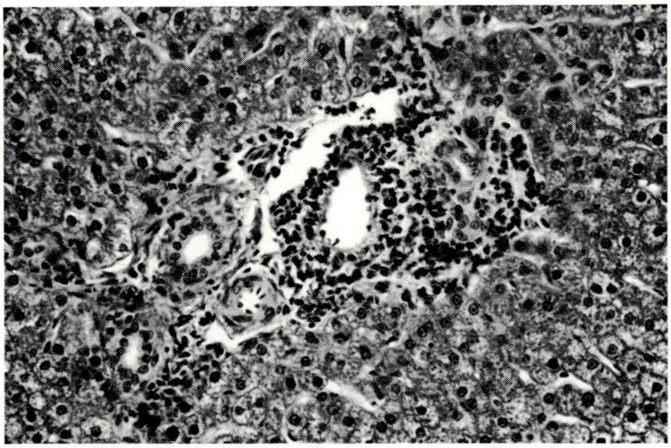

Figure 3 Hepatic histology of UDCA-treated monkey (40 mg/kg/day)

Figure 3 shows the liver histology in a comparable UDCA-treated animal: the magnification is different but you can see that the liver architecture is perfectly normal. Note the central vein and the portal area and no inflammation is present.

The formation of lithocholic acid (LCA) from CDCA and two doses of UDCA are shown in Table 1. In the 40 mg/kg/day CDCA-treated animal over 80% of the bile acids were CDCA and 10% were lithocholic acid while in the 100 mg/kg/day CDCA-treated animals (not shown) the proportion of lithocholic acid increased to 15% of the total bile acid. In the UDCA-treated animals, the proportion of

Table 1 Biliary bile acid composition after CDCA and UDCA treatment (% total bile acids)

Treatment	*LCA*	*DCA*	*CDCA*	*UDCA*	*CA*
Control	1.1	21.3	17.3	—	60.2
40 mg/kg, CDCA	10.3	2.1	82.7	3.4	3.1
40 mg/kg, UDCA	3.8	8.5	12.7	32.5	42.5
100 mg/kg. UDCA	3.4	2.2	15.3	73.8	5.4

UDCA in the bile was dose dependent and accounted for 33% and 74% of the total bile acid respectively. However, unlike the CDCA-treated animal, *the proportion of lithocholic acid in the bile did not increase significantly* (between 3% and 4% of total bile acids). Further, no sulphated lithocholic acid was found in any animals. Of course, we believe that the reduced amounts of biliary LCA reflects decreased formation from UDCA and is the reason for the lack of toxicity. I would like to support this concept by showing the results of bacterial incubation with CDCA and UDCA.

In these experiments, we examined the rate of 7-dehydroxylation of (lithocholic acid formation) both CDCA and UDCA. Intestinal bacteria from faeces were incubated together with (7β-^{3}H)CDCA and (24-^{14}C)UDCA and the rate of disappearance of both bile acids was measured along with the formation of lithocholic acid. The results are shown in Figure 4.

Within 1 hour, about 80% of the CDCA had disappeared and was replaced by lithocholic acid. At the end of 2 hours only 9% of chenodeoxycholic acid remained. In contrast, after 1 hour 70% of the UDCA was left and after 2 hours 50% remained. Lithocholic acid was the main product formed. Therefore, if UDCA and CDCA are in the

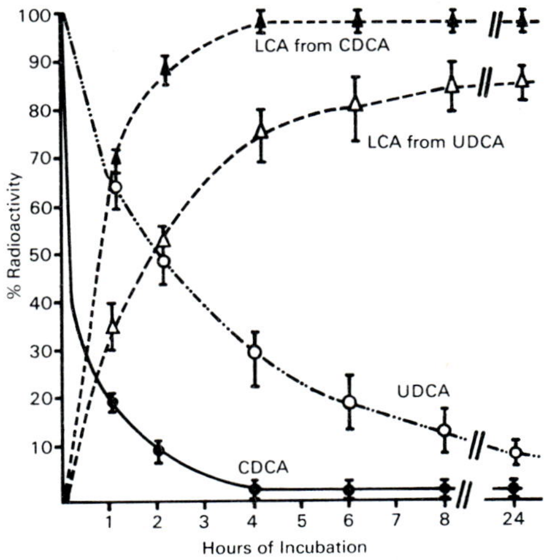

Figure 4 The bacterial degradation of CDCA and UDCA and the formation of lithocholic acid after incubation of intestinal bacteria with (7β-^{3}H)CDCA and (24-^{14}C)UDCA

intestine, lithocholic acid will be produced from either bile acid by intestinal bacteria but because the lithocholic acid is formed more slowly from UDCA there is a greater chance for the intact UDCA molecule to be reabsorbed. This may be an important mechanism why UDCA is safer (less lithocholic acid formed) and also why a smaller dose seems to be effective (less is destroyed).

Dr Fromm A previous study by Federowski *et al.* indicated that the two gallstone dissolving bile acids, chenodeoxycholic acid (CDCA) and ursodeoxycholic acid (UDCA), differ in their hepatotoxic potential. These investigators reported that, in the rhesus monkey, UDCA causes, in contrast to CDCA, no liver damage and no increase of lithocholic acid in bile. The results of a controlled toxicity study, which we conducted in the same primate species, disagree with the findings of Federowski *et al.* Today I would like to give a summary of our toxicity study in 20 rhesus monkeys, which has now been published in this month's issue of *Gastroenterology*.

Five groups of rhesus monkeys, each consisting of two male and two female animals, were treated with 40 mg/kg/day of CDCA, 120 mg/kg/day of CDCA, 40 mg/kg/day of UDCA, 120 mg/kg/day of UDCA and placebo, respectively. After 6 months, CDCA and UDCA treatment was discontinued and the bile acid treated animals were placed on placebo for 6 months.

Liver function tests were performed monthly. Liver histology and biliary as well as serum bile acids were studied before the treatment and 6 and 12 months after initiation of the treatment. Half of the animals were sacrificed after 6 months of treatment with CDCA, UDCA and placebo, respectively, and an autopsy was performed. Both CDCA and UDCA induced comparable abnormalities of liver function and structure, which appeared to be more pronounced on the 120 mg than on the 40 mg/kg/day dose. The histological changes were characterized by inflammation, bile duct proliferation and fibrosis. On the 120 mg/kg/day dose, cirrhosis was observed both in CDCA and UDCA treated animals.

All CDCA and UDCA treated monkeys showed, in contrast to the placebo treated animals, comparable increases in lithocholic acid in bile. All lithocholic acid was unsulphated. Measurements of serum bile acids, which were carried out by Drs Franco Bazzoli and Aldo Roda from the University of Bologna showed considerable increases of lithocholic acid in serum, which paralleled those in bile.

Presently it is not known, whether conditions of decreased or inadequate sulphation also exist in man. Yesterday we heard from Dr Schoenfield that gallstone patients who, during CDCA treatment, develop increases in the activity of GPT and/or GOT in serum, sulphate a lower proportion of an administered tracer dose of radiolabelled lithocholic acid than patients in whom these enzymes remain normal. Further studies would be of interest to determine, in CDCA and UDCA treated patients, the relation between liver function and sulphation, in particular, the relation between liver function abnormalities and serum levels of unsulphated and sulphated lithocholate.

At the end of my presentation I should like to acknowledge the important contributions of Dr R. P. Sarva and Dr S. Farivar to the toxicity studies in the rhesus monkeys.

Dr Dowling I am going to direct this discussion towards the topic of this session which is about bile acid and biliary lipid metabolism. Although we have heard an interesting controversy about hepatotoxicity in animals that is not strictly our brief and I think Dr Fromm's last point that animals behave differently in the capacity to sulphate makes it rather difficult to interpret these hepatotoxicity studies. So can we focus please on bile acid and biliary lipid metabolism.

Dr Northfield Dr Stiehl mentioned two possible mechanisms of action of CDCA and UDCA, that is to say their effects on HMG-CoA reductase and effects on cholesterol absorption and I would like to draw attention to a third possible mechanism, that is to say an effect on the membrane, the bile canalicular membrane, and the possibility that effects on HMG-CoA reductase might be secondary to this. I would like to draw attention to a poster on this subject by my colleague John Graham, in which he showed that CDCA removes less cholesterol from isolated bile canalicular membranes than does cholic acid but removes more phospholipids. There does seem to be a third possible mechanism that warrants further investigation.

Dr Mazer I would like to continue on with the line that was just presented because on the basis of our theoretical analysis of the biliary lipid secretion, this is indeed a further mechanism that must be considered in order to explain the differential effects of bile salts on cholesterol desaturation. In fact one can appreciate why different bile salts could differentially bring less cholesterol into micellar solutions in bile by a revision of the model of the mixed micelle that was shown in Dr Stiehl's lecture. Specifically I want to emphasize that we have in the past years through studies of model systems suggested that bile salts not only coat the edge of the mixed micelle as was shown in the picture, but that bile salts can also be present in the interior of the lecithin bilayer. When one realises the possibility that specific bile salts can interact differently with the cholesterol molecules that go into the micelle, it is apparent that different bile salts can have important effects at the membrane solubilizing level as was pointed out. So I think that this is an effect that must be looked at. It is very possible in fact that the observation of a reduced HMG-CoA reductase is simply a secondary effect of allowing less cholesterol to come out into the bile and thereby turning off its own synthesis.

Dr Dowling Is this pure hypothesis based on your experimental model or is there any evidence that it actually happens in life?

Dr Mazer I would say that on the basis of our interpretation of the existing biliary lipid secretion data one can come to the conclusion that the detergent capacity of different bile salts to solubilize cholesterol provides a quantitative explanation of the data.

Dr Hofmann I think that it is a very difficult thing to go from physical properties *in vitro* to *in vivo* animal studies, including man, because in work that Dr Gilmore has done in the dog and what we have done in the hamster, CDCA and UDCA make bile much worse. They pull out much more cholesterol and lecithin than does cholate and I just cannot see how, when we have totally opposite secretory effects, we can explain this by any simple physical model.

Dr Mazer The answer to this question is indeed complicated because we have not only physical mechanisms in operation but biochemical mechanisms that are delivering cholesterol and lecithin to the canalicular membrane with different control mechanisms. It is possible to understand the differences in species by postulating that the physical mechanisms in each case are the same, but that the regulatory mechanisms which are at least half of the story are different in the different species. I think that we will certainly have to agree that it may not be only physical mechanisms that are pertinent here. We can probably hope to find a unified explanation of the data assuming that the same physical mechanisms operate in all species and that the difference is referred to the regulatory effects.

Dr Salen Yes. I would like to go along with that idea. If you study it within the *in vitro* systems you are dealing with something that is very static and there are no dynamic things going on as in the intact animal.

Dr Gilmore I was not planning to enter into the thorny problem of cholesterol secretion. I wish to make a comment about Dr Stiehl's beautiful overview and his comment on the small spill-over into peripheral blood of the two therapeutic agents. I would just like to make a short plug for our poster which shows that there is a small but definite difference emerging between CDCA and UDCA. The first pass extraction measured directly in normal subjects by hepatic vein catheterization is about 65% for CDCA and definitely lower, less than 50%, for UDCA. This is unlikely to be of any significance in terms of therapeutic dissolution, but I think it does explain why you are seeing higher serum levels with UDCA; and it is relevant to people who are using bile acids as an oral tolerance test looking at liver disease.

Dr Paumgartner We have done studies of first pass extraction of UDCA in normal subjects and in patients with liver disease. We have given UDCA intravenously and orally and have determined first pass extraction by the classical method. It was about 50% in healthy subjects. This would agree with your values for UDCA. You and others have found about 65% for CDCA. This indicates that there is less first pass extraction for UDCA than for CDCA.

Dr Stiehl I am happy that you and Dr Paumgartner have found the reason why the UDCA levels are higher than the CDCA levels. The spill-over of UDCA apparently is a little bit higher. I might add that Dr Götz of our group has shown in the isolated liver cell that indeed there is a slight difference between uptake of UDCA and CDCA. UDCA uptake is somewhat smaller than CDCA uptake.

Dr Dowling There is a practical application to the first pass clearance of UDCA and CDCA. It has been suggested by Jim Watts in Adelaide, Australia that serum UDCA levels can be used to monitor compliance in patients taking UDCA.

Dr MacDonald I just want to address a point that I do not think has been emphasized very much. It seems to me that whether or not you believe how much more toxic CDCA is than UDCA, litho formation is common to both of them. If one could possibly prevent litho formation during the administration of either of these substances by one mechanism or another, one could not only overcome the problem of potential hepatotoxicity, one could increase the pharmacological efficacy of the bile acid, because less is going into useless litho. I think that it is important to consider the work of Dr Mosbach, for example, who showed that tetrol could stop 7 β-hydroxylation in the rat and work by Dr Hyleman who is examining 7 β-hydroxylating organisms and maybe specific inhibitors of these organisms. If one could come up with a pharmacological agent like a tetrol that was not well absorbed and providing it did not interfere in any way one could improve the matter. I would be interested to hear what people have to say about this proposal.

Dr Stiehl First, Dr Fromm brought this up already: the formation of lithocholic acid in these patients treated with chenodeoxycholic acid and the spill-over of litho into the peripheral blood. We have studied this and we could not find a correlation between elevated transaminases and the amount of unsulphated lithocholic acid in the peripheral blood. We heard yesterday from Dr Schoenfield that apparently there are only very few patients with more than 2% of lithocholic acid in the bile who had elevated transaminases. This raises some doubt whether these increases of lithocholic acid, which are really very small, have anything to do with these elevations of transaminases, but I think your second point is really a point that we have to take into consideration.

Dr Dowling I suppose it is worth emphasizing again that although we have been talking about hepatoxicity and preventing it in humans, in the doses used with both CDCA and UDCA, we really have no histological evidence of toxicity as yet.

Dr Thistle A brief question to Dr Stiehl. I think all of us are struggling with deciding what the most effective dose of UDCA might be and I do not think we are ready this year to come to a conclusion. Dr Stiehl illustrated to us that, in fact, looking at efficacy data there really is not any perceptible difference between 3 mg and 15 mg/kg/day in terms of efficacy. Therefore, would not a dosage in the range of 5 or 6 be more suggestible than 10 to 12 as your conclusion slide suggested or had you other factors in mind?

Dr Stiehl So far we can only say that a dose above 12 mg/kg is certainly not good. I agree with you that we have to do some more work to define accurately the optimal dose. We think it is around 10 to 12 mg/kg/day but there are others that are convinced that a dose of 10 mg leads to better dissolution rate than a dose of 5 mg/kg/day. This very low dose in some hands was not very effective.

Dr Dowling I think we are all making the tacit assumption so far that it is appropriate to do the correction, that it does have some predictive value on hypothetical grounds and that taurine feeding might help. We badly need solid information from different dose–response studies in terms of absolute gallstone dissolution rates, that is, speed of dissolution and efficacy of dissolution.

Dr Tint has indicated that he wants to make a comment on that because I think he has actually got some hard data.

Dr Tint We have the results from 51 gallstone patients who were fed three different doses of ursodeoxycholic acid for periods from 6 months to 2½ years. 17 patients were fed about 1000 mg/day which averages out at about 14 mg/kg, 19 patients at 500 mg/day which is about 7.5 mg/kg, and 15 patients at 300 mg/day 250 mg/day which averages about 3.7 mg/kg. At the high dose (14 mg/kg/day) in 53% of the patients the gallstones were completely dissolved; in 29% a 50% reduction in gallstones size occurred; at the dose of 7.5 mg/kg/day 32% completely dissolved, 26% became smaller; at the low dose (3.7 mg/kg/day) 33% dissolved and 20% became smaller. Thus, there is no difference between 3.7 mg/kg/day and 7.5 mg/kg/day, but a very distinct difference at the high dose level. The length of treatment was actually longer at the lower dose level. This is because the people were not dissolving the gallstones. Actually, the three groups were very well matched. The dissolution was very much faster and much more efficacious at the high dose.

Dr Erlinger I also would like to comment briefly on this dose–response problem. In a controlled prospective multi-centre trial, the results of which will be presented in detail next week in Paris, we have observed that with doses increasing from 2 to 4 to 8 to 16 mg/kg body weight per day, there was a clear and significant increase in efficacy from about 25% total efficacy for the dose of 2 mg/kg/day to about 30% for the dose of 4 mg/kg/day, to about 50% for the dose of 8 mg/kg/day and then thereafter there was no further increase in efficacy for the dose of 16 mg/kg/day. So we think that the optimal dose is in the order of 8 mg/kg/day.

Dr Bateson I want to make one statement and two observations. We have also used serum UDCA levels as a test of compliance. We have been able to prove in one patient that it is a reliable test of compliance with a lady whose gallstone got bigger on treatment, whose serum UDCA level after 6 months was 0.2 μmol/l and whose bile contained less than 1% of UDCA. So we think this is a jolly good test of compliance. The separation of pretreatment UDCA level and post-treatment UDCA levels is complete and this can be done on postprandial spot samples just when people turn up in the clinic without even making them lose their breakfast. That is my statement. I would like to challenge two things that Dr Stiehl has said. We and many other workers, have found no increase in UDCA in bile in humans after CDCA therapy, and we found that there was less than 2% both before and after CDCA therapy. Secondly we have shown a clear increase in unsulphated lithocholic acid in bile after treatment with UDCA and at a dose of 14–15 mg/kg this increase was from 1.9–4.1 moles % of the bile acids which was statistically significant. So I think that the differences between urso and cheno cannot be explained by this particular phenomenon.

Dr Dowling Just before Dr Stiehl answers this, can you remind us of your methods for measureing serum UDCA and then the percent of UDCA in bile.

Dr Bateson The serum UDCA has been measured both by radioimmunoassay and by gas–liquid chromatography. The biliary UDCA acid has been measured by gas–liquid chromatography without solvolysis. I cannot say what happens to the sulphates.

Dr Stiehl As far as the transformation of CDCA and UDCA is concerned, there are really many others who have confirmed the data of Dr Salen that CDCA can be transformed to UDCA. In some patients you find it, and in others you do not.

As far as lithocholic acid is concerned there are also data from the Japanese, who have shown that there is no significant increase in lithocholic acid. I could only speculate why in your patients there was an increase; but in our patients there was really a decrease of lithocholic acid in bile. This is in agreement with what others find, like Dr Salen and the Japanese.

Dr LaRusso I would like to make two comments. When we study the metabolism of bile acids and when we are looking at something that bacteria make, all the rules break down and the whole system becomes very erratic.

When Dr Thistle and I reviewed the literature of say 300 people in whom biliary bile acid analysis had been done during CDCA, we found about five people with these enormous increases in urso: two of Dr Stiehl, one of Dr Salen, two of Dr Fromm, but if you look at 100 people you find that the UDCA goes up in about 2% to 4%. The average increase in UDCA is very small, and some do not go up at all. Can I get you to agree with that Dr Bateson?

Dr Bateson I agree. I think the increase is idiosyncratic and I think overall we certainly cannot confirm it.

Dr LaRusso I think even you, Dr Stiehl, would agree that it is not routine: the striking increase in UDCA during cheno.

Dr Stiehl Well I can only say again that in some patients you find it and not in others. If you study enough patients you will find it in some and then on the average you will get an increase of let's say up to 10%. For example, in the groups we studied recently we found only slight increases during CDCA treatment up to 5%.

Dr Dowling Well, I think we really have not grasped the nettle about this whole problem of cholesterol solubilization and its quantitative importance in determining whether or not saturation indices are of predictive value. I hope we will address this question in the next session.

PART III
Medical Treatment of Gallstones with CDCA and UDCA

Medical treatment of gallstones with CDCA and UDCA

R. HERMON DOWLING

The introduction to this workshop on gallstone dissolution attempts to provide a 'state-of-the-art' based largely on our own experience which is, I think, reasonably representative of that in other centres. This acts as a framework to indicate difficulties, unresolved problems and areas of controversy in the gallstone dissolution field. To set the scene, I shall start with some old data which summarize the importance of patient selection and management, on efficacy. A fairly detailed comparison of CDCA and UDCA follows and the discussion ends with a consideration of two specialized topics – diarrhoea and its mechanism, and dyspepsia and its relief, during bile acid treatment.

Figure 1 was prepared in collaboration with Paul Maton nearly 3 years ago. It depicts the efficacy of CDCA treatment, defined as the percentage of patients showing complete gallstone dissolution (the solid bars) or partial

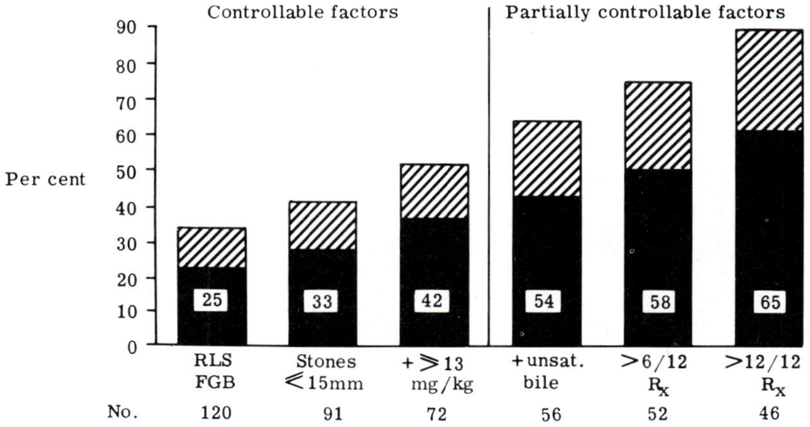

Figure 1 Influence of patient selection and management on efficacy of CDCA in producing complete (solid bars) or partial (cross-hatched bars) gallstone dissolution. The results are expressed as percentages with the numbers of patients in each group shown below the appropriate columns. RLSFG = Radiolucent gallstones in functioning gallbladders. $>6/12\ R_x$ $>12/12\ R_x$ = greater than 6 and 12 months treatment. (From Maton *et al.*[11])

dissolution (the cross-hatched bars) for different categories of patients where the results were grouped into factors which, through patient selection and management, we could control completely and factors over which we had only partial control.

We started with 120 patients, all of whom had radiolucent stones in functioning gallbladders, and a rather low efficacy rate (25% complete and 34% partial plus complete gallstone dissolution). We arbitrarily found, as others have done, that patients with large stones respond poorly to treatment and if we exclude from the analysis those with stones measuring more than 15 mm in diameter and insist on a minimum dose of 13 mg CDCA $kg^{-1}day^{-1}$, the efficacy improved to 42% complete and 53% partial plus complete. The 13 mg dose usually, but not always, produces unsaturated bile and if we take the trouble to monitor this, the additional benefit in efficacy at that stage of the analysis is about 12%. (It varies between 10 and 20% depending on how the results are analysed.) It is reasonable to suggest that a patient should have completed at least 6, and preferably 12, months treatment with X-rays, before one can assess the response to therapy. And when we did that, efficacy rose to 65% complete and 90% partial plus complete gallstone dissolution.

This is what Woody Fisher calls a 'gardening slide', because it progressively weeds out those who do not respond, so that the increasing efficacy is 'bought' at the expense of diminishing patient numbers. However, it was not designed simply to produce good efficacy figures but to teach us, retrospectively, which patients, when selected prospectively, are most likely to benefit from therapy. We have now tested this prospectively in patients selected for treatment since 1976 and find that with careful patient selection and management, we get comparable efficacy figures (78% complete; 93% partial + complete) to the maximum shown in the figure.

This then is the basis for suggesting that we ought to confine our treatment (and our discussion) to patients with radiolucent stones measuring less than 15 mm in diameter in functioning gallbladders. We should also consider one other factor – obesity – which renders patients relatively resistant to the charms of chenodeoxycholic acid[1]. With this in mind, we next attempted to compare, retrospectively, dose and efficacy, a possible mechanism of action, symptoms and side-effects of CDCA and UDCA in two comparable groups of gallstone patients ideally suited for medical treatment. Even in retrospect, the mean age, sex ratio, weight and ideal body weight were comparable in the two groups.

(i) Dose (Figure 2)

In the past, we suggested that there was a linear relationship between saturation index and the dose of CDCA plotted on the upper panel (data from a paper published by Henry Mok)[2] and for UDCA plotted below (the data of Paul Maton[3], Gareth Williams[4] and others in our unit). The logical corollary of these results is that, by extrapolation, the bigger the bile acid dose, the better should be the saturation index response. Clearly this does not happen. There must come a point where the linear relationship between the

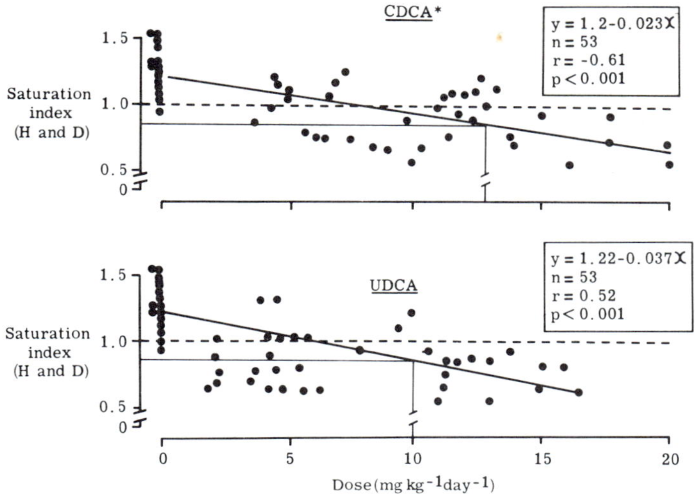

* Mok et al Lancet 1974, ii, 253.

Figure 2 Relationship between the fasting cholesterol saturation indices (SI) in duodenal bile (according to the limits of cholesterol solubility of Hegardt and Dam) and bile acid dose in mg kg^{-1} day^{-1} for CDCA (above) and UDCA (below)

two variables breaks down with a plateau effect. This is particularly true for UDCA. Indeed, from a study of the individual data points in Figure 2, it is obvious that many patients will desaturate their bile with quite small bile acid doses. Despite this objection, based on the linear regressions in Figure 2, we have drawn lines which link a post-treatment saturation index of 0.8 (the level at which gallstones dissolve[5]) with the mean dose required to produce this effect – 10 mg for UDCA and 13 mg kg^{-1} day^{-1} for CDCA. But if we exclude the pretreatment data for UDCA (0 mg kg^{-1} day^{-1}), this linear relationship no longer holds true. Indeed, when we examined the SI response in individual patients given multiple UDCA doses, we found that in many cases the relationship was curvilinear with a plateau effect, so that with increasing UDCA doses, there was no further reduction in SI[4].

Now these results were calculated ignoring Carey's correction factor[4] for UDCA-rich bile[6], but when the correction was applied, many of the patients who had unsaturated bile during treatment, had supersaturated bile after applying the Carey factor[6]. Despite this, their gallstones still dissolved!

This raises the question, therefore, is there any predictive value in measuring the saturation index, and in patients treated with UDCA, should one apply the Carey correction before doing so? In our experience, the on-treatment SI is of value in predicting which patients will subsequently respond with gallstone dissolution[5] – but *not* after applying the correction factor[7]. Indeed, the demonstration by Corrigan and Higuchi[8] that there is non-micellar solubilization of cholesterol in UDCA-rich bile casts further doubt on the validity of any correction factor for the amount of UDCA in bile.

Table 1 shows the lowest bile acid doses found to desaturate bile in patients

Table 1 Mean bile acids doses (mg kg^{-1} day^{-1}) found to change bile lipid composition in patients treated with UDCA or CDCA

	UDCA	*CDCA*
(i) Minimum dose found to produce unsaturated bile	2.0	4.0
(ii) Minimum dose found to produce unsaturated bile consistently	9.5	14.5
(iii) Minimum dose found to produce a mean post-treatment saturation index of 0.8 (See text)	9.9	14.4

treated with UDCA and CDCA. They were very low – the sort of doses that Rudy Danzinger has shown will *occasionally* dissolve gallstones in patients from Canada[9]. More important is the minimum bile acid dose which will desaturate bile consistently. At the time of this analysis, it was about 10 mg kg^{-1} for UDCA and about 15 mg kg^{-1} for CDCA but these data, based only on bile lipids, are of limited value. More important, is the bile acid dose required to dissolve gallstones and Figure 3 illustrates not only dose but indicates the sort of efficacy seen at different times after starting UDCA.

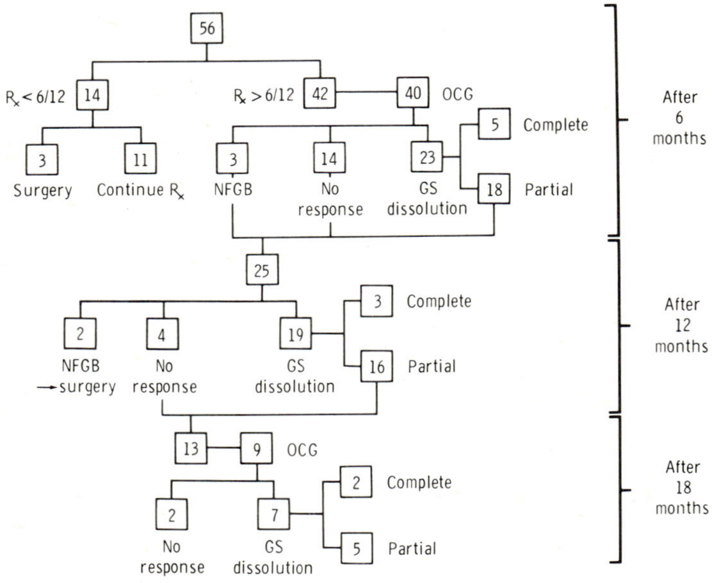

Figure 3 Outline results of 6, 12 and 18 months UDCA therapy in 56 patients with radiolucent gallstones and functioning gallbladders. $R_x < 6/12$ = treated for less than 6 months; OCG=oral cholecystogram; NFGB=non-functioning gallbladder; GS=gallstone

(ii) Efficacy (Figure 3)

Of 56 patients treated to date with UDCA at Guy's Hospital, 14 have had less than 6 months treatment – three because they required surgery for biliary colic whilst 11 continue treatment and await their first follow-up X-ray.

Of the 42 who have completed 6 months treatment, 40 have had oral cholecystograms which showed the development of a non-functioning gallbladder in three and no response in 14 while the remaining 23 (58% of the 40 X-rayed) have shown either complete or partial gallstone dissolution. Twenty-five patients (two of those with non-functioning gallbladders, eight of the non-responders and 15 of the partial responders) went on to complete 12 months treatment and of these, the two who had shown non-visualizing gallbladders at the 6-month X-ray, showed persistent non-opacification of the gallbladder and went on to surgery, four showed no response and 19 (76% of the 25 X-rayed) showed complete or partial gallstone dissolution.

Table 2 Liver structure and function in patients treated with UDCA or CDCA

	UDCA	*CDCA*
Hypertransaminasaemia	1/56(2%)	17/48(35%)
Liver biopsies 'within normal limits' during treatment	6/6(100%)	46/46(100%)

If we express this as cumulative efficacy (including in the analysis patients who had shown complete gallstone dissolution at 6 months), depending on whether or not the patients who stopped treatment are excluded from, or included in, the analysis, overall efficacy rises to 69–80% (23–27% complete and 46–53% partial).

The data at 18 months are too limited to permit any firm conclusions, but of the 13 patients treated for 1½ years, nine had cholecystograms which showed: two further patients with complete gallstone dissolution, five with partial and two with no response, giving a maximum cumulative efficacy of 90%.

Considering the overall results in all 56 UDCA-treated patients, there are four additional points:

First, there was a relatively high 'success' rate, with partial or complete gallstone dissolution in 29 patients.

Secondly, in agreement with results by Bateson *et al.*[10], the X-ray taken at 6 months is a remarkedly accurate predictor of what will happen subsequently. We found only 4 out of 35 patients in whom the first, on-treatment, X-ray gave misleading information. Nearly all those who are going to dissolve their stones showed evidence of doing so at 6 months: only three patients who showed no response at the 6 month X-ray, went on to show partial or complete gallstone dissolution at 1 year. Therefore, although one gets a good indication about the response to therapy at the 6 month cholecystogram, one should be prepared to go on for at least 1 year before deciding whether or not the treatment is going to be effective.

Thirdly, the mean time required to produce complete gallstone dissolution was 10 months – pretty close to the 12 months which we found previously for CDCA. So, if the stones are going to dissolve, they will probably do so fairly quickly, but of course this relates, in part, to gallstone size and to the initial patient selection.

Fourthly, and most important of all, the mean UDCA dose required to produce partial or complete gallstone dissolution in this series was 7.9 mg/kg (although this figure is artefactually lowered because some of these patients had initially participated in a dose–response study using lower UDCA doses.) These results, therefore, support our earlier recommendation[3] that a dose of about 8–10 mg UDCA kg^{-1} day^{-1} should effectively dissolve suitable stones.

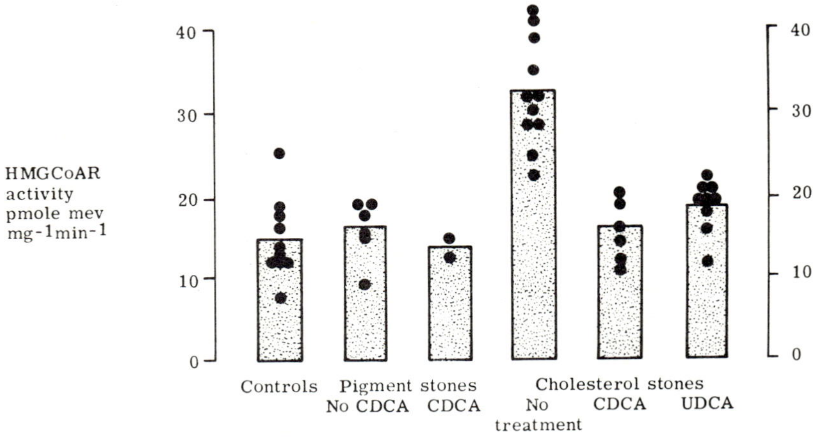

Figure 4 HMG-CoA reductase activity (pmoles mevalonate formed mg microsomal $protein^{-1}$ min^{-1}) in control subjects and different groups of gallstone patients. (From Maton *et al.*[11] by permission of the publishers of the Europ. J. Clin. Invest.)

(iii) Mechanism of action (Figure 4)

We have already discussed HMG-CoA reductase activity *ad nauseam* but Figure 4 summarizes Paul Maton's results from our unit[11]. In our experience, CDCA and UDCA both depress the activity of this enzyme, UDCA doing so at a relatively small dose[11]. Similar results have been obtained by Gerry Salen[12] and we have already heard that Kurt Einarsson finds a 25% reduction in this enzyme's activity during ursotherapy even though this is not a statistically significant fall[13]. Yet Carulli[14] from Modena, finds that the activity of this enzyme *increases* during treatment with urso, but he examined his patients after only 8 days UDCA treatment and his studies should probably be repeated after longer therapy.

(iv) Side-effects (Table 2; Figures 5 and 6)

(a) *Liver structure and function.* We have also discussed the liver at length and therefore I will not dwell on this, because everyone finds a similar pattern of results in patients treated with CDCA and UDCA. Table 2 summarizes our findings of liver structure and function in CDCA- and UDCA-treated patients. We saw hypertransaminasaemia in only one patient treated with UDCA (he had had biliary colic). With that exception, we never saw the modest, dose-related and usually transient rise in transaminase seen in 30%

of our CDCA-treated patients[15] although other groups have reported a 0–2% incidence of raised transaminase levels in patients treated with UDCA. However liver biopsies are usually 'within normal limits' in patients studied before and during both CDCA and UDCA treatment. From the patient's point of view, the most important difference between the two bile acids in terms of acceptability of treatment is the incidence of diarrhoea.

(b) *Diarrhoea.* Figure 5 shows the incidence of diarrhoea in gallstone

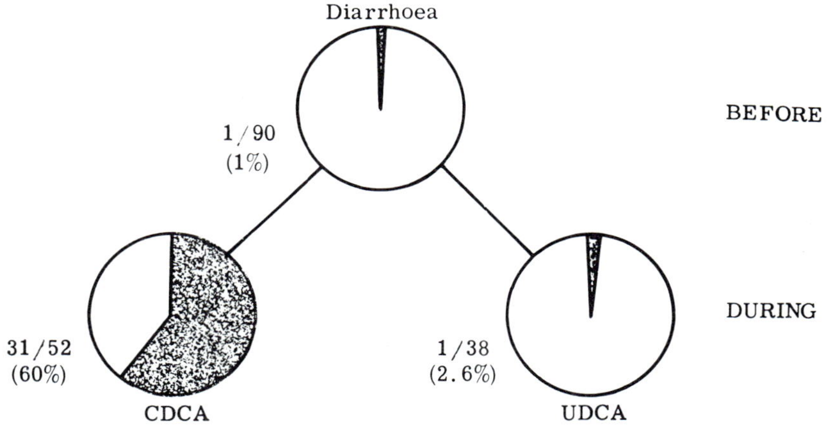

Figure 5 Incidence of diarrhoea before and during bile acid treatment. The numerators refer to the number of patients with diarrhoea and the denominators, the number of patients studied

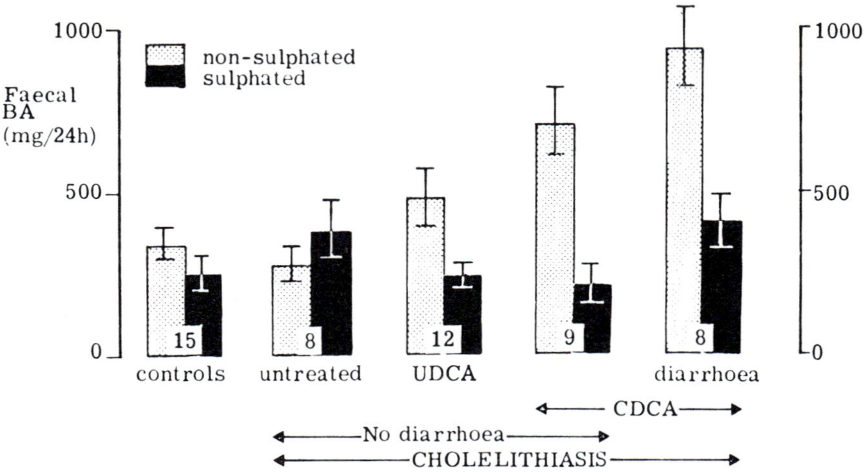

Figure 6 Faecal bile acid excretion (mg/day) in control subjects and gallstone patients with and without diarrhoea, sub-divided into the sulphated and non-sulphated fractions. (From Podesta *et al.*[16])

patients studied before treatment and during CDCA and UDCA therapy. Before treatment, only one out of the total of 90 patients had diarrhoea. On clinical grounds, he was considered to have a spastic colon. He was treated with UDCA and his diarrhoea got no better and no worse. With that exception we never saw diarrhoea during UDCA treatment. However, in this particular series, there was quite a high incidence (60%) of diarrhoea in the CDCA-treated group although this was seldom a major problem.

I would like to digress, for a moment, to discuss some new results from our unit on the mechanism of diarrhoea during CDCA treatment. At this meeting 2 years ago, my colleague, Marie Podesta[16], presented some controversial data on faecal bile acid output subdivided into non-sulphated and sulphated fractions (Figure 6) in controls and different groups of gallstone patients – untreated, those given UDCA and those given CDCA sub-divided into results for patients with and without diarrhoea. Now from a consideration of these results, it is not possible to say whether the non-sulphated or the sulphated fraction is responsible for the diarrhoea. And so, in our unit, Norbert Breuer (from Essen in Germany) turned to rats and using an *in vivo*, single-pass colonic perfusion technique, he studied the effects of both sulphated and non-sulphated bile acids on the colon[17]. He began with an isotonic electrolyte control solution made up to simulate ileal effluent, studied steady state net water and sodium transport and then changed to a solution containing 5 mM non-sulphated deoxycholate (DCA) or 5 mM sulphated deoxycholate. During the control perfusion, there was net absorption of both water and sodium but not surprisingly (given the results of many previous studies), perfusion with either 5 mM non-sulphated DCA or 5 mM non-sulphated CDCA changed net absorption to net secretion and produced histological damage in the colonic mucosa. However, at concentrations ranging from 5 to 15 mM, perfusion with *sulphated* DCA or CDCA had no such cathartic effect: there was no change in net water or electrolyte transport and by histology, the colonic mucosa remained unscathed.

Why do the non-sulphated bile acids cause diarrhoea? There are many possible mechanisms but the one which Breuer and David Rampton in our unit explored in some depth, was prostaglandin synthesis and production[18]. They measured prostaglandin output (PGE_2) into the perfusion effluent of rats perfused with a control solution followed by 1, 2 or 5 mM deoxycholate and showed a huge increase (700 fold) in prostaglandin output in the animals treated with 5 mM deoxycholate. Could this be the mechanism whereby bile acids induce diarrhoea? To study this, they went on to perfuse prostaglandins themselves and showed a modest, but significant, reduction in water and electrolyte absorption only with PGE_2 concentrations above those found previously in the perfusion effluent. Next repeating the 1, 2 and 5 mM deoxycholate perfusions but this time with the prostaglandin synthesis inhibitor indomethacin, they clearly showed that indomethacin pretreatment reduced prostglandin output quite drastically. But when we came to match the changes in PGE_2 output with the changes in fluid and electrolyte transport, there was a marked dissociation. For example, with the 2 mM deoxycholate perfusion, prostaglandin output was reduced by indomethacin pretreatment, but the use of the PG synthesis inhibitor made no difference to delta water transport. And when we compared PGE_2 output using 5 mM deoxycholate with indomethacin and 2 mM deoxycholate without, we found comparable PGE_2 output, but a huge difference in net water transport. This dissociation suggests to us, that prostaglandins cannot be the major mediators of bile acid-induced diarrhoea seen during treatment with CDCA and that indomethacin treatment is *not* likely to help the diarrhoea seen in patients treated with CDCA.

(v) **Symptoms during treatment**

Finally, I would like to discuss symptoms and the frequency of non-specific dyspepsia and biliary pain occurring before and during treatment with CDCA and UDCA. In open, unblinded studies, both bile acids show a comparable benefit – an observation which has been made repeatedly but one which is vulnerable to a placebo effect. It seems essential, therefore, that these phenomena should be confirmed (or denied) by carefully controlled, double-blind studies[19,20].

I would like to deal further with the question of dyspepsia in untreated gallstone patients and its relief during CDCA and UDCA treatment – topics which have been poorly studied to date. Our postulate was this: the dyspeptic symptoms in these patients were due to duodeno-gastric reflux with bile acid-mediated gastritis. We argued that only those bile acids which remained ionized in the stomach would be capable of mediating mucosal injury. We further hypothesized that before treatment, at normal gastric pH, say around 3.0 or less, the glycine-conjugated bile acids (which make up about 2/3 of the total) would precipitate out as inert crystals leaving the taurine conjugated bile acids in solution, ionized, surface active and capable of damaging the gastric mucosa. During treatment, we know that the glycine conjugates predominate with a reciprocal reduction in the surface active, taurine conjugates which might thereby diminish mucosal injury and the dyspeptic symptoms.

To study this, Tim Meredith in our unit correlated symptoms and endoscopic findings, with the degree of duodeno-gastric reflux measured by scintigraphy using both biliary (^{99m}Tc-HIDA) and gastric (^{111}In-DTPA) markers and by gastric bile acid concentrations. We also looked at the physical chemistry of the refluxed bile acids aspirated from the stomach[21]. Based on preliminary results in ten patients with dyspeptic symptoms and endoscopic evidence of biliary reflux and 'gastritis', he found that up to 25% of the imaged HIDA refluxed into the area of the stomach (as defined by the indium marker). He also found very high bile acid concentrations (up to 9 mM) in the aspirated gastric contents – confirming duodeno-gastric reflux.

He then went on to study the effect of treatment with 600 mg UDCA/day for 4 weeks. As predicted, there was no change in gastric pH before and during treatment but there was a marked increase in the gastric bile acid glycine : taurine ratio and in the percentage of gastric bile acids in the precipitate phase. At the same time, seven out of the ten patients claimed a marked reduction in their dyspeptic symptoms and there was an improvement in the endoscopic findings – preliminary results, but at least they give us a clue about the way ahead in our studies of that debated entity – gallstone-associated dyspepsia.

References

1. Iser, J. H., Maton, P. N., Murphy, G. M. and Dowling, R. H. (1978). Resistance to chenodeoxycholic acid (CDCA) treatment in obese patients with gallstones. *Brit. Med. J.*, **1,** 1509
2. Mok, H. Y. I., Bell, G. D. and Dowling, R. H. (1974). The effects of different doses of chenodeoxycholic acid and of withdrawing treatment on bile lipid composition and liver function in patients with gallstones. *Lancet*, **2,** 253
3. Maton, P. N., Murphy, G. M. and Dowling, R. H. (1977). Ursodeoxycholic acid treatment of gallstones. Dose–response study and possible mechanism of action. *Lancet*, **2,** 1297
4. Williams, G. W., Maton, P. N., Meredith, T. J., Murphy, G. M., Saxton, H. M. and Dowling, R. H. (1981). Will "Urso" replace "Cheno" in the medical treatment of gallstones? A retrospective comparison and up-date of results with ursodeoxycholic acid therapy. (Submitted for publication)
5. Iser, J. H., Dowling, R. H., Mok, H. Y. I. and Bell, G. D. (1975). Chenodeoxycholic acid treatment of gallstones – a follow-up report and analysis of factors influencing response to therapy. *N. Engl. J. Med.*, **293,** 378
6. Carey, M. C. (1978). Critical tables for calculating the cholesterol saturation of native bile. *J. Lipid Res.*, **19,** 945
7. Williams, G. W., Tanida, N., Maton, P. N., Murphy, G. M. and Dowling, R. H. (1979). Ursodeoxycholic acid (UDCA) therapy of gallstones. Is correction of biliary cholesterol saturation index according to percentage UDCA in bile necessary for prediction of gallstone dissolution? *Clin Sci.*, **57,** 27p
8. Corrigan, O. I., Su, C. C., Higuchi, W. I. and Hofmann, A. F. (1980). Mesophase formation during cholesterol dissolution in ursodeoxycholate-lecithin solutions: new mechanism for gallstone dissolution in humans. *J. Pharm. Sci.*, **68,** 869
9. Danzinger, R. G., Kurtas, T. K. and Torchia, M. G. (1980). Low-dose chenodeoxycholic acid for gallstone dissolution: a randomized trial in poor operative risk patients. *Dig. Dis. Sci.*, **25,** 785
10. Bateson, M. C., Trash, D. B. and Bouchier, I. A. D. (1980). Can a six-month cholecystogram predict eventual response to gallstone dissolution therapy? *Gut*, **21,** A443
11. Maton, P. N., Ellis, H. J., Higgins, M. J. P. and Dowling, R. H. (1980). Hepatic HMG-CoA reductase in human cholelithiasis: effects of chenodeoxycholic and ursodeoxycholic acids. *Eur. J. Clin. Invest.* **10,** 325
12. Salen, G., Colalillo, A. and Verga, D. *et al.* (1980). Effect of high and low doses of ursodeoxycholic acid on gallstone dissolution in humans. *Gastroenterology*, **78,** 1412
13. Einarsson, K., Angelin, B., Ahlberg, J. and Ewerth, S. (1981). Bile acids and hepatic HMG-CoA reductase in man. This volume, Chap. 9
14. Carulli, N., Ponz de Leon, M., Zironi, F. *et al.* (1980). Hepatic cholesterol and bile acid metabolism in subjects with gallstones: comparative effects of short term feeding with chenodeoxycholic and ursodeoxycholic acid. *J. Lipid Res.*, **21,** 35
15. Bell, G. D. Mok, H. Y. I., Thwe, M., Murphy, G. M., Henry, K. and Dowling, R. H. (1974). Liver structure and function in cholelithiasis: effect of chenodeoxycholic acid. *Gut*, **15,** 165
16. Podesta, M. T., Murphy, G. M., Sladen, G. E., Breuer, N. F. and Dowling, R. H. (1979). Fecal bile acid excretion in diarrhoea: Effect of sulfated and non-sulfated bile acids on colonic structure and function. In Paumgartner, G., Stiehl, A. and Gerok, W. (eds.) *Biological Effects of Bile Acids*, pp. 245–256. (Lancaster: MTP Press)
17. Breuer, N. F., Tammar, A., Murphy, G. M. and Dowling, R. H. (1979). Sulphation of bile acids abolishes their cathartic effect on the colon. *Eur. J. Clin. Invest.*, **9,** 5
18. Breuer, N. F., Rampton, D. S., Vaja, S. G., Sladen, G. E. and Dowling, R. H. (1980). The role of prostaglandins in bile acid-induced alterations of water transport in the rat colon. *Eur. J. Clin. Invest.*, **10,** 4

19. Frigerio, G. (1979). Ursodeoxycholic acid (UDCA) in the treatment of dyspepsia: Report of a multicenter controlled trial. *Curr. Ther. Res.*, **26**, 214
20. Polli, E. *et al.* (1979). Effect of ursodeoxycholic acid (UDCA) on dyspepsia in patients with gallstones or other biliary tract anomalies. *Curr. Ther. Res.*, **26**, 230
21. Meredith, T. J., Hilson, A., Murphy, G. M. and Dowling, R. H. (1981). An explanation for bile-acid mediated gastritis and the relief of dyspepsia with chenodeoxycholic (CDCA) and ursodeoxycholic (UDCA) acid therapy. *Clin. Sci.*, **60**, 22p

Discussion

Dr Schoenfield I will tell you about the status of the National Cooperative Gallstone Study, and then comment on some specific aspects of Dr Dowling's elegant lecture.

As you know, the National Cooperative Gallstone Study (NCGS) is evaluating 1000 patients receiving one of two doses of CDCA or placebo. The data currently are being analysed. I expect that the analyses of the major results pertaining to efficacy and safety will be completed by February of 1981. The first presentation of the data to the scientific community will be at the meeting of the American Gastroenterological Association in New York in May of 1981.

Regarding the comments that I now will make on Dr Dowling's presentation, I want to clarify that I am not speaking from the results of the NCGS because these are not yet available. Rather, my discussion will be based on our work in Los Angeles as well as on my interpretation of the literature. The first point that I would like to make – about which we have heard little so far at this meeting – is the importance of the validation of the techniques for assessing dissolution of gallstones. I am speaking particularly about the importance of showing the validity and reproducibility of the roentgenographic techniques for determining progressive or partial dissolution. In the entire world's literature only 20% of all patients that have been treated with CDCA or UDCA have had complete dissolution of gallstones. Higher percentages, of course, are obtained by careful selection of patients as Dr Dowling indicated, or by omission of dropouts from the calculations of efficacy. Much of the efficacy of both CDCA acid and UDCA described in the literature, therefore, is due to partial dissolution, emphasizing the importance of validating the technique for assessing partial and progressive dissolution.

The next point I want to consider is the choice between CDCA and UDCA. On the basis of all of the available current data, I do not think that the choice between these two agents has yet been established. Experience with UDCA still is relatively small. The third point that I want to make relates to the value of monitoring biliary lipid composition during therapy. I am inclined to agree with Dr Dowling's conclusion. We probably will have definitive information on this when these results of the NCGS are available.

When should therapy be stopped? Here again, I agree with Dr Dowling. In Los Angeles, if we find no dissolution after one year of therapy, then we discontinue therapy. What is the mechanism of action? We, too, have found that CDCA in patients, and CDCA or UDCA in hamsters, inhibits the activity of HMG-CoA reductase and that CDCA in the patients decreases biliary cholesterol secretion.

Side-effects: We still do not know the significance of the elevations of serum transaminases in patients treated with CDCA. Yesterday, I presented data showing that the sulphation fraction can predict subsequent elevations of the serum transaminase in patients treated with CDCA. Well, of course, this test is meaningful only if in fact CDCA or UDCA does cause clinically significant hepatic injury in humans. The diarrhoea with CDCA in our experience also usually has been only a minor problem.

Finally, I want to comment on the response of symptoms to therapy. Dr Dowling's presentation of the proposed physiology was fascinating. What must be stressed in addition to mechanisms, however, is the importance of *controlled* trials in assessing the symptoms, particularly dyspepsia, such as reported by Dr Frigerio with UDCA.

I mentioned earlier that the results of the NCGS will be presented next May.

Dr Weis

After such brilliant talks from my predecessors it is very hard now to present anything new to you.

So I will just have to stick to the meat of our data which we have collected together with Prof Holtermüller and I would like to show you some highlights first of the study which we did using 750 mg CDCA in patients.

The influence of CDCA dosage on the dissolution rate, a point which was emphasized already by Dr Dowling; of 16 patients taking less than 10 mg CDCA per kilogram body weight over 1 year, only two patients dissolved their gallstones.

Now in the group taking 10–13 mg consisting of 30 patients eight had successful dissolution. However in the group of 29 patients taking 13 mg or a higher dose of CDCA 20 patients dissolved their gallstones. So there seems to be at least in the treatment with CDCA a definite correlation between dissolution rate and the dosage of CDCA. Another important factor is the size of the stone.

In 25 patients in whom the stones had a diameter of 2 cm or more, we did not see any complete dissolution. There was one patient having a partial dissolution, but none showed complete dissolution over 1 year of treatment. In 52 patients having stones less than 2 cm in size, 30 patients showed positive results, partial or complete dissolution of their stones. Now it was already mentioned that patients respond very well with their subjective symptoms, especially that the rate of biliary colics went down.

We asked the patients how many colics they have had in the last 12 months before we started our study. Over 1 year of treatment these patients reported their biliary colics in a little diary. In the group who dissolved their stones there was a marked decrease in biliary colic. However, the other group without dissolution also showed a decrease in their biliary colics. Apparently this decrease of biliary colic is not related at all to gallstone dissolution and you cannot take this as an indication of future dissolution of the stones. Why should the rate of biliary colic go down? Is it just a placebo effect? I would like to explain this by the following observation and hypothesis.

We measured the gallbladder area on the X-ray pictures of these patients. Before the treatment was started in 25 patients with gallstone dissolution, and in 34 patients with failure, we found the same size of gallbladder areas. After 12 months of treatment with CDCA there was a significant increase of gallbladder areas in both groups. Between the two groups there was no statistically significant difference after therapy. The enlargement of the gallbladders might be due to the increase of the bile acid pool which also increases gallbladder volume. The stones have now more space to move and do not get stuck in the cystic duct so often as they did before. This might be an explanation for the decreased rate of biliary colics under therapy.

Some observations of our UDCA study:

We have treated three groups: 11 patients in the first group, with 5 mg UDCA/kg, 12 patients in the second group treated with 10 mg and 13 patients treated with 15 mg/kg UDCA over 12 months. They were well controlled.

During that time, more than 20 laboratory tests were checked every 3 months. Just let me mention that none of these tests changed significantly. There were especially no increases of serum transaminases observed in any of these patients.

We also asked for their subjective symptoms like heartburn, pressure in the abdomen, etc. Some patients were unchanged, many reported an improvement, but there was one patient in each group who said that he felt worse.

The result on the lithogenic index can only contribute here to the confusion because, as you see, the administration of 5 mg UDCA in five patients did not lower the lithogenic index according to Hegardt and Dam. Only one patient came below, i.e., he desaturated his bile after 3 months of medication. Now in the next group, receiving 10 mg, almost all the patients except one desaturated their bile.

In the 15 mg group most of the patients had desaturated their bile after 3 months. Now the results:

In the first group receiving only 5 mg/kg UDCA we started with 11 patients; after 1 year only seven were left. Three of these had a partial gallstone dissolution and one had completely dissolved his stones, even though we had only found desaturation of bile in one patient. In the next group finishing with 11 patients, three had partial dissolution, four complete dissolution of their gallstones. In the last group with 15 mg/kg body weight finally comprising 12 patients five had dissolved their stones partially and two completely. Overall, of 30 patients 18 showed a positive response of their gallstones with regard to dissolution.

An interesting observation was that during the dissolution of gallstones, we found that four patients suddenly had calcium in their gallstones which was not visualized before the start of therapy; so there was a kind of demasking effect of the treatment. Relating stone size and dissolution rate we found that of ten patients with stones over 20 mm in diameter only one had partially dissolved. Of the stones measuring 15 – 20 mm only 3 showed partial dissolution. Most of the success was observed with stones below 15 mm in diameter. I like to emphasize that point which Dr Schoenfield raised, that is the diagnosis and the following up of gallstones. A recent study of Goodmann and co-workers showed that even i.v. cholangiograms give a wrong diagnosis in 40% and that really should stimulate us to look for better diagnosis of gallstones early enough to treat these people.

Dr Hofmann Before you go can you tell us, in both the 10 and 15 mg you had some people who persisted in supersaturated bile. Did they achieve dissolution of their stones?

Dr Weis No, these did not dissolve their stones, but I must say on the other hand dissolution was found in the first group on 5 mg and there was only one which went below. So I am sure you can still dissolve stones independent of their lithogenic index.

Dr Hofmann So a single sample showing supersaturated bile did not preclude dissolution at low dose UDCA?

Dr Weis That is right.

Dr Fisher In a randomized double-blind trial essentially the same if not identical to the American National Cooperative Gallstone Study, to which we express our sincere thanks, Canada Packers Ltd and Sunnybrook Medical Centre, University of Toronto, entered 175 more or less asymptomatic patients with radiolucent gallstones into one of three groups, a placebo group, a low dose CDCA group receiving 375 mg daily and a high dose CDCA group receiving 750 mg daily. There were 11 post-randomization pretreatment withdrawals leaving a data base of 164 subjects.

The study is not yet complete but it is sufficiently advanced for this presentation. 136 subjects, 85% of those on bile acid treatment, have completed the 2-year programme and 28 subjects are still in progress. There have been 42 dropouts, 75% of them programme related, that is due to cholecystectomy (justified or not), lack of compliance (in spite of our best efforts) or diarrhoea. Approximately two-thirds of the programme related dropouts have been due to surgery and one-third to lack of compliance. There have been only two dropouts due to diarrhoea and one of these was in a subject on placebo who was afraid of developing diarrhoea.

On completion of the study our programme related withdrawal rate will be a minimum of 18%, a maximum of 35% and certainly closer to the former.

Only four patients felt worse on treatment and 40% actually felt better. A representative 25% of the latter were on placebo.

Diarrhoea was a problem in only 13 patients but three of these subjects were on low dose CDCA and three were on placebo. Furthermore, three of the seven subjects on high dose CDCA achieved complete dissolution of their gallstones and one achieved partial dissolution. Only one patient on CDCA withdrew from the study because of diarrhoea and only one had her dose of CDCA compromised by diarrhoea.

(1) To date 17 patients, more than 10% of the study population, have developed non-functioning gallbladders and bile acid treatment offered no protection in this regard.

(2) Three patients on bile acid therapy *probably* and five patients, two of them on bile acid therapy, *possibly* developed calcified gallstones during the course of the study.

(3) Of the 13 patients achieving radiologically complete dissolution, as determined on the basis of two oral cholecystograms at least 1 month apart while therapy continued, four still had calculi on ultrasound examination of the gallbladder.

We do not believe that we should consider efficacy on the basis of only those ideal patients who take the optimum dose of bile acid for the entire length of study during which they feature non-calcified floating stones of less than 1.5 cm diameter in radiologically functioning gallbladders. Dropouts do occur, the uninvited does arrive.

13 patients have achieved complete radiological dissolution, 8 of 63 patients receiving high dose CDCA and 5 of 53 receiving low dose CDCA. There have been 7 partial dissolution, 6 having completed the 2-year study and all in the high dose group.

Our minimum efficacy, if no further dissolutions occur, will be 17.2%. Our maximum efficacy, if all patients still on bile acid therapy achieve a significant degree of dissolution, will be 46.6%. Obviously the figure will be in between and probably in the region of 20%.

These are raw data. The success rate could be made a bit higher and perhaps justifiably. But the facts are, that in a very stable, relatively homogeneous and highly selected population of patients studied in one committed academic institution, the programme-related dropout rate has been about 20% and the development of non-visualizing gallbladders about 10%. Furthermore, stones became calcified during the course of therapy and stones which apparently dissolved radiologically were found, on ultrasound examination, to be still present.

On the other hand, over a 2-year period of study, most patients remained asymptomatic or actually felt better, CDCA related diarrhoea was not a problem, clinical or biochemical hepatotoxicity sufficient to promote withdrawal from the study did not occur and there were successes. And of particular interest with regard to the successes is the observation that, with 85% of the treatment group analysed, complete dissolution was observed in 12.1% of the low dose group and 13.8% of the high dose group, a remarkably small difference.

Within the confines of this clinical study on gallstone dissolution, we conclude that chenodeoxycholic acid therapy is safe. But the efficacy of such therapy is unacceptably low, a more rigorous assessment of gallstone dissolution is necessary, and breakthroughs, particularly in the area of patient selection, are urgently required.

Dr Hofmann Before you sit down, Dr Fisher, did people on high dose or low dose have a greater incidence of surgical complications than people on placebo?

D. Fisher No they did not.

Dr Hofmann Is there anybody in the room who has observed any important new side-effects that are clearly related to CDCA or UDCA that are not reported in the literature? I ask this because this is one of the larger groups of users and it is very important that we should know if anything bad is happening.

Dr Maudgal During dose–response studies using UDCA, one of the patients who had radiolucent gallstones before he was started on UDCA was found to have calcified grains around his radiolucent stones after 6 months of treatment with UDCA.

Dr Hofmann Well, this is an observation which several people have been making. We do not yet know whether this is a specific UDCA effect. Does that calcium dissolve subsequently or does it stay there?

Dr Maudgal It is too early to say, Dr Hofmann. We have not yet repeated the study after 12 months of treatment.

Dr Möckel I have the same question. I saw in one case of 37 UDCA patients calcification during treatment with UDCA, but in 150 CDCA patients no calcifications were observed.

Dr Hofmann Does the calcium-coated stone respond or does it become resistant?

Dr Mockel At the beginning we did not find any calcium. The calcium developed during the treatment and it remained resistant.

Dr Hofmann The question is: is UDCA better than CDCA? I would like to know if there are any people here who have well-designed studies with comparative information for partial or complete dissolution comparing CDCA versus UDCA. The literature, to my knowledge, if you review it, does not answer this question. Clearly, UDCA has less problems with diarrhoea and transaminasaemia but is it a better gallstone dissolving agent?

Dr Dowling I do not think that there is yet a prospect of a random allocation trial comparing CDCA and UDCA which would provide you with the sort of information that you need. In retrospect, efficacy is comparable in comparably selected patients. You can get as high as 80% partial and complete dissolution at 6 months and 90% at 1 year with both forms of treatment. Different doses will produce that response.

I think we will not improve on that degree of efficacy because it is an absolute maximum, but whether high dose UDCA will produce more rapid dissolution is a different matter. I do not know of any information on that.

Dr Kern I would like to commend Dr Dowling on his remarkably comprehensive, logical, literate and elegant presentation. For the sake of your less literate American colleague could you please define dyspepsia?

Dr Dowling One is talking about fat intolerance, epigastric distension, bloating and heartburn. It is a totally non-specific thing which one sees in many other conditions which often might arise from spastic colon. It cannot be quantitated and it is the most difficult imprecise area to work in: I cannot define it, we associate it with a beefy red stomach at endoscopy, with histological changes of gastritis, with frothy bile in the stomach, with up to 25% reflux of visualized HIDA and with concentrations of bile acids up to 9 mmolar, but that is only one facet. It completely ignores other things like lysolecithin, it completely ignores alternative mechanisms. I cannot take it further.

Dr Iser Question to Dr Dowling. In the presentation of your results you mentioned the advantage of being non-obese and also the dubious benefit of measuring bile lipid composition. Now it is some years since we looked at the resistance of obese patients to dissolution therapy. I wonder if you could suggest how we should approach the management of the obese patient today.

Dr Dowling I can only give you a limited answer. It is really based on Adrian Reuben's work. Adrian Reuben looked at the effect of increasing the dose of CDCA in obese patients in two ways. First maintaining weight and increasing the number of capsules, secondly maintaining the number of capsules and decreasing weight by dietary restriction. There was a response in both cases, but there was a better response marginally but not significantly with weight reduction.

Dr Scherstén A brief comment on Dr Weis's data concerning the discrepancy between response in saturation index and dissolution at the low dose. I think it is important to remember that there could be a difference between the bile composition in the gallbladder and in duodenal bile, and I assume that these analyses were performed in duodenal bile. It was shown a couple of years ago by van der Linden that the saturation index differs between gallbladder bile and duodenal bile, mainly because of a decrease in the lecithin content in duodenal bile due to a rapid hydrolysis of lecithin to lysolecithin, which is rapidly absorbed. I think this might be of importance when bile is collected in the duodenum and related to the effect of therapy.

Dr Weis There are on the other hand studies that have shown that the duodenal aspirate is absolutely the same in respect to the lithogenic index as gallbladder bile. I do not think that there is much difference in the lecithin content.

Dr Dowling Just to supplement what Dr Weis has said. I think that there have been at least four studies where people have compared fasting bile ex duodenal fluid with gallbladder bile. We did it, the Mayo group did it, and some others did it. Dr Bell in our unit extended that and confirmed it; but there is a problem in terms of the assay system you use and whether or not phospholipid is extracted before you measure it. I think that there is another question and that is whether you are dealing with a dilute or a concentrated sample; there is a considerable margin of error if you do not make absolutely certain that you are dealing with a concentrated sample of bile. We have found on arbitrary grounds that unless you have got at least 20 mmol of bile acid concentration as a marker of concentration you get very spurious results.

Dr Ostrow Has anybody operated on the patient who did not respond and can tell us how many of the stones that did not dissolve turned out not to be cholesterol stones? I have not heard anything on that at all today. Is the lack of success due to failure of treatment or due to the wrong kind of stone being treated?

Dr Dowling Well there are three problems. There are radiolucent stones, which are not cholesterol in type, there are stones which dissolve partially but never completely because of a non-cholesterol residue, and there is a tiny group of patients who are resistant to treatment, that is, they have CDCA or UDCA-rich bile but they never desaturate bile. They have been studied by Paul Maton and the results will appear in *Gut*. Radiolucent non-cholesterol stones, I think, were found in about five patients out of 140, and partial dissolution that never became complete in three or four out of the same numbers.

Dr Hofmann We have detected a few new points about UDCA since our last meeting. We certainly have less enrichment, more spill-over into plasma, the required dose is less, we are not seeing transaminase elevations, and we are not seeing diarrhoea. Key questions remain with respect to dissolution efficacy, the total lack of correlation of changes in saturation index with UDCA and response to gallstone dissolution rate. Finally new differences emerge between CDCA and UDCA with respect to the levels of HDL and LDL lipoproteins in blood.

WORKSHOP ON DISSOLUTION OF GALLSTONES

PART IV
Treatment of Bile Duct Stones

Treatment of bile duct stones

J. L. THISTLE

Biliary duct stones are of particular interest to cholelithologists because they have a wide range of aetiologies and composition and they present a broad spectrum of therapeutic problems for the clinician. In contrast to stones in the gallbladder which can usually be removed easily surgically, biliary duct stones, particularly intrahepatic stones, represent a major therapeutic problem. Clearly the most common type of gallbladder stone and therefore duct stone is the cholesterol stone. Pure pigment stones may also occur in the gallbladder however, and get into the duct, and these two types of stone characterize the retained stones which represent the vast majority of stones in the bile duct we have to deal with.

Among patients who had common duct explorations in one collected series from five clinics comprising 4000 patients the incidence of retained stones was 4.4%. This is a problem, therefore, that many different therapeutic efforts have been directed towards, other than surgery. Adding to the depth of interest in biliary duct stones are so-called primary duct stones. The definition of these is controversial. They are often described as being earthy and may have a central nidus which is usually also pigment. Occasionally they may be just a muddy mass comprised of multiple separate stones. Perhaps the most convincing sort of evidence that primary duct stones occur are those formed around foreign bodies such as silk sutures from a previous cholecystectomy. Primary duct stones, for some reason tend to form in the left main hepatic duct twice as often as in the right hepatic duct. Intrahepatic stones are a particular therapeutic challenge because of the difficulty of their surgical management. Unfortunately, these stones that form in the duct system are most often calcium bilirubinate and this material seems to be unresponsive to either chenodeoxycholic and ursodeocycholic acid treatment or direct contact cholesterol solvents such as mono-octanoin.

A number of therapeutic options are available, however, to deal with duct stones. Certainly, small stones may pass within a period of a few weeks of observation with the T-tube clamped. A simple flushing procedure of, e.g. 100 ml an hour of saline, perhaps with an anticholinergic, often suffices for stones less than ½ cm and this has been done by surgeons for decades. When that is not sufficient, what other considerations are there? Basket extraction as popularized by Dr Burhenne is very successful with a success rate of about 95%, and a very low level of morbidity of about 4%. Variants of this such as using a choledochoscope, basket or scoop are also very successful and this clearly is the most commonly used method for approaching most of the biliary duct stones. I will not comment in detail about endoscopic papillotomy; Dr Safrany who is with us today is one of the World's experts in this procedure and many others in the audience have experience with this. This is successful in perhaps 90% of patients with a morbidity of about 8½% and mortality perhaps 1%. So that is a very effective therapy also, even though it is invasive with some morbidity and mortality.

I will now turn to a discussion of the dissolution of duct stones, the major topic of today's workshop. Certainly the most common situations are multiple stones in the common bile duct system. If stones are cholesterol stones UDCA and CDCA therapy can be expected to be effective. The problem is that more often than in the gallbladder these stones are not cholesterol stones. Another situation where oral CDCA and UDCA therapy can be effective is illustrated by a patient who was postoperative and had a catheter in the duct system. This patient was treated first with basket stone extraction, successfully removing a number of stones, then a catheter was placed up into the left main hepatic duct and a number of stones were able to be dissolved with mono-octanoin. However, she still had residual stones up in tertiary branches of the hepatic ducts both superior and inferior. She was put on CDCA therapy and 6 months later endoscopic retrograde cholangiography illustrated complete disappearance of all of the intrahepatic stones. She has since remained stone free. One last example of where bile acid dissolution therapy is almost the only option with reasonable hope of success in getting rid of the stone problem is in a patient with Caroli's syndrome who may have cholesterol stones. The Bologna group has reported one such case with cholesterol stones successfully treated with CDCA. Oral CDCA or UDCA therapy, therefore, clearly has a place in the management of duct stones, recognizing that we do have a higher possibility of pigment stones which are unlikely to respond.

Efforts to directly perfuse a stone dissolving agent have been going on for decades initially using chloroform, ether or other potentially toxic substances. More recently bile acid infusions, especially sodium cholate solution, have been studied. Using a constant infusion, monitoring the pressure and keeping it within the 15–25 cmH^2O pressure that is physiological for the biliary tree, this therapy has been evaluated in a number of centres around the world with varying success. Dr N. F. LaRusso and I studied this in Rochester, using a cross-over technique with saline and cholic acid and we were not impressed that cholate had a very rapid effect, in fact was any more effective than saline alone. Dr A. F. Hofmann and I worked with Dr W. Higuchi and G. Flynn at the University in Michigan trying to find some better way to treat these patients. With these collaborative efforts we settled on an agent, mono-octanoin which is an 8-carbon monoglyceride, and in fact *in vitro* is an excellent solvent for cholesterol. This solubility for cholesterol is similar to that of ether, it is a digestive product of medium chain triglycerides which has had a large clinical experience, and it is easily available and inexpensive.

In *in vitro* studies we measured the amount of cholesterol dissolved from cholesterol stones using matched pairs of stones from 15 different patients in mono-octanoin and in sodium cholate at concentrations usually used in patients. We found that mono-octanoin dissolved $2\frac{1}{2}$ to 3 times as much cholesterol as cholate. This study was confirmed by Dr T. R. Gadacz in Baltimore showing almost identical findings. In a gross representation comparing the effect on gallstones of 200 mmol/l sodium cholate, which is the highest concentration which has been perfused in man to my knowledge, with mono-octanoin one can see during a 6 day period a marked difference in the dissolution rate of these cholesterol stones all initially of the same size and from the same patient.

A variety of ways have been successful in getting mono-octanoin to the stones. Certainly the easiest situation is when one has a T-tube in place and the stones are downstream from the lower limb of the T-tube. Another situation which can be successful, if one has a radiologist highly skilled with cardiovascular catheters, is demonstrated by a patient with multiple moderate size stones in the common bile duct. A catheter was placed through his cholecystostomy and manipulated through the cystic duct and treatment was successful within a few days. Another example is a patient with multiple stones out in the peripheral ducts of the liver. These were multiple cholesterol stones some of which had been analysed, and the catheter was placed well out into one of the ducts containing the stones. Over a period of several days, the stones completely dissolved. With skilful radiologists, therefore, one can get the catheters in many places in the liver. Another way to get mono-octanoin to the stones is by means of a percutaneous transhepatic catheter which we placed in the patient illustrated who had one large stone and multiple other small stones not only in his common duct but intrahepatic ducts as well. One other approach of course is to use endoscopic retrograde placement through the papilla and this has been reported by Dr Cotton in London and others.

Our initial therapeutic effort with mono-octanoin was using a constant infusion pump connected in-line with a central venous pressure manometer to keep pressure within the biliary tree within 15–20 cm of solvent. Continuous infusion sometimes is not possible however because of obstruction or a small catheter lumen and one can then use an exchange procedure by withdrawing bile and replacing it with an equal volume of mono-octanoin usually in the 2 to 10 ml range. Dr Duncan Bell has had experience with 24 patients with success in the majority of them, and he has tried using a pump which the patient can carry. Such patients, instead of being restricted to bed for a week or two or three, can use a portable pump to slowly infuse mono-octanoin at 2–4 ml/hour. This interesting innovation can only be used in patients who are capable of cooperating and can be closely monitored. Among 118 patients from a variety of centres, treated with mono-octanoin the incidence of total disappearance of all stones was 45%. Partial reduction in size occurred in 20%, and in most of these patients the stones had decreased in size so that they could then be removed with basket extraction, or had moved out of the liver so that a simple choledochotomy would suffice for surgery. In a third of the patients treatment failed and a number of these were subsequently found to have pure pigment stones which were insoluble in mono-octanoin.

Mono-octanoin has generally been well tolerated, although some patients get mild discomfort, nausea or diarrhoea. One patient has reportedly developed gastritis and one severe diarrhoea during mono-octanoin but the relationship to the treatment, if any, is unclear. We have had no serious problem and a variety of laboratory studies have been normal.

How does stone dissolution fit in with the management of these patients? One rather simplistic way to look at this is in an algorithmic form (Figure 1). If stones happen to be downstream from the T-tube and the patient is

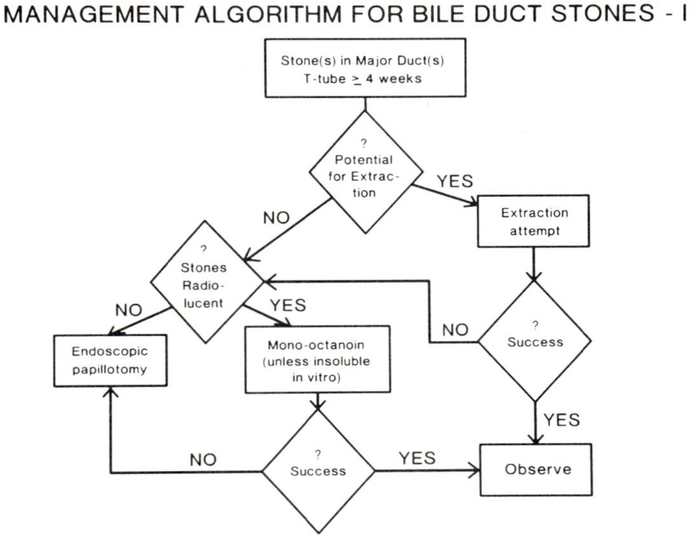

Figure 1

10 days to 2 weeks from surgery, one may be able to use mono-octanoin first before the T-tube tract is firm. However, most of the time these patients are doing well and anxious to go home, and we usually wait 4 or 5 weeks from surgery until the T-tube tract is firm. If the stones have the physical potential for extraction and the T-tube is large enough and well placed, we usually go first to extraction because of the very high success rate and low morbidity. If that is successful the problem is solved within a day or two or three, if not and the stones are radiolucent, mono-octanoin I think is a very reasonable consideration. I emphasize here that it is important in these patients to save any gallstones obtained at surgery so that they can be incubated in mono-octanoin. Within 3 to 7 days we should see unequivocal signs of *in vitro* dissolution and therefore be able to predict if they are going to respond *in vivo*. There is obviously no sense in treating the patient with mono-octanoin if the stones are insoluble *in vitro*. If *in vitro* dissolution is unsuccessful or the stones are radiopaque and the patient needs to have therapy then endoscopic papillotomy would be the reasonable next choice. Some patients one might prefer just to observe, for example, if the patient is elderly and the stones are non-obstructive and asymptomatic.

MANAGEMENT ALGORITHM FOR BILE DUCT STONES - II

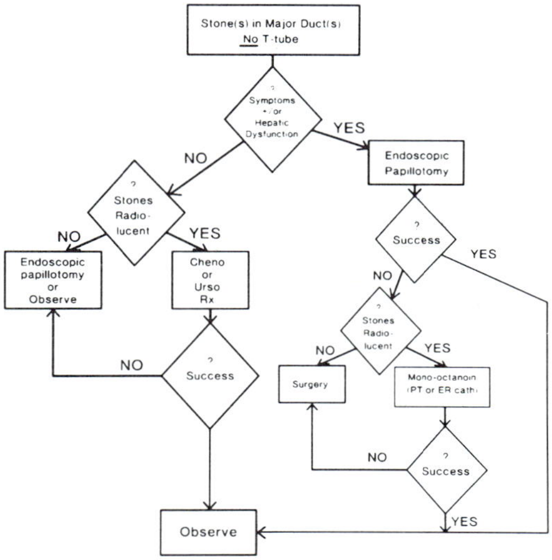

Figure 2

In the patient without T-tube access (Figure 2) I have discussed some of the options one might use. The important question here is whether these stones are causing trouble. Other considerations include the patient's age and surgical status. Clearly if the stones are obstructing, if liver function is abnormal or symptoms are present one needs to do something active therapeutically. An endoscopic papillotomy would usually be the first choice and if that is successful that solves the problem. If it is not effective one can then ask whether the stones are radiopaque or not. If they are radiolucent monoactanoin can be considered either by percutaneous transhepatic catheter placement or endoscopic retrograde placement and that may well be successful. If it is not these symptomatic stones probably will need surgical treatment. Stones that are asymptomatic, however, if they are radiolucent would be candidates for UDCA and CDCA therapy. If that is unsuccessful or the stones are radiopaque, endoscopic papillotomy would often be the next step, although again some of these patients may be selected for observation. Although we have very limited natural history data on this a number of patients can have many stones in their bile duct system for years with no cholangitis and no obstruction.

Finally, there are patients with stones such as in Caroli's syndrome in whom the stones simply are inaccessible to any mechanical procedure or direct perfusion procedure (Figure 3). If they are symptomatic one needs to do something and surgical approaches as you know often are heroic with a significant mortality and often with a low rate of real long term success. If these patients are not severely symptomatic UDCA or CDCA therapy is a reasonable consideration providing the stones are radiolucent. If the stones are not or dissolution is ineffective we are back to where we were 10 years ago with observation plus antibiotics as needed as the only remaining options.

Biliary duct stone disease represents a very challenging heterogenous problem and a number of areas clearly need further investigation. Some efforts have been made at trying to fragment stones so that they can be extracted more easily with the basket or balloon. Attempts to do this ultrasonically or with electrical impulse-hydraulic effects, seem to require direct contact with the stone by the instrument. External efforts at fragmentation have not been promising to my knowledge. Ways to break up these stones not only if they are cholesterol stones but in particular if they are pigment stones is an important area for investigation. Many pigment stones, particularly those developing within the liver, e.g. above strictures, are recurrent stones often requiring repeated operations. We know too little about the pathogenesis of these stones although stasis and bacterial infection is the most suspected relationship. We also know too little about bilirubin solubilization. We obviously have much to learn about why these patients get stones and what to do to get rid of them and prevent them.

Although we have talked in some detail about dissolving cholesterol stones, in fact, dissolution of many of these with mono-octanoin takes 1–3 weeks, often in hospital and it takes considerable patient tolerance. We note some interesting work on cholesterol stone solvents going on in some laboratories, including some with mono-octanoin in Germany and I think we will soon hear about some ways in which we might speed up solubilization of these stones. One other minor factor which could facilitate duct stone therapy is effective chronic relaxation of the sphincter mechanism so that resistance to mechanical flushing could be minimized during a several day period.

MANAGEMENT ALGORITHM FOR BILE DUCT STONES - III

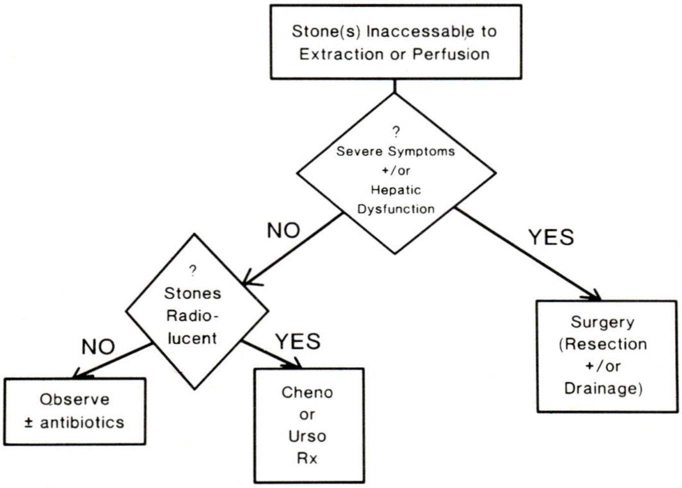

Figure 3

New aspects of conservative treatment of bile duct stones

U. LEUSCHNER AND H. BAUMGÄRTEL

The dissolution of cholesterol bile duct stones may be attempted by the infusion of a bile salt solution via T-tube. Side-effects are considerable and the success rate is approximately 20–40%.

Capmul 8210 (glycero-1-mono-octanoin) may dissolve cholesterol concrements 2.5 times faster. Side-effects are also considerable; and sufficient therapeutical experience is still lacking[1–3].

Why are the results still unsatisfactory? There are six possible contributing factors:

(1) date of commencement of therapy;
(2) stone composition;
(3) stone architecture;
(4) treatment scheme;
(5) side-effects of therapy;
(6) topography of biliary system.

DATE OF COMMENCEMENT OF THERAPY

Up to now infusion therapy was possible only in the presence of a T-tube. After removal of the T-tube there was only recourse to surgery. If we introduce endoscopically an indwelling nasobiliary tube, which is successful in 90%, then time-restrictions are no longer a problem.

STONE COMPOSITION

Three components of stone composition can inhibit dissolution: mucoproteins; calcium salts (Cu, Fe); and pigments. As we have learned from stone analysis, bile duct stones differ from one another considerably. Therefore every stone requires individual treatment.

Our method of dissolving the three separate layers is as follows:

(1) By means of lipid solubilizer, a special Capmul preparation (GMOC: glycero-mono-octanoin-carnosine) we were able to demonstrate in several

stones a coat, consisting of a mucoprotein layer, that could be dissolved neither by bile salts nor GMOC. We could degrade this layer by means of proteolytic enzymes *in vitro* (Figures 1 and 2).

(2) Calcium salts are resistant to the usual infusion media. We could extricate calcium salts from cholesterol stones *in vitro* and *in vivo* by a bile salt–EDTA solution (Ursodeoxycholic acid 0.5%; cholic acid 0.5%; EDTA–Na (ethylenediamine tetracetic acid) 1.0%; carnosine (β-alanyl-L-histidine) 0.27%. Buffered to pH 9.4 with NaOH and carnosine. Equilibrated to an osmolarity of 320–360 mosmol/l with 0.5% NaCl.)

(3) With this solution we finally succeeded in dissolving a pigment stone with a water- and mucoprotein-containing matrix (Figures 3 and 4).

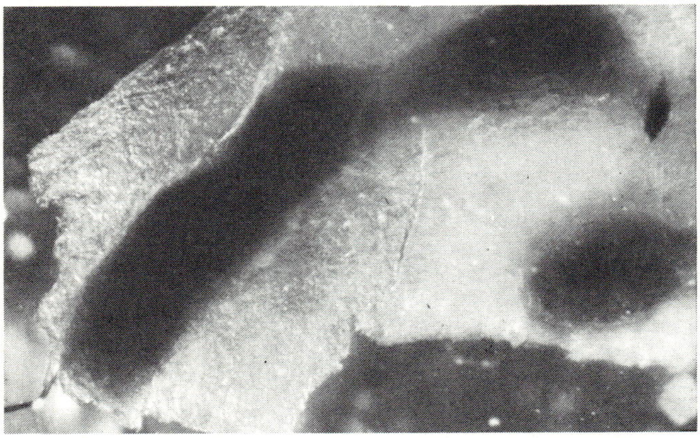

Figure 1 Membrane-like layer of an organic matrix, containing pigment occlusions of varying density that do not dissolve in GMOC or in bile acid–EDTA solution

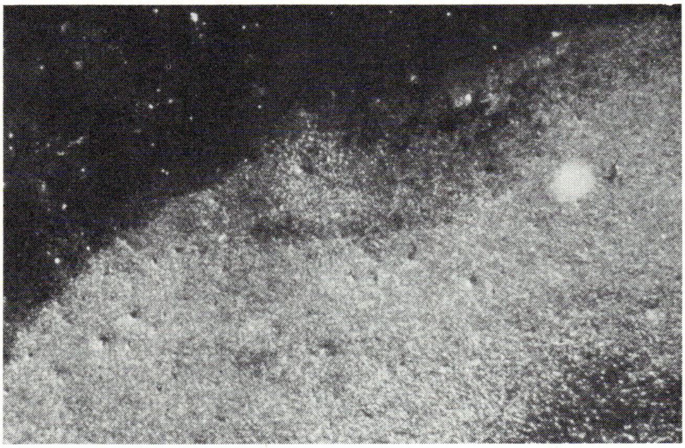

Figure 2 In a trypsin solution or SH-activated papain solution in bile acid–EDTA pigment was extracted and the organic matrix disaggregated

STONE ARCHITECTURE

Stone architecture is more important than data on the average distribution of certain substances in the concrement. For example we have found in several stones that about 80% of the calcium content is concentrated in one or two shells while only about 20% is distributed in the rest.

TREATMENT SCHEME

Monotherapy with a lipid solubilizer such as Capmul therefore may not always prove effective. In more than 20 patients we have performed an alternating treatment using a nasobiliary tube with a special preparation

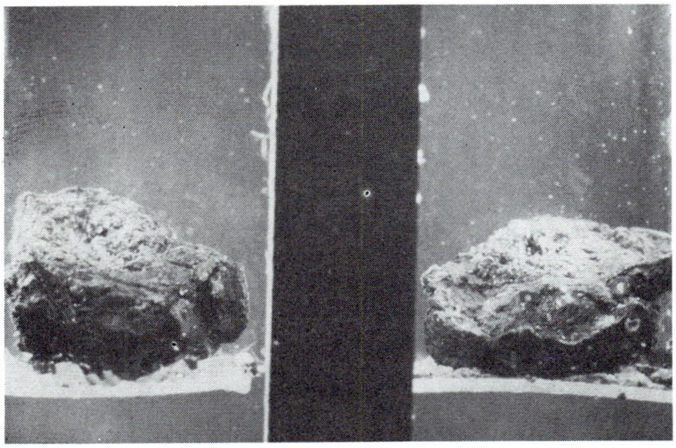

Figure 3 Two pigment matrix stones of identical weight; on the left in Capmul 8210, on the right in bile acid–EDTA (cholesterol: 8.8%)

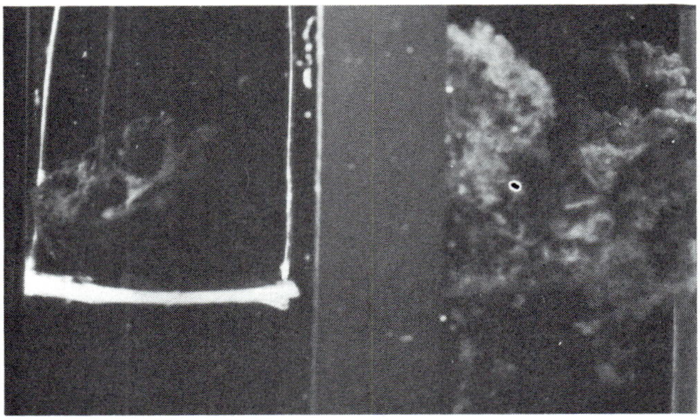

Figure 4 State after approximately 36 h. The left stone lies in Capmul 8210; on the right is shown a loose heap of brownish pigment sedimenting as mud

of Capmul (GMOC) and the above-mentioned bile salt–EDTA solution and were successful in 64% of the cases[4]. *In vitro* our treatment scheme produced a faster stone dissolution than Capmul 8210[5] (Figures 5 and 6).

TOLERANCE AND TOPOGRAPHY

We have also tried to improve the tolerance of Capmul 8210. This was achieved partly by enhancing the emulsifiability and making the pH value more alkaline.

The topographical conditions present us with an obstacle to bile duct stone dissolution. Although this will always prove to be a barrier to success, we hope nevertheless that, by improvement of infusion media and therapeutic schemes, better results will be obtainable.

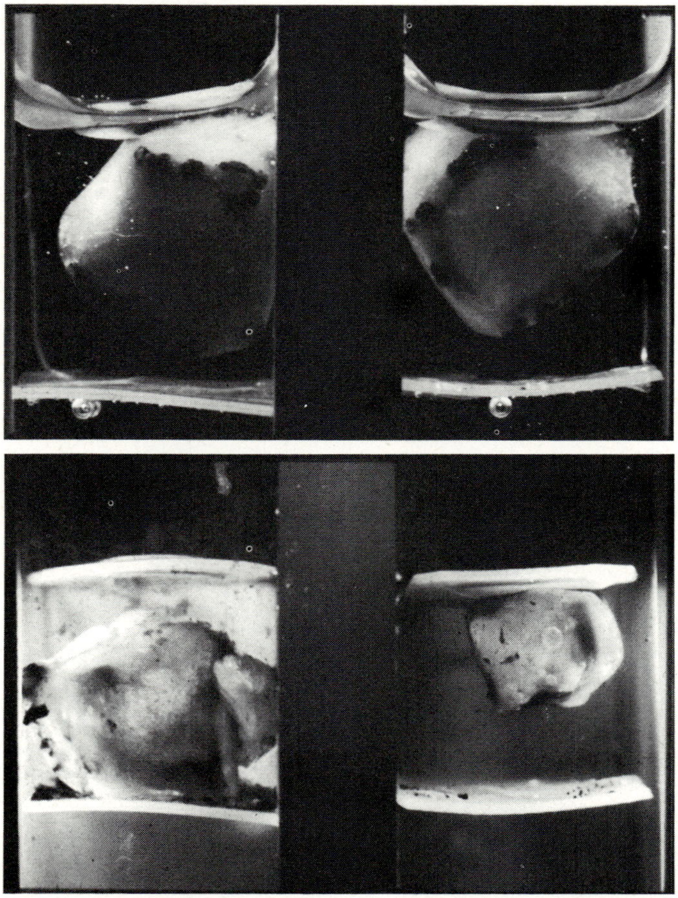

Figures 5 and 6 Two cholesterol concrements of identical weight (cholesterol: 84%). After 28 h treatment with Capmul 8210 (left) and GMOC and bile acid–EDTA alternatingly (right) the right stone has decreased markedly in size. After 88 h the right stone was completely dissolved; the left one only slightly reduced in size

References

1. Thistle, J. L., Carlson, G. L., Hofmann, A. F. *et al.* (1980). Monooctanoin, a dissolution agent for retained cholesterol bile duct stones: physical properties and clinical application. *Gastroenterology*, **78,** 1016
2. Schenk, J., Schmack, B., Rosch, W. *et al.* (1980). Spülbehandlung von Choledochussteinen mit Octanoat (Capmul 8210). *Dtsch. Med. Wochenschr.*, **105,** 917
3. Uribe, M., Uscanga, L., Sanjurgo, J. L. and Lagarriga, J. (1980). Medium chain glycerides for the dissolution of retained gallstones: success and side effects. *Gastroenterology*, **78,** 1281 (abstr.)
4. Leuschner, U., Wurbs, D., Baumgärtel, H. *et al.* (1981). Alternating treatment of common bile duct stones with a modified glyceril-1-monooctanoate preparation (GMOC) and a bile acid-EDTA solution (BA-EDTA) by nasobiliary tube. *Scand. J. Gastroenterol.* (In press)
5. Leuschner, U., Baumgärtel, H. and Wurbs, D. (1980). Auflösung von Cholesterin-Gallengangssteinen mit einer modifizierten Capmul 8210-Emulsion und einer EDTA-Gallensalzlösung. *Leber Magen Darm*, **10,** 284

Treatment of common bile duct stones

P. CZYGAN, A. STIEHL, R. RAEDSCH, R. GÖTZ, S. WALKER AND B. KOMMERELL

Gallstones are retained in the biliary tree after cholecystectomy in approximately 0.5–5.0%[1,3] and after choledochus revision in approximately 5.9–11.9%[4] of patients or are new formed by recrystallization on thread material[5]. Beside a choledochotomy[6], a transduodenal papillotomy[7] or an endoscopic papillotomy[8], where the mortality rate is 1.8%, 3.6% and 1.4% respectively, a dissolution of common bile duct stones can be performed by bile acids[2,9–17] or glyceryl-1-mono-octanoate[5,18,19] over a T-tube or an endoscopically introduced choledochal tube.

Eleven females and five males ageing from 28 to 83 years with intrahepatic stones (n = 2) or common bile duct stones (n = 14) were treated by sodium cholate (n = 11) or by glyceryl-1-mono-octanoate (n = 5). The dose of sodium cholate was 10–15 g/day (in addition 4–6 g cholestyramin) and of

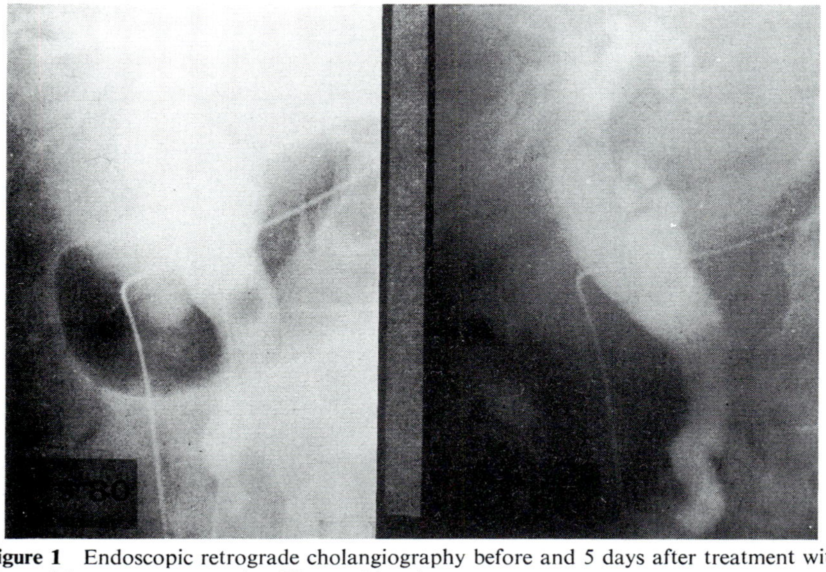

Figure 1 Endoscopic retrograde cholangiography before and 5 days after treatment with glyceryl-1-mono-octanoate in a 79 year old male

glyceryl-1-mono-octanoate 6–8 ml/h. Glyceryl-1-mono-octanoate or sodium cholate were applied via a T-tube ($n = 9$) or an endoscopically introduced choledochal tube ($n = 7$) over a period of 2–7 days or 1–25 weeks respectively.

The indications for the treatment with sodium cholate or glyceryl-1-mono-octanoate were intrahepatic stones in two patients, retained common bile duct stones after cholecystectomy in six patients and common bile duct stones in eight patients with high risk for surgery (a cholecystectomy was performed between 3 and 17 years prior to the treatment in five patients).

In four out of eleven patients treated by sodium cholate the gallstones were dissolved, in two diminished and in five patients not dissolved. From the patients treated by glyceryl-1-mono-octanoate in two patients the gallstones were dissolved (Figure 1), in one diminished and in two patients not dissolved.

Side-reactions observed in the 16 patients were vomiting, diarrhoea and colics (Table 1). Complications were observed as cholangitis in one patient of each group (Table 1).

Table 1 Side-reactions and complications in 16 patients treated by sodium cholate or glyceryl-1-mono-octanoate

	Cholate	*Glyceryl-1-mono-octanoate*
Side-reactions		
● vomiting	4/11	3/5
● diarrhoea	6/11	2/5
● colics	2/11	2/5
Complications		
● cholangitis	1/11	1/5
Mortality	0/11	0/5

In all patients with unsuccessful gallstone dissolution an endoscopic papillotomy ($n = 3$) or a surgery ($n = 4$) was performed. In six out of seven patients bilirubin stones were detected. This supports the finding that only 50% of the gallstones in the common bile duct contain more than 90% cholesterol[5], which explains why only 50% of the common bile duct stones are dissolved by treatment with bile acids[9–12,14–15,17].

References

1. Burhenne, H. J. (1976). *Adv. Surg.* **10,** 121
2. Way, L. W., Admirand, W. H. and Dunphy, J. E. (1972). *Ann. Surg.*, **176,** 347
3. Glenn, F. (1973). *Ann. Surg.*, **179,** 528
4. Andreassen, M., Holm-Bentzen, M. and Christiansen, L. A. (1976). *Scand. J. Gastroenterol. Suppl.*, **11,** 7
5. Koch, H., Schenk, J., Schmack, B. and Stolte, M. (1979). In Demling, L. and Rösch, W. (eds.) *Operative Endoskopie*, pp. 151–156. (Berlin: Acron Verlag)
6. Glenn, F. (1967). *Surg. Gynec. Obstet.*, **124,** 974
7. Gall, F. P. and Franke, F. (1979). In Demling, L. and Rösch, W. (eds.) *Operative Endoskopie*, pp. 157–164. (Berlin: Acron Verlag)
8. Safrany, L. (1978). *Lancet*, **2,** 983

9. Lansford, C., Metha, S. and Kern, F. (1974). *Gut*, **15,** 48
10. Britton, D. C., Gill, B. S., Taylor, M. R. and James, O. (1975). *Br. J. Surg.*, **62,** 520
11. LaRusso, N. F., Thistle, J. L. Hofmann, A. F. and Fulton, R. E. (1975). *Gastroenterology*, **68,** A-75/932
12. Toouli, J., Jablonski, P. and McK Watts, J. (1975). *J. Surg. Res.*, **19,** 47
13. Dihos, P. E., Borster, H. and Dihos, A. (1976). *Med. Welt.*, **27,** 2072
14. Schmidt, G. F. and Bauer, H. (1976). *Med. Klinik*, **71,** 1849
15. Way, L. W. and Motson, R. W. (1976). *Adv. Surg.*, **10,** 99
16. Czygan, P., Stiehl, A., Fröhling, W. and Kommerell, B. (1977). *Dtsch. Med. Wochenschr.*, **102,** 518
17. Sobrabi, A., Max, M. H. and Herstey, C. D. (1979). *Arch. Surg.*, **114,** 1169
18. Thistle, J. L., Carlson, G. L., LaRusso, N. F. and Hofmann, A. F. (1978). *Gastroenterology*, **74,** 1103
19. Witzel, L., Wiederholt, J. and Wolberg, E. (1980). *N. Engl. J. Med.*, **303,** 465

Treatment of bile duct stones

W. RÖSCH

Mono-octanoin (Capmul 8210) was used in our clinic to dissolve retained common bile duct stones in a total of 11 patients. In five the solvent was infused via an endoscopically placed indwelling catheter and in six via a T-tube (Table 1). In the first group (2 men, 3 women; age 27–89) the biliary catheter was introduced through the intact papilla in three and after a small cut (precutting manoeuvre) in two patients. An overflow valve kept the intraductal pressure during infusion of 5 ml/h constant below 25 cmH_2O. A mean of 100 ml of Capmul 8210 (30–150 ml) was instilled for 3–10 days ($\overline{m}$ 6 days). The patients were placed on enzyme substitution and received spasmolytics on demand, GPT, GOT, γ-GT, aP and amylase were checked every other day. Complete dissolution did not occur; three stones became soft after 3–6 days' treatment with 90, 550 and 700 ml octanoate solution so that they could be cracked with the Dormia basket, the fragments passing spontaneously. In one patient 10-day-treatment was unsuccessful and the stone had to be removed by EPT, in one patient severe side-effects caused discontinuation after 5 days. In two patients dislocation of the indwelling catheter occurred, in two other patients marked peripapillary erosions were noted after 5 and 7 days' treatment which healed spontaneously within 2 days after discontinuation of infusion.

Table 1 Dissolution of common bile duct stones

	Dissolution	*Softening*	*Failure*	*Side-effects*
T-tube (n = 6) 6 ml/h – 120 ml/d 5 days	3	—	3	2
Naso-biliary tube (n = 5) 5 ml/h – 100 ml/d 6 days	0	3	2	1

Out of the six patients (age 55–82) in whom dissolution was attempted via T-tube, stones were dissolved or spontaneously expelled in three after 3, 5, and 6 days and the instillation of 250, 440 and 530 ml of solvent.

In one patient a 10-day-treatment was unsuccessful, in two patients therapy had to be discontinued because of severe side-effects (colicky pain and diarrhoea in one, stone impaction in the other).

The success of dissolution therapy depends on four factors which have to be reconsidered before this treatment can be generally recommended. When using the retrograde way a preformed catheter according to Wurbs should be used to guarantee constant bathing of the concrement in the solution. The composition of stones in the common bile duct apparently varies considerably compared to the ones in the gallbladder. Analysis of endoscopically extracted concrements by Dr Wosiewicz from the Institute of Medical Physics at Muenster revealed that 41% were pigment stones which are unsoluble in Capmul 8210 (30%, by the way, contain retained suture material as crystallization point for stone formation). This figure of 41% compares favourably with the recently compiled figures of Hofmann *et al.* with no or uncertain clinical utility of mono-octanoate in 44.1%.

Taking this observation into account the ideal solvent would be an alternating instillation of mono-octanoin and alkaline EDTA solution, since Nakamura *et al.* could successfully dissolve calcium bilirubinate concretions *in vitro* with the latter substance.

Table 2 Results of animal experiments with solvents (tissue damage)

Organ	*Infusion 0.6 ml/h – 4 × 4 hours* Capmul 8210* pH 4.24	Cholate† pH 7.35	EDTA‡ pH 10.0	*0.9% NaCl*
Gallbladder	+++	+	(+)	—
Common bile duct	+++	(+)	(+)	—
Papilla	+++	(+)	(+)	—
Pancreas	+	—	—	—
Liver	+	(+)	(+)	—

*glyceryl mono-octanoate
†100 mM sodium cholate
‡EDTA Na 1.2% + 0.5% heparin 5000 U/ml

Finally, the biological side-effects are to be considered. The low pH of the original Capmul solution (pH 4.24) may be responsible for the tissue damage seen in animal experiments (Table 2) and in our two patients with periampullary erosions. The subjective symptoms like nausea, vomiting, diarrhoea and abdominal pain are not bearable over a longer period of time in these bed-ridden high-risk patients who prefer endoscopic sphincterotomy if offered a choice. Nevertheless further attempts seem justified to improve substances and modalities of litholysis in the common bile duct.

References

1. Harmon, J. W., Gadacz, T. R., Weichbrod, R. H. and Hofmann, A. F. (1980). Effect of mono-octanoin (MO) on canine gastric mucosa. *Gastroenterology*, **78,** 1179
2. Hofmann, A. F., Schmack, A. F., Thistle, J. L. and Babayan, V. K. (1981). Clinical experience with mono-octanoin for dissolution of bile duct stones: an uncontrolled multicentre trial. *Lancet*, **1** (In press)
3. Schenk, J., Schmack, B., Roesch, W., Riemann, J. F., Koch, H. and Demling, L. (1980). Spülbehandlung von Choledochussteinen mit Octanoat (Capmul 8210). *Dtsch. Med. Wochenschr.*, **105,** 917

4. Thistle, J. L., Carlson, G. L., Hofmann, A. F., LaRusso, N. F., MacCarthy, R. L., Flynn, G. L., Higuchi, W. J. and Babayan, V. K. (1980). Mono-octanoin, a dissolution agent for retained cholesterol bile duct stones. Physical properties and clinical implication. *Gastroenterology*, **78,** 1016
5. Wurbs, D. and Classen, M. (1977). Transpapillary long standing tube for hepatobiliary drainage. *Endoscopy*, **9,** 192

Discussion

Dr Stiehl Before we start the general discussion I would like to discuss those patients with a T-tube. Are there any questions or discussion remarks concerning patients with T-tubes?

Unidentified discussant We have had the opportunity to study 12 patients with indwelling T-tubes, and ten of these (all of the patients had their stones analysed for cholesterol content prior to Capmul dissolution) had stones with a high cholesterol content and dissolved their stones in periods ranging from 4 days up to 15 days, most of them within the first week.

Dr Bell Really, as far as mono-octanoin treatment in patients with T-tube is concerned, I would just like to make one or two comments. We have now treated 24 patients. We never go above a dose of 5 ml per hour in any patient and most of our patients are treated with 2 or 3 ml per hour and as Dr Thistle showed earlier we have been able to treat some of our patients, in fact nine of the 24 patients as outpatients. I think one of the reasons for problems with diarrhoea and nausea and so on are the high infusion rates of 6–8 ml per hour. All of our patients are given instructions as soon as they have any pain at all, they must stop their constant infusion which is done with a battery operated pump. I think we have 15 complete and five partial dissolutions out of 24, using the smaller infusion rates and that dissolution rate compares very favourably with the response rate that was reported for the higher rates. I would say that if you are going to use mono-octanoate there is no point in going above 5 ml per hour and probably 2 or 3 ml per hour is more than adequate.

Dr Stiehl And how long does it take with 3 ml per hour?

Dr Bell Our experience is that if the stones are going to dissolve they are going to dissolve in 5–6 days, although we have had one or two patients whom we have treated as outpatients for up to 110 days with many stones in the duct and they have gradually dissolved. Most patients' stones dissolve in a period of about 1 week.

Dr Stiehl So you have outpatients on mono-octanoin?

Dr Bell Yes. We have treated nine patients as outpatients. They visit hospital 2 or 3 days to learn how to use the battery operated constant infusion pump. If they are getting colic they are taught how to aspirate the bile each hour. As long as the patients know that they can just unclamp the tube or aspirate bile if they get pain they seem quite happy to be treated as an outpatient.

Dr Czygan May I ask Dr Thistle how pure the commercial available mono-octanoin is, because I put it on a thin layer plate and found a lot of bands. Perhaps these impurities have some bearing on the side-effects.

Dr Thistle The Capmul or as we refer to it, the mono-octanoin is about 70% mono-octanoin, the rest predominantly dioctanoin with a little bit of trioctanoin and some fatty acid. I think it is possible that some of the side-effects with higher doses might be related for example to fatty acid.

Dr Ostrow What bothers me is the definition or the use of the term pigment stones. This is important because some of the stones that were shown by some of the speakers are not pigment stones, they are still 30, 40 or 50% cholesterol. To say that you can dissolve those stones with EDTA sodium and so forth makes sense. But real pigment stones, the ones that have virtually no cholesterol, less than 10% and usually less than 5%, those that are the black ones and are predominantly a polymer of bilirubin will not dissolve either *in vitro* or in anything. I think you may be able to break up some of the matrix in the mixed stones, but the true black stones will not dissolve. The orange ones I think will dissolve because those are not polymerized.

Dr Hofmann We have been making new esters and I think that we have some compounds which will work about three times as fast as mono-octanoin. We cannot put them into man until we do toxicity studies. When we have something that you all can use we will tell you. I would like to ask Dr Leuschner if there have been any major complications from the use of bile acid EDTA solutions because this is the first we have heard about it.

Dr Leuschner We had a few complications similar as under the treatment with Capmul: that is diarrhoea, and in two patients hypokalaemia. If our patients had diarrhoea this was usually under the treatment of GMOC and not under bile acid EDTA. We know that the lethal dose of EDTA is 50–7000 mg, but it is not absorbed in the intestine. Our concentration is about 1% and that is below the concentration in other preparations already used in medicine.

Dr Stiehl Dr Leuschner, may I ask you how long it takes to dissolve a calcified stone?

Dr Leuschner The mean in our 24 patients has been 15 or 16 days, but the longest time was 86 days and after this we stopped therapy because there was only a partial success. The stone became smaller but did not disappear.

Dr Stiehl Could you repeat what is your indication for giving Capmul and what is your indication for giving your solution with EDTA and bile salts?

Dr Leuschner We hope that by alternating treatment with bile acid EDTA and Capmul we have a more successful therapy.

Dr Fromm A question to Dr Thistle. Before you do your treatment, do you do *in vitro* tests of gallstone dissolution? I think that would be very important before you go through all the difficulties of infusing gallstone dissolving agents.

Dr Thistle It is an established criterium to first test the gallstones *in vitro* before you go through the treatment.

Dr Fromm In my experience, most of the stones are already lost when you start to treat, since the surgeon in general does not collect the stones he has taken out.

Dr Thistle I think it is very important to preserve the stones before you are sure that the repeated cholangiogram is free of stones.

Dr Stiehl We take this as a recommendation and now I would like to hand over to Dr Paumgartner.

Concluding remarks

G. Paumgartner

To summarize in the time left is impossible. I know that many of you have to leave soon. If I would have made a summary, I would have stressed that it became clear that in staging of gallstone disease it is insufficient to look at the saturation index of bile. We should know much more about factors which influence nucleation. We can expect more information about this in the future. I feel that there is a strong need to develop methods to measure nucleation time in a given patient, as we measure cholesterol saturation index. Such developments may help us to increase our knowledge about factors that influence formation and dissolution of gallstones. Furthermore, we have to improve our methods to assess the calcium content of stones prior to treatment. There was some indication that new radiological methods such as computerized tomography may be helpful.

In the second and third section of this workshop certain advantages of UDCA over CDCA for the dissolution of cholesterol gallstones were discussed and I do not want to repeat all this. There was still some controversy about whether or not an increase in the dose of UDCA above 10 mg/kg/day would further increase the efficacy of this bile acid to desaturate bile and to dissolve gallstones. Taking all statements together it seems to me that there is an optimal dose of UDCA between 8 and 12 mg/kg/day and that more UDCA does not necessarily mean more rapid dissolution. An important point was raised by Dr Dowling, when he indicated that in uncontrolled studies with UDCA in gallstone patients there was, independent of stone dissolution, decreased frequency of colic and dyspeptic symptoms. He showed preliminary studies which were designed to investigate the mechanisms which might be responsible for the effect of UDCA on dyspepsia. I think that this represents an important new development in the research on the clinical effects of UDCA and CDCA in gallstone patients.

You have just heard a very clear presentation by Dr Thistle about the dissolution of duct stones including an algorithm for the management of these patients. I do not want to repeat anything of this. I want not to forget that in the near future Dr Hofmann is going to tell us more about a new compound which will dissolve common duct stones three times as fast as mono-octanoin.

The 6th Bile Acid Meeting has now come to its end. It was a 10th anniversary and it was an outstanding meeting from its scientific quality. For this I want to thank all of you who have contributed. I want to thank also those who have worked behind the scene to make this meeting a success. All this would not have been possible without our host and patron Dr Herbert Falk. I speak not only on behalf of myself but also on behalf of Dr Gerok and Dr Stiehl when I say that working together with Dr Falk was a pleasure and that we want to thank him for that.

Index